Cultural Competence
A Lifelong Journey to Cultural Proficiency

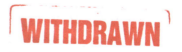

Cultural Competence
A Lifelong Journey to Cultural Proficiency

Ronnie Leavitt, PhD, MPH, PT
Associate Clinical Professor
University of Connecticut
Storrs, CT

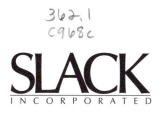

SLACK
INCORPORATED

www.slackbooks.com

ISBN: 978-1-55642-876-0

Published by: SLACK Incorporated
                 6900 Grove Road
                 Thorofare, NJ 08086 USA
                 Telephone: 856-848-1000
                 Fax: 856-853-5991
                 www.slackbooks.com

Contact SLACK Incorporated for more information about other books in this field or about the availability of our books from distributors outside the United States.

Library of Congress Cataloging-in-Publication Data

Cultural competence : a lifelong journey to cultural proficiency / [edited by] Ronnie Leavitt.
    p. ; cm.
  Includes bibliographical references and index.
  ISBN 978-1-55642-876-0 (alk. paper)
  1. Transcultural medical care. 2. Cultural competence. 3. Physical therapy--Practice. 4. Occupational therapy--Practice. I. Leavitt, Ronnie Linda.
  [DNLM: 1. Cultural Competency. 2. Physical Therapy Modalities. 3. Cross-Cultural Comparison. 4. Cultural Diversity. WB 460 C968 2010]
  RA418.5.T73C845 2010
  362.1--dc22
                                    2009048300

Printed in the United States of America.

Last digit is print number: 10 9 8 7 6 5 4 3 2 1

Contents

Acknowledgments

I would like to express my deep appreciation to the many people who have led me to believe in the importance of this book and to those who have helped me become the person I am.

To my patients who have taught me how important it is to consider their cultural way of life and worldview.

To my professional colleagues who have either contributed to this book or stood by me and encouraged me over the many years it has taken to bring this content area to the profession of physical therapy.

To SLACK Incorporated (John Bond, Publisher; Brien Cummings, Acquisitions Editor; Debra Toulson, Managing Editor; and Dani Karaszkiewicz, Assistant Project Editor) for their continued efforts in bringing this book to fruition.

To my dear personal friends, many of whom have been "with me" for decades. I recognize how lucky I have been to know you. You have always been incredibly supportive of my professional and personal life. Without you, I could not have accomplished so much or received such satisfaction from life.

Lastly, I acknowledge the abiding support of my family. My children, Alan and Kenny Leavitt; my sister Leslie Lawrence; and most of all my parents, David and Frieda Lawrence. The idea that I must always pursue knowledge and social responsibility has been passed from generation to generation. I feel blessed to have all of you in my life.

About the Editor

Ronnie Leavitt has been instrumental in bringing the socio-cultural and public health perspective to the profession of physical therapy. Dr. Leavitt began her career as a physical therapist at Harlem Hospital (1968) where she quickly learned that her "life of privilege" is not universal. In 1971, she embarked on the first of her many trips to developing nations that further reinforced her thirst for exploring different ways of life and cultural perspectives.

Dr. Leavitt pursued her graduate work in public health and medical anthropology. These areas of study matched her interests in people from diverse cultures, global health, and social justice. Her doctoral dissertation, *Health Beliefs and Behaviors of Families With Disabled Children in Rural Jamaica*, led to the beginning of her expertise in cultural competence and international rehabilitation. During the early 1980s, these areas were rather new to most physical therapists.

Highlights of Dr. Leavitt's professional accomplishments include being a co-founder of the Cross-Cultural and International Special Interest Group (CCISIG) of the APTA and Physical Therapy Overseas (PTO), a component of Health Volunteers Overseas (HVO). She has published extensively regarding cultural competence and international rehabilitation, has had professional presentations throughout the U.S. and internationally, and has volunteered as a physical therapist in developing nations. Dr. Leavitt has been honored to receive recognition for her work by both lay and professional groups, including the APTA CCISIG and the APTA Department of Minority and International Affairs.

Dr. Leavitt was a faculty member in the Department of Physical Therapy at the University of Connecticut from 1979 to 2009. She has recently retired and is continuing to pursue clinical, academic, and volunteer experiences.

Contributing Authors

Jill Black Lattanzi, EdD, PT (Chapter 6)
Clinical Assistant Professor
Institute for Physical Therapy Education
Widener University
Chester, PA

Kristin Lefebvre, PhD, CCS, PT (Chapter 6)
Assistant Professor of Physical Therapy
Institute for Physical Therapy Education
Widener University
Chester, PA

Christine A. Loveland, PhD (Chapter 2)
Professor of Anthropology
Sociology-Anthropology Department
Shippensburg University
Shippensburg, PA

Helen L. Masin, PhD, PT (Chapter 9)
Associate Professor of Physical Therapy
Department of Physical Therapy
Miller School of Medicine
Miami, FL

Rebecca Reviere, PhD (Chapter 7)
Professor and Director of Graduate Studies
Department of Sociology & Anthropology
Howard University
Washington, DC

Pamela J. Reynolds, EdD, PT (Chapter 10)
Professor, Doctor of Physical Therapy
    Program
Gannon University
Morosky College of Health Professions and
    Sciences
Erie, PA

Susan E. Roush, PhD, PT (Chapter 5)
Professor of Physical Therapy
Department of Physical Therapy
University of Rhode Island
Kingston, RI

Joseph W. Smey, EdD, PT (Chapter 8)
Professor, Physical Therapy
Neag School of Education
University of Connecticut
Storrs, CT

Valerie R. Stackman, MA (Chapter 7)
Doctoral Student
Department of Sociology & Anthropology
Howard University
Washington, DC

Preface

The new millennium has arrived, and the world is in a state of transformation. The United States is experiencing considerable demographic shifts along with an increasingly wide range of ethnic identification, religion, material reality, beliefs, and behaviors—all leading to rich diversity and cultural complexity. At the same time, health professionals (physical therapists specifically) are becoming more aware of the need to become culturally competent in order to be most effective in their interaction with patients and their families. The time is ripe for emerging subspecialties within physical therapy (and rehabilitation); that is, to study the causes and effects of ethnic and racial disparities, disability studies in a cross-cultural environment, and physical therapy in a global context. Working toward effective and efficient public policy to address these issues is also within our means.

As my professional career has expanded to include physical therapy, public health, and medical anthropology, I have been frustrated by the way medical and rehabilitation professionals generally focus solely on their area of clinical expertise and rarely pay adequate attention to the socio-cultural context in which our clients live. Too many still believe that such areas of inquiry are not relevant or our business. This frustration has been exacerbated by the dearth of accessible literature and resources linking these professional areas of expertise.

My interest in these areas began in earnest when I worked at Harlem Hospital upon graduation from a physical therapy school. Harlem, as many of you undoubtedly know, is a Black neighborhood in New York City. Although some of Harlem has been gentrified and there are lovely areas, it is known to be impoverished and many of the people living there are faced with greater-than-expected health problems and limited access to high-quality health care. During my time in Harlem, my world expanded in ways I never anticipated. As a White Jewish woman from the suburbs, I was surely in the minority, which was a new experience for me. I realized that my physical therapy clinical skills, although important, would not alone make me an effective therapist. Over the years, I have found myself drawn to travel throughout the world and work or volunteer experiences in environments that have increased my awareness and knowledge of people from very different walks of life. With increasing clarity, I continue to learn and embrace the wonderful differences of so many cultures and recognize that to be a truly effective health care practitioner, one must know and understand where and how the patient lives, works, and socializes.

The election of Barack Obama shows us the rich possibilities for all of us. Yes, we are now a people with a renewed commitment to the promises of our founding ancestors. The promise of our future is one of optimism—everything is possible in America. Yet racism, health disparities, poverty, and ethnocentrism have not disappeared. There has undoubtedly been upward mobility for some, but there has been downward mobility for many more. Segregation in the United States is worse now than during the 1960s, and it is the worst in parts of the country with the highest level of Black people participating in public life. There is public mingling but not social mingling (Patterson, 2008). For children, inner city schools' conditions and segregation are at a level no better than 50 years ago (Kozol, 2005). Blacks, more than other ethnic groups, are the most endogamous (i.e., least likely to mix). This is unfortunate as it keeps people cut off from each other. It does not foster the ability to take advantage of what we each bring to the table (Patterson, 2008).

We are faced with economic turmoil, the likes of which most of us have never witnessed. Poverty rates are going up for all groups of people. I fear that individuals will seek a "scapegoat" (i.e., someone to blame for our misfortune). Historically, it has been minorities who, through no fault of their own, have been unjustly blamed and persecuted. With regard to health disparities, poverty, racism, and other topics discussed in this book, I worry that things may get worse before they get better. We need to remain vigilant as to how this economy will impact our beliefs and behaviors.

The struggle for equality remains as does the struggle for a health care system that makes health care a right, not a privilege. Today we count single victories, but single victories do not lead to systemic change, and systemic change is what we need. Cultural competence should help us to achieve change more quickly and to a greater degree.

I challenge myself and my colleagues to travel the path of intercultural learning toward cultural competence and cultural proficiency. We must move away from ethnocentrism and cultural incapacity toward acceptance and respect for difference, continuing self-assessment, ongoing expansion of cultural knowledge and resources, and adaptations of services. We should revel in our enjoyment of doing so; we will be enriched with the many additional life experiences we encounter.

To quote the words of Anna Deavere Smith (an African American writer and actress) with regard to the election of Barack Obama (2008):

> "We need a narrative that is full of wildly different strands, firmly woven, so…that we have the confidence to even break a central thread or two to make the design more interesting. We need a narrative that gives us the confidence to work on behalf of more than our individual families. We know it's not right to have such a wide gap between the rich and the poor, the educated and the uneducated, the ones with means and the ones without… The time is ripe…to set about weaving a new narrative, for a new country. We need a dynamic weave…the world around us is in flux and full of the unknown…that's the possibility we see…"

As further inspiration, I quote part of the prayer given by Gene Robinson (the Episcopal Bishop of New Hampshire who has "come out" as a gay man) from the inauguration of Barack Obama on January 18, 2009. It seems apropos to the goal of cultural competence:

> O God of our many understandings, we pray that you will…
>
> Bless us with tears—for a world in which over a billion people exist on less than a dollar a day. Where young women from many lands are beaten and raped for wanting an education, and thousands die daily from malnutrition, malaria, and AIDS.
>
> Bless us with anger—at discrimination; at home and abroad; against refugees and immigrants, women, people of color, gay, lesbian, bisexual, and transgender people.
>
> Bless us with discomfort—at the easy, simplistic "answers" we've preferred to hear… instead of the truth about ourselves and the world, which we need to face if we are going to rise to the challenges of the future.
>
> Bless us with patience—and the knowledge that none of what ails us will be "fixed" anytime soon…
>
> Bless us with humility—open to understanding that our own needs must always be balanced with those of the world.
>
> Bless us with freedom from mere tolerance—replacing it with a genuine respect and warm embrace of our differences, and an understanding that in our diversity, we are stronger.
>
> Bless us with compassion and generosity—remembering that every religion's God judges us by the way we care for the most vulnerable in the human community…

It is truly a privilege and honor to make this contribution to the physical therapy profession.

REFERENCES

Kozol, J. (2005). *The shame of the nation: The restoration of apartheid schooling in America.* New York, NY: Crown Publishing.

Patterson, O. (2008). The new mainstreaming. *Newsweek*, Nov. 10, 40-42.

Robinson, G. (2009). Barack Obama Inauguration, Lincoln Memorial, Washington DC, January 18, 2009.

Smith, A. D. (2009). What Obama means to me. *Newsweek*, Jan. 21, 127.

1

Introduction to Cultural Competence

Ronnie Leavitt, PhD, MPH, PT

INTRODUCTION TO COMPETENCE

Does the duck that quacks the loudest get shot or does the squeaky wheel get the grease? The answer to this question might depend upon how you view the world, what assumptions you make about the nature of reality, and what cultural value system you hold dearest. Today, with the recognition that we increasingly live in a multicultural world with a wide range of life-ways, it becomes apparent that there is no one correct answer.

The modern Western medical and rehabilitation paradigm assumes a very biomedical, clinical orientation toward health and illness. It presumes that illness is due to abnormalities within the body, without consideration for potential social or psychological factors. Furthermore, physical therapists have historically worked primarily within their own socio-cultural communities. As the United States of America (U.S.) has experienced demographic shifts and increased diversity, rehabilitation personnel have not likely appreciated the importance of considering differences in the cultural way of life of co-workers or patients. When faced with less familiar multicultural or cross-cultural settings within our professional and private lives, we are not likely to know the best ways to alleviate obstacles thwarting care or positive relationships.

This book represents an effort to facilitate the development of cultural competence and cultural proficiency of physical therapists. The premise is that diversity is a positive thing and that diversity within the U.S. is a given. John Stuart Mill, in his treatise *On Liberty* (1859), stressed the need for diversity of opinion and noted the importance of being in the actual presence of people who are dissimilar from oneself in significant ways to learn from them. In 1869, Charles Eliot, the president of Harvard University after the Civil War, promoted diversity in education (regional, social, economic, religious, racial, and ethnic) as a defining cornerstone of American democracy and the foundation of responsible citizenship and leadership (Siantz & Meleis, 2007).

This book covers theory, practice, and professional development areas of study that have been, more often than not, omitted from the traditional curriculum for rehabilitation professional students or continuing education for the practitioner. This book hopes

R. L. Leavitt (Ed.).
Cultural Competence: A Lifelong Journey to Cultural Proficiency (pp. 1-18).
© 2010 SLACK Incorporated

to convince rehabilitation professionals to be more oriented to socio-cultural domains—areas that are typically found within the social science and public policy arenas. This orientation will include a greater appreciation of material conditions, social relationships, and aspects of the non-material culture (i.e., values and beliefs), specifically culture, ethnicity, economic status, political environment, religion, gender, sexuality, disability status, and other such variables clinicians often ignore. With greater insight into the variability of social, cultural, and economic conditions that others experience, attempts to improve the life situation of our clients are likely to be more successful. There is a presumed goal of health equity (i.e., increased access, improved quality of services, and fewer health disparities) for those who might not otherwise receive ideal, or even any, rehabilitation services. At the same time, if rehabilitation professionals truly consider social and cultural domains, social scientists (e.g., medical anthropologists and medical sociologists) are likely to pay more attention to people with disability and the field of physical therapy. In summary, within the health care system, a greater understanding of how or why people think or behave in a particular manner can lead to more positive outcomes. These outcomes include improved patient outcomes with regard to functional ability and/or quality of life, as well as improved levels of professional and personal satisfaction for the health care professionals who feel more competent at their job.

Chapters 1, 2, and 3 specifically address the salient domains of culture and cultural competence from a broad perspective, yet they also address these domains as they specifically relate to physical therapy. Chapter 4 identifies the special considerations that need to be addressed when doing an ethnography of a client. Chapter 5 is the only chapter devoted to a specific cultural group. By definition, we as physical therapists most typically work with people with disabilities and bear a special responsibility to understand more about the "culture of disability."

Chapter 6 focuses on the present-day circumstances of disparities in health status, health care, and physical therapy. Chapters 7 and 8 are about poverty and racism. Arguably, these two topics are most important in helping a physical therapist understand how to move away from disparity toward health equity in the U.S.

Chapter 9 is included in this book because communication is recognized as perhaps the key to improving cultural competence. It is through communication that we learn about other peoples' beliefs and ways of life. The way in which we communicate with people from different cultures will impact our ability to elicit information and relate to other people.

Chapter 10 introduces the concept of service learning and explores the relationship between service learning and cultural competence. Physical therapists have recently begun to recognize the importance of service learning for both students and clinicians. Chapter 11 is important because most physical therapists have little or no knowledge of the social construction of disability outside of the industrialized world or alternative models of rehabilitation, yet individually and at the level of the profession (i.e., the American Physical Therapy Association [APTA]), are increasingly interested in global health and international physical therapy and rehabilitation. Our ability to be culturally competent across the globe will have a great impact on our capacity to be involved in international rehabilitation education and service.

Chapter 12 provides specific strategies (e.g., in education, research, and health promotion) to enable individual physical therapists and the profession of physical therapy to work toward the pinnacle of cultural competence.

The main target audiences for this text are physical therapists, physical therapy assistants, and other rehabilitation personnel. However, the principles elucidated are relevant for anyone (health care professional or not) interested in improving the outcomes associated with cross-cultural encounters. In the next millennium, world and national population patterns will continue to shift, and health care professionals will increasingly be required to share and practice their knowledge and skills in diverse settings. Professionally, the challenges of delivering effective and humanistic care are evident.

Words of caution are in order. First, some colleagues will argue that a concern for our patients' socio-cultural way of life is neither pertinent nor appropriate. In fact, some may resent its inclusion in the curriculum or practice environment. Nevertheless, an analysis of the literature reveals that stakeholders in the health care system are requiring initiatives in cultural competence. The perspective of the authors represented in this text is that physical therapists must understand the essence of an individual's culture to be effective.

Second, it may be argued that using broad categories to teach about culture is practical for descriptive purposes but can perpetuate culturally biased racial or ethnic stereotyping and prejudices. Clearly, this is not the intent. Rather, the intent is to incorporate knowledge about the people one is working with, considering the broad cultural landscape in which they live as well as their individual characteristics in order to recognize inter- and intra-ethnic diversity. It is necessary to take into account all of the variables that might influence the professional-patient interaction. Ethnicity, socioeconomic status, and religion are but a few. One may need to consider broad categories as a starting point from which to delve deeper into the life of the individual patient. One should not generalize about an entire ethnic group any more than one should not generalize about a patient based on the diagnosis of stroke or Parkinson's disease. A health professional would ask a multitude of questions and keenly observe the patient for clues to the person's full situation. That is, one would measure functional capabilities, range of motion, muscle strength, movement patterns, and more during the examination of each individual patient, rather than make a general assumption. If a client came to you with a diagnosis with which you were unfamiliar, you would access information about the problem to learn more. Similarly, it is appropriate to access information about the client's cultural ways of life if it is not familiar to you. It should be no different.

Third, in this text, the goal is to present theoretical and practical examples of beliefs and behaviors from a wide variety of cultures that specifically relate to the disciplines associated with the rehabilitative process. These examples, however, are just that—examples. In this complex world, it is impossible to provide details for all groups of people, let alone individuals, or for all topics of study (e.g., cultural explanations/definitions of anatomy and physiology, pain, stress, diet, sexuality, etc.). Yet, it is necessary to learn from the examples and extrapolate the concepts to provide insight into the larger principles at hand. One can usefully generalize or learn from one context (specific population group or geographic region) and apply the lesson to another context. This is true even though each culture may have specific culturally defined differences.

Nevertheless, as noted above, there are two exceptions within this book where a specific culture and a specific "-ism" are addressed. First is the cultural group of people with disabilities. Naturally, people with disabilities simultaneously belong to many other cultural groups (e.g., ethnic or religious), and their primary identification will vary (see discussion on subcultures for more). The specific "-ism" included is racism. Prejudice and discrimination come in many forms: real or imagined; covert or overt; individual, cultural, or institutional. In no way is the inclusion of racism meant to imply that sexism, ageism, homophobia, anti-semitism, or any other "-ism" is less important or not worthy of study by physical therapists or of action by physical therapists to diminish their presence in society.

CULTURAL COMPETENCE: WHAT IS IT?

In the beginning of this new millennium, the field of cross-cultural health has begun to flourish and the idea that cultural competence is desirable, and necessary, has become more widely accepted. Demographic transitions, substantial disparities in health outcomes among ethnic and cultural groups, and the moral imperative to treat individuals by a gold standard have led to the development of regulatory and accreditation standards regarding cultural competence by groups such as the Joint Commission on Accreditation of Healthcare Organizations (JCAHO) and APTA. In the 31st APTA Mary McMillan Lecture, Ruth Purtilo (2000) called for cultural competence to be a non-negotiable skill, tested as rigorously as competence in pathokinesiology or any other field of study.

There is an increasing body of literature on definitions and theoretical models describing cultural competence. See Chapter 3 for a more in-depth discussion of alternative definitions, models, and assessments. Arguably, the most relevant and thorough definition of cultural competence is that developed by Cross, Bazron, Dennis, and Isaacs (1989):

> "Cultural competence is a set of behaviors, attitudes, and policies that come together in a continuum to enable a health care system, agency, or individual rehabilitation practitioner to function effectively in trans-cultural interactions. In practice, cultural competence acknowledges and incorporates, at all levels, the importance of culture, the assessment of cross-cultural relations, the need to be aware of the dynamics resulting from cultural differences, the expansion of cultural knowledge, and the adaptation of services to meet culturally unique needs."

For physical therapy practitioners, cultural competence is an essential element in making effective and efficient examination, evaluation, diagnosis, prognosis, and intervention possible. Developing rapport, collecting and synthesizing patient data, recognizing personal functional concerns, and developing the plan of care for a particular patient requires cultural competence. The physical therapist who sees a wide range of functional impairments is expected to meet the needs of a patient within the context of that patient, the patient's family and community, and the broader cultural setting. By reviewing information on some of the unique characteristics associated with the patient, a physical therapist may gain insight and adapt the patient-therapist interaction and the rehabilitation services provided to create the best plan of care possible.

Understanding the concept of culture is the key to understanding cultural competence. The concept of culture has been defined in dozens of ways going back to the 19th Century. Chapter 2 provides a more thorough discussion of the concept of culture. Tylor (1958) defined culture as "that complex and whole which includes knowledge, belief, art, morals, law, custom, and any other capabilities and habits acquired by man [sic] as a member of society" (p. 1). Lynch and Hanson (1998) describe culture as the framework that guides and bounds life practices. People do not biologically inherit a culture, they learn it. People may share cultural tendencies and pass these tendencies to the next generations. However, cultural frameworks are never rigid, and they are constantly evolving. Many factors including ethnic identification, socioeconomic status, migration history, gender, age, religion, and physical capabilities have a profound impact on a person's way of life. A person's culture is closely interrelated to value systems, health beliefs and behaviors, and communication styles. Based on these variables, people may be members of several subcultures, which are smaller, but in some ways distinct, units within a larger culture (Loveland, 1999) (see Chapters 2 and 5). Cultures may have many similarities and differences between them, and a specific culture is not inherently better or worse than any other.

In every interaction, the physical therapist will need to consider, minimally, four broad but specific cultural milieus: the physical therapist's own culture, the patient's culture, the culture of the profession of physical therapy, and the culture of the health care system/organization in which the interaction is taking place. To be culturally competent, a practitioner must (Cross et al., 1989; Leavitt, 1999):

1. *Acknowledge the immense influence of culture.* This, in my opinion, is the most important concept to explore. It is essential to understand that all people are immersed in their own culture—with its associated beliefs, attitudes, and behaviors—that guides their

personal and professional interactions. Human nature, however, is such that everyone tends to be ethnocentric, believing that their own cultural way of life is the norm and the standard by which all others are judged. What we forget is that the next person, who may be from another culture, is probably also ethnocentric. Thus, the relevance of this self-awareness (or lack of it) is especially critical when physical therapists work with patients who come from different cultures. I do not believe that one can properly succeed at steps two through four if this step is passed over. (See sidebar discussion of "Body Ritual Among the Nacerima.")

2. *Assess cross-cultural relations and be vigilant concerning the dynamics that result from cultural differences.* With cross-cultural interaction comes the possibility that the other person's intentions and actions may be misjudged. Each party brings a specific set of experiences and personal and communication styles to an interaction. Physical therapists must be vigilant to minimize misperception, misinterpretation, and misjudgment through improved communication and thoughtfulness. With more insight into the patient or client's perspective (and fewer stereotypes) the ability to develop a mutually advantageous relationship is bound to be enhanced.

3. *Expand our cultural knowledge and incorporate this knowledge into our everyday practice.* If the assumption is that health care professionals can work effectively with people from other backgrounds, increased knowledge about the patient or client's socio-cultural context can only improve the relationship. Physical therapists must seek out socio-cultural information about the patient or client that will then help them appropriately modify an interview or history (i.e., what questions to ask and how to ask them) and modify interventions based on a person's cultural reality. Physical therapists should ask patients questions about their culture and lifestyle and indicate their willingness to learn about that culture. In that way, each party in the interaction can presume the desire to both give and receive information. Clinicians must be aware of the ethnographic makeup of the local community and the relevant beliefs and behaviors of their patients and the patients' families.

4. *Adapt to diversity.* Physical therapists need to develop culturally sensitive examination and intervention practices that facilitate a patient's comfort. The physical therapy department or health care environment should be adapted to create a better fit between the needs of the people requiring services and the needs of the clinicians and staff. Chapter 12 has specific suggested adaptations that may be considered.

It is important to remember that cultural competence is *NOT*:

- Abandoning our own culture and becoming a member of another culture by taking on all of the attitudes, values, and behaviors of that culture
- Asking our patients to abandon their culture and take on the attitudes, values, and behaviors of your culture
- Learning everything about all cultures and subcultures. This is impossible and unnecessary
- Assuming one person speaks for an entire group of people
- Assuming that a person's health concern is attributable only to socio-cultural factors and that it is not necessary to examine the patient for physiological pathology
- Agreeing with cultural relativism; it is unrealistic to presume that one will not make judgments about other cultural practices. Few would deny that there can be cultural practices that are deemed by some to be detrimental to others with regard to health
- Being "politically correct." Cultural competence is not a passing phase
- A quick fix

BODY RITUAL AMONG THE NACIREMA

To understand culture and ethnocentrism a bit better, I have included some excerpts from a classic article, "Body Ritual Among the Nacirema" by Horace Miner. As you read this description, please ask yourself, "Who are the Nacirema?"

"...the focus of this activity [daily rituals] is the human body, the appearance and health of which loom as a dominant concern in the ethos of the people...its ceremonial aspects...are unique... The fundamental belief underlying the whole system appears to be that the human body is ugly and that its natural tendency is to debility and disease. Incarcerated in such a body, man's [sic] only hope is to avert these characteristics through the use of the powerful influences of ritual and ceremony. Every household has one or more shrines devoted to this purpose...

"The focal point of the shrine is a box or chest...[in here] are kept the charms and magical potions without which no native believes he could live. These preparations are secured from a variety of specialized practitioners. The most powerful of these are the medicine men, whose assistance must be rewarded with substantial gifts...

"[Some medicine men] are specialists...[referred to as] "holy-mouth-men". The Nacirema have an almost pathological horror of and fascination with the mouth, the condition of which is believed to have a supernatural influence on all social relationships...

"The daily body ritual performed by everyone includes a mouth-rite. Despite the fact that these people are so punctilious about care of the mouth, this rite involves a practice which strikes the uninitiated stranger as revolting. It was reported to me that the ritual consists of inserting a small bundle of hog hairs into the mouth, along with certain magical powders, and then moving the bundle in a highly formalized series of gestures...

"The medicine men have an imposing temple, or *latipso*, in every community of any size. The more elaborate ceremonies required to treat very sick patients can only be performed at this temple, these ceremonies involve...a group of vestal maidens who move sedately about the temple chambers in distinctive costume and head-dress...

"The supplicant entering the temple is first stripped of all his or her clothes. In everyday life the Nacirema avoids exposure of his body and its natural functions. Bathing and excretory acts are performed only in the secrecy of the household shrine, where they are ritualized as part of the body-rites. Psychological shock results from the fact that body secrecy is suddenly lost upon entry to the *latipso*. A man, whose own wife has never seen him in an excretory act, suddenly finds himself naked and assisted by a vestal maiden while he performs his natural functions into a sacred vessel... The excreta are used by a diviner to ascertain the course and nature of the client's sickness...

"Our review of the ritual life of the Nacirema has certainly shown them to be a magic-ridden people..."

Do you think the Nacirema are foreign, exotic, possibly from the jungles in Latin America? Do you have an initial impression that these people are "strange" and that it might be difficult to treat them in a physical therapy department? How might the Nacirema view you as the physical therapist?

Well, if you haven't already guessed, the Nacirema are likely you! Nacirema is American spelled backwards. *Latipso* is hospital backwards, without the "h." The vestal maidens are nurses.

Please take a moment to rethink your ideas about who the Nacirema are, how we perceive people from a different cultural background, and how they might perceive us.

Excerpts reprinted from Miner, H. (1956). Body ritual among the Nacirema. *American Anthropologist, 58*(3), 503-507.

Although some relatively small actions such as changing the décor of a waiting area or hiring a person of color can make a difference in a client's comfort level, this alone is not cultural competence. Rather, the lifelong journey of achieving cultural proficiency requires changes that go deeper—a systematic appraisal and attempt to meet the requirements discussed above. Furthermore, even if all health professionals become culturally competent, it will not eradicate the myriad problems facing the health care system.

Cross et al. (1989) described six stages along a continuum of cultural competence ranging from cultural destructiveness to cultural proficiency (Table 1-1). In my view, and based on my 40 years of experience in this area, many physical therapists (and health care institutions) today are moving from Stage 3 (cultural blindness) to Stage 4 (cultural pre-competence). In the specific cohort studied by Wong and Blissett (2007), physical therapy students were rated most often as being culturally pre-competent. In cultural blindness, clinicians and health care institutions assume that they are unbiased. This assumption, however, is based on an incorrect belief that all people are the same. In this stage, facility policies and practices do not recognize the need for culturally specific approaches to solve problems. Cultural pre-competence moves toward the more positive end of the continuum. In this stage, therapists recognize weaknesses in the health care delivery system or in their personal cultural knowledge base, and they explore alternatives. They are also committed to responding appropriately to cultural differences. Cultural competence is Stage 5, and the last stage is cultural proficiency, where physical therapists recognize the need to conduct research, disseminate the results, and develop new approaches that might increase culturally competent practice.

CULTURAL COMPETENCE AND THE PHYSICAL THERAPY PROFESSION

The APTA steadfastly works to ensure that the physical therapy profession excels as health care providers. The *Guide to Physical Therapist Practice* (APTA, 2001), the *Normative Model of Physical Therapist Education* (APTA, 2004), and the Evaluative Criteria for Accreditation of Education Programs for the Preparation of Physical Therapists (APTA, 2009) all directly refer to cultural competence. See Chapter 3 for more on the history of cultural competence in the medical, nursing, and physical therapy profession.

CULTURAL COMPETENCE AND THE "CORE VALUES" OF PHYSICAL THERAPY

Professionalism in Physical Therapy: Core Values (APTA, 2003) identifies seven core values that are essential for physical therapy practice, education, and research. For each value, the APTA has defined the term and provided indicators to measure the presence of the value. The concept of cultural competence is embedded in each of the values. Below are the core values and an example(s) of an indicator that can relate to cultural competence (APTA, 2003):

1. *Accountability*: Responding to patient/client's goals and needs

2. *Altruism*: Providing patient/client services that go beyond expected standards of practice

3. *Compassion/caring*: Communicating effectively, both verbally and nonverbally, with others, taking into consideration individual differences in learning styles, language, cognitive abilities, etc.; demonstrating respect for others and considering others as unique and of value

4. *Excellence*: Engaging in acquisition of new knowledge; demonstrating a tolerance for ambiguity

5. *Integrity*: Using power (including avoidance of use of earned or unearned privilege) judiciously

6. *Professional duty*: Demonstrating beneficence by providing "optimal care"

7. *Social responsibility*: Advocating for the health and wellness needs of society, including access to health care and physical therapy services; promoting cultural competence within the profession and the larger public

	TABLE 1-1	

THE CONTINUUM OF CULTURAL COMPETENCE

STAGE	NAME	DEFINITION
1	Cultural destructiveness	People are treated in a dehumanizing manner and are denied services on purpose.
2	Cultural incapacity	Health care systems are unable to effectively work with patients from other cultures; bias, paternalism, and stereotypes exist.
3	Cultural blindness	The presumption is that all people are the same and that no bias exists; policies and practice do not recognize the need for culturally specific approaches to problem solving; services are ethnocentric and encourage assimilation; patients are blamed for their problems.
4	Cultural pre-competence	Health care system is committed to using appropriate response to cultural differences; weaknesses are acknowledged and alternatives are sought.
5	Cultural competence	Cultural differences are accepted and respected; continuous expansion of cultural knowledge and resources and continuous adaptation of services occur; continuous self-assessment about culture and vigilance toward the dynamics of cultural differences exist.
6	Cultural proficiency	Cultural differences are highly regarded; the need for research on cultural differences and the development of new approaches to enhance culturally competent practice are recognized.

Reproduced with permission from Cross, T. L., Bazron, B. J., Dennis, K. W., & Isaacs, M. R. (1989). *Towards a culturally competent system of care volume 1: A monograph on effective services for minority children who are severely emotionally disturbed.* Washington, DC: National Technical Assistance Center for Children's Mental Health, Georgetown University.

CULTURAL COMPETENCE AND "GENERIC ABILITIES" REQUIRED BY PHYSICAL THERAPISTS

Recognizing that it takes more to be an excellent physical therapist than technical skills alone, May, Morgan, Lemke, Karst, and Stone (1995) identified generic abilities that are considered essential for success. Listed below are the generic abilities and examples of criteria that might demonstrate the possession of such ability by being congruent with the notion of cultural competence (May et al., 1995):

- *Commitment to learning*: Accepts the challenge of new experiences; accepts the need to be a lifelong learner
- *Interpersonal skills*: Is respectful regarding others' lifestyle and cultural and personal differences; demonstrates acceptance of limited knowledge base
- *Communication skills*: Modifies communication to meet the needs of different audiences
- *Conflict resolution skills*: Approaches others to discuss differences in opinion
- *Effective use of time and resources*: Demonstrates flexibility
- *Use of constructive feedback*: Modifies own feedback style when needed
- *Clinical problem solving*: Considers all factors in selection of solution
- *Professionalism*: Demonstrates knowledge regarding all environmental factors that affect patient care
- *Responsibility*: Makes appropriate referrals to other health care providers
- *Critical thinking*: Feels compelled to examine new ideas
- *Stress management*: Seeks assistance as needed

CULTURAL COMPETENCE AND "EVIDENCE-BASED PRACTICE" AND "PATIENT-CENTERED CARE"

Physical therapy, along with the other health professions, is promoting the use of evidence in clinical decision making. *Evidence-based practice* (EBP) or *evidence-based physical therapy practice* (EBPT) are the terms most often used by physical therapists. This concept presumes "'open and thoughtful clinical decision making' about the physical therapy management of a patient/client that integrates the 'best available evidence with clinical judgment' and the patient/client's preferences and values, and that further considers the larger social context in which physical therapy services are provided, to optimize patient/client outcomes and quality of life" (Jewell, 2008, p. 8). Thus, within the definition itself, the socio-cultural context is recognized as a fundamental component of EBP. Contrary to general belief, EBP is not solely based on published research evidence because the interaction of past experience, beliefs and values, and preferences of the client and physical therapist must be taken into account for there to be true EBP.

According to Jewell (2008), once the validity of a test/measure or treatment is established, one must still consider whether the evidence is appropriate for use with a given patient. It is at this time that the PT will consider personal expertise and judgment in addition to the patient's preferences and values. For example, the cultural and social norms for the patient/family may impact the feasibility of a particular intervention. Thus, the challenge is to collect evidence from three sources: research-based clinical evidence, clinician judgment, and patient need. The final decision-making process integrates these factors. This model of clinical practice reinforces that health care interventions cannot be reduced merely to "science." Evidence-based research is done on populations, but physical therapists treat individuals.

Patients and families need an opportunity to have input on preferences (deciding between perceived desirability of two or more options) and values (personal concepts of beliefs about desirable behaviors or states of being that are prioritized relative to one another). This concept, referred to as *patient-centered care*—another emerging principle of the physical therapy profession—is "characterized by informed, shared decision making, development of patient knowledge, skills needed for self-management of illness, and preventive behaviors" (Knebel, 2008, p. 3 as cited in Jewell, 2008, p. 379). Patient-centered care rejects the traditionally practiced bio-medical model whereby health care professionals alone, based solely on "scientific" evidence, make decisions for the patient without consideration of a shared decision-making partnership with the patient and their unique perspective. The presumption is that patient-centered care may enhance biological and psychological outcomes through increased patient satisfaction, adherence to prescribed regiments, and acceptance of changes in life-ways.

CULTURAL COMPETENCE AND CROSS-CULTURAL ETHICS: A CHALLENGE TO ETHNOCENTRISM

APTA has a Code of Ethics within which all physical therapists are expected to practice. The first principle of the code requires that physical therapists respect the rights and dignity of all individuals and shall provide compassionate care (APTA, 2006). This presumes cultural competence.

With regard to the broader domain of health care, physical therapists are duty bound to accept the major health care ethical principles of autonomy, beneficence, and justice. Autonomy—the right to personal choice and self-determination—assumes the existence of individual values. It requires that one is fully informed. To be informed, one must be knowledgeable, reasoned/competent, and able to make a voluntary decision.

This principle is the most important at the individual or patient level. Non-maleficence/beneficence, is considered the most important principle for the health professional. To "do good," the health professional must abide by the four components of this standard:

1. One should not do evil/cause harm

2. One should prevent evil or harm

3. One should remove evil or harm

4. One should promote good

The third ethical principle, justice (i.e., fairness), is the most important ethical code in determining public health policy. The idea of distributive justice evaluates how the burdens and benefits of society should be distributed (Morrison, 2009).

Based on a review of the cultural value systems associated with different populations, it is possible to imagine how ideas concerning these ethical principles might not be the same for different people (see Chapter 4). For example, autonomy may be held in high esteem by people from individualistic cultures, and potentially not much at all in a collectivist culture. Also, paternalism, gender inequality, or the valuing of elders may impact who is supposed to make a decision for someone in the family. The idea of telling the truth to a patient, something that health professionals are taught, may be secondary to allowing someone to "save face" or not be embarrassed. What if, according to the principle of self-determination, a patient refuses a treatment that they really know very little about? What is considered evil or good are certainly not universal concepts. In a hierarchical society, concern for justice may be deemed not important as compared to a society that thinks of itself as egalitarian. Thus, one of the real challenges facing someone who is working toward becoming culturally competent is to be able to evaluate a situation without focusing solely on your own ethical perspective and decision-making process. One must recognize the potential for inherent conflicts and the idea that these conflicts may be difficult to resolve to your personal satisfaction.

In summary, as we begin the 21st Century, the notion of cultural competence is now firmly embedded into the requirements for being a physical therapist. The professional core values, therapist generic abilities, evidence-based practice, and professional ethics each require an understanding of the nature of culture and of the cultural competence paradigm.

TERMINOLOGY: THE USE OF LABELS WHEN DISCUSSING CULTURAL GROUPS

Terminology identifying people and groups of people is often confusing and controversial. The world contains a kaleidoscope of individuals and cultures: people self-identify or are categorized by a wide range of terms based on such things as race, ethnicity, religion, material reality, beliefs and behaviors, geography, and more. Cultural competence requires that one critically analyze the actual and perceived meaning of language.

In this book, we are often speaking about people from a particular ethnic group. From a socio-cultural perspective, ethnicity is a better label than race. Ethnic identification is classified by common traits or customs. It is based on a person's self-identification (i.e., it is subjective) as belonging to a distinct behavioral or ideational group that has a presumed shared cultural heritage. Ethnicity may be based on color, religion, place of origin or ancestry, language, or territory. Common categories of ethnic groups in the U.S. representing the above respective categories include but are not limited to White Anglo-Saxon Protestant (WASP), Black, Jewish, Italian American, Navajo, and Inuit. The degree of ethnic identification is fluid, depending upon such things as age, acculturation status, or stage of life.

Race, a concept historically used to divide the world's population into three biological/ genetic species (Caucasian, Negroid, and Mongoloid), was used to differentiate people by physical characteristics such as skin color. Today, it is an increasingly meaningless concept as people from different groups intermarry and reproduce, and people with similar genetic background have very divergent socio-cultural ways of life. For example, people who may have historically been identified as Negroid have black skin, yet people with black skin in the U.S. may consider themselves from very different ethnic groups, (e.g., African [Nigerian], African American [born and raised in Mississippi], Caribbean American [Jamaican], etc.). These differentiations are associated with cultural heritage and geography, and not race. Similarly, there is an enormous variety of individuality among Caucasian cultures as well. Caucasians may identify as noted above by varying key demographic features such as country of ancestor's origin (Irish American) or religion (Muslim). The term *Euro-American* encompasses people whose ancestors come from many European nations, including but not limited to England, Italy, Greece, and Poland. However, this tendency to identify with a particular country of origin was more pronounced prior to the mid 1950s. Now, people who have European ancestry are typically labeled "White."

I prefer to use terms relating to ethnic identity rather than race when possible because I consider it more relevant and meaningful. Nevertheless, it is critical to not minimize the impact of race and racism on health (see Chapters 6 and 8) and remember that race may relate to drug metabolism or predisposition to certain diseases (see Chapter 4). Race should not be used as a proxy for genetic individuality. The U.S. Census Bureau uses the terminology *racial and ethnic designations,* and the phrase "racial and ethnic disparities" is typically used in the associated literature published by the U.S. government and health-related journals. APTA policies and literature use the following designations: American Indian or Alaskan Native; Asian; Pacific Islander or Native Hawaiian; White (which indicates people of European ancestry or origin); African American or Black; and Hispanic/Latino.

Labels are often problematic because it is recognized that broad categories fail to represent subgroups and the presence of intra-cultural diversity. For example, the category "Asian" represents at least 18 subgroups, and there are over 500 American Indian tribal groups in the U.S. The "Hispanic" or "Latino" ethnic identification encompasses over 20 subgroups. Furthermore, the terms *Hispanic* or *Latino* are often used interchangeably in the literature to refer to persons of any race living in the U.S. whose origins can be traced to the Spanish-speaking countries of Europe, Central and South America, and the Caribbean. They may be born in the U.S. or in their homeland and be naturalized citizens or recent immigrants (legal or undocumented). More typically, people on the West Coast self-identify as "Latino" or "Chicano" (specifically for those of Mexican-American descent) and on the East Coast as "Hispanic." However, my observation is that, in recent years, the term *Latino* has become more prevalent because of its connection to people of Latin America. Also, people born to parents of two distinct ethnic groups increasingly prefer to identify themselves by using a multi-ethnic category, a trend that should continue to grow as the frequency of inter-ethnic relationships increases.

Terminology can also be complicated by the subliminal messages and implications that are associated with words. For example, I do not like the term *minority* as a designation for a group of people, who are, in fact, sometimes the majority. *Minority* can imply inferior or lesser and the subliminal message is that this person is less important. Conversely, in the global context, Caucasian people, though the minority, generally speaking have far greater economic resources and political power. Hence, they have more access to health and rehabilitation services and are more likely to be the ones providing services to others in a multi-cultural environment.

Thoughtful individuals struggle in trying to determine appropriate language and terminology so that no one is offended. The phrase "people of color" is often the preferred terminology used in the U.S. today for non-White individuals. Yet, the term *of color* often evokes a visual image of someone that is false. Some Native Americans, Hispanics, or very light skinned Black people may appear White. In many ways, this term merely implies that one belongs to a group of individuals who are not descended from Northern Europe. In any case, careful attention should be paid to using language that conveys inclusion. In real life circumstances, one needs to ask a person to self-identify. If someone prefers a particular label, then that is the obvious choice to use.

Finally, it bears repeating that the use of broad categories is practical for descriptive purposes but should not be used to perpetuate culturally biased racial or ethnic stereotyping and prejudices. Stereotyping is assigning the characteristics of a group to a person without regard for individual differences. It is the process by which people use social categories (e.g., race or sex), often unconsciously, in acquiring, processing, and recalling information about others. Stereotyping is an end point, that is, no effort is made to learn more and determine if a person/group fits the statement. Negative stereotypes can exert a powerful influence on self-fulfilling prophecies. Even so-called positive stereotypes should be recognized for their potential damage to a person. If "all blacks are great basketball players," or "all Asians are good in math," what happens to individuals who do not fit that stereotype? They may be more likely to have a negative self-image or feel pressure to conform. Stereotypes can lead to prejudice and discrimination and serve as obstacles in getting to know other people for whom they are.

Although most people do not believe that they stereotype, research shows otherwise. Research on social categorization and stereotyping supports the fact that people universally apply stereotypes when trying to know and understand other people (van Ryn & Fu, 2003). It is a natural function of the human mind: It is an efficient, unconscious, and automatic response to simplify cognitive processing in our very complex world. Stereotypes are acquired from the world around us or from cultural mediators such as the media rather than from personal experiences, and they are resistant to change. Thus, it is unrealistic and not useful to expect people to be immune from stereotyping. But, as an individual and as a physical therapist, we must admit to this tendency. We must always use the perception as a starting point from which to gather more information.

In contrast, a "generalization" is a beginning point to classify someone as it acknowledges that additional information is needed to determine whether the information presumed relevant applies to a particular person. Generalizations can be used when looking for common patterns that might be shared by a group. Children are taught to generalize at an early age—animals are one category, things that move are another, and things we eat are a third. However, all individuals are distinguished by many personal characteristics and by being a part of many subgroups. Variation in any one of these, such as innate personality type, degree of acculturation, socioeconomic status, sexual orientation, and disability status can cause an individual to not fit a particular pattern.

Lastly, as critical thinkers and lifelong learners, physical therapists must recognize statistical data analyses as being based on categorical facts and not stereotypes. That is, as described in detail in Chapter 6, it is a fact and not a stereotype that, for example, African Americans have higher rates of hypertension.

Authors in this book come from different academic disciplines. These authors typically use terminology that is preferred for their field of study, and thus terminology will vary somewhat chapter to chapter. The contributors to this book are primarily physical therapists, but there are also social scientists represented. In the case of material quoted or summarized from another source, the racial/ethnic designations used in that source will be used to avoid altering data from that source.

In summary, broad categories and labels are sometimes used out of necessity, but there is a wide range of *interethnic* diversity and *intra-ethnic* diversity. Physical therapists manage individual patients or clients and not a population. Clinicians should not make general assumptions about an entire ethnic group any more than they would with a patient with a stroke, Parkinson's disease, or joint degeneration.

THE CHANGING DEMOGRAPHIC LANDSCAPE IN THE UNITED STATES

In the U.S., changing demographics provides a major reason why cultural competence has become so critical. From the beginning of nationhood, the U.S. has been made up of Native Americans and immigrants, albeit with varying governmental policies that encouraged or discouraged groups of people from around the world settling here. During the early 1900s, most of the immigrants coming to the U.S. were from European nations. In 1965, a major change in the U.S. immigration policy occurred that led to a substantial increase in diversity within this land. The Immigration and Naturalization Act of 1965 ended the previous quota system. Most immigrants from that time on have been from the Caribbean, Asia, or South and Central America (LeMay, 2004).

The future can be imagined by reviewing the recent past. Between 1980 and 1990, the total U.S. population increased by 9.8%. The rate of growth, however, varied widely. The Asian/Pacific Island population rate of growth was 107.8%, the Hispanic/Latino was 53%, the Native American was 37.9%, the Black was 13.2%, and the White was 6% (U.S. Census Bureau, 1990).

Between 1990 and 2000, the historical course that was most sharply defined during the previous decade continued. Understanding the 2000 Census is somewhat complicated, however, by the fact that it used 63 ethnic categories instead of the five categories used previously. This more complex scheme was created to accommodate people who identify themselves in ways that are different from older classifications or who consider themselves multiracial (U.S. Census Bureau, 1996). In 2000, approximately 75% of the U.S. population was White; 12.5% was Black or African American; 12.5% was Hispanic or Latino; 1% was American Indian and Alaska Native; 3.7% was Asian or Native Hawaiian and Other Pacific Islander; 2.4% identified themselves as part of two or more ethnic groups; and 5.5% identified themselves as "Other" (U.S. Census Bureau, 2000).

Statistics from the 2006 census (U.S. Census Bureau, 2006), demonstrate a continuation of the aforementioned trends. The Hispanic population, demonstrating the fastest rate of growth, has grown to 15.1% of the U.S. population (45.5 million people), and is the largest "minority" group. Blacks are reported to be 13.9% (40.7 million), Asians 5.04% (15.2 million), American Indian/Alaska natives 1.49% (4.5 million), and Pacific Islanders .33% (1 million). The population of Whites (non-Hispanic) totaled 66% (199.1 million) down from the 75% reported in 2000.

Further analysis of census data reveal that California, Texas, Florida, New York, and Illinois are the states with the largest numbers of Hispanic people (U.S. Census Bureau, 2000). However, Hispanics in the U.S., both recent immigrants and people born here, are moving away from the traditional immigrant strongholds to rural and suburban areas and to states such as North Carolina, Tennessee, Georgia, and Indiana in search of jobs (Frey, 2008).

A more in-depth look at the aforementioned numbers is required to understand the demographic picture in the U.S. Using the category "Hispanic" or "Latino" as an example, there is substantial intra-ethnic diversity. Approximately 64% of the Hispanic population in the U.S. are Mexican American, 11% are Puerto Rican, 13% are from Central and South America (excluding Brazil), 5% are Cuban American, and 8% are other (Therrien & Ramirez, 2001). The concepts of "mixed race" or multi-ethnic identity continue to evolve as more people from different backgrounds produce offspring (Navarro, 2008).

Of special interest to the physical therapist working in geriatrics is the unprecedented growth of the older Hispanic population. Hispanics are the fastest growing subpopulation of those over 65 years old. The elderly Hispanics will grow from 1.1 million in 1990 to 4.7 million in 2020 and are expected to reach 12 to 14 million by 2050. Fifteen and one half percent of older Americans will be Latino, and most will live in Southwest U.S. At 20%, Cuban Americans have the greatest percentage of their total population over 65 years old (Aguirre-Molina, Molina, & Zambrana, 2001; Huff & Kline, 1999). Overall, the largest percentage of the Latino elderly is Mexican (50%), followed by Cubans (17%), Puerto Ricans (11%), and South and Central Americans (22%). Similar to other groups, the relative increase among those over 85 years old is greatest. In addition to the aging population in general, the U.S. immigration law's favorable stance on family reunification encourages the entry of older family members (Villa & Torres-Gil, 2001). In summary, the relative increase in the population over 65 years of age will be greatest for people of color, specifically people of Latin origin. Of special interest to the physical therapist working in pediatrics, is the estimate that 45% of children under the age of five are from a racial or ethnic group other than White (U.S. Census Bureau, 2008).

Furthermore, for most socio-cultural domains, the statistics associated with subgroups vary. Puerto Ricans as a group are the most impoverished Hispanics, whereas Central and South Americans are the least impoverished (Therrien & Ramirez, 2001). However, one cannot assume that all subgroup statistics are similarly proportional. For example, there is also a range for those with health insurance coverage among Hispanic subgroups. Those without health insurance include 37.6% of Mexicans, 20.4% of Puerto Ricans, 22.8% of Cubans, and 32.3% of other Hispanic groups (MacDorman & Mathews, 2008). Infant mortality rates for people of Hispanic origin vary widely as well with Puerto Ricans having the highest rate. For all Hispanics, the infant mortality rate is 5.6%. It is 5.5% for Mexicans, 8.3% for Puerto Ricans, 4.4% for Cubans, 4.6% for people from Central and South America, and 7.1% for other and unknown Hispanic/Latino groups (MacDorman & Mathews, 2008, Table 3). For the variable of high school graduation rates, there is intra-ethnic variation again. The percent of individuals of Hispanic origin age 25 and older who graduate from high school is 57% overall (compared to 88% for Non-Hispanic Whites), 73% for Cuban, 64% for Central/South American, 64% for Puerto Rican, and 51% for Mexican (Therrien & Ramirez).

To conclude, based on immigration patterns (there are especially high numbers of Asian and Hispanic immigrants) and fertility rates (birth rates are generally higher for Hispanics, especially Puerto Ricans), the U.S. Census Bureau has been projecting that, by the year 2050, White non-Hispanic Americans will represent approximately 52% of the total population, demonstrating a continuous downward trend. Hispanic Americans are expected to account for 22% of the population, with African Americans at 16% and Asian/Pacific Island Americans at 10% (Figure 1-1). The 2008 estimate, however, is that Whites will no longer be in the majority by 2042, eight years ahead of the earlier predictions (Frey, 2008).

HEALTH PROFESSIONAL DEMOGRAPHICS

An additional consideration when addressing population patterns is the substantial disparity between the number of people from particular ethnic groups who are health professionals or enrolled in health care education and their representation in the society as a whole. In general, people of color are underrepresented in all of the health professions. In 2007, the following data were reported for Blacks and Hispanics respectively: physicians—9.9% and 5.2%; dentists—5.4% and 3.4%; pharmacists—5.9% and 2.5% (U.S. Department of Labor, 2008).

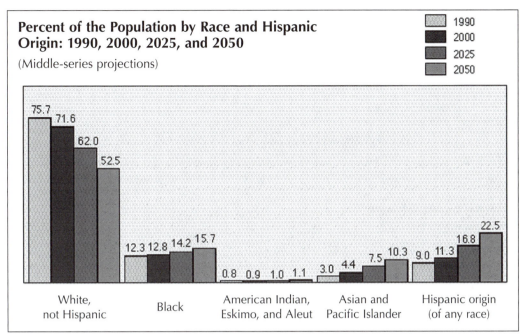

FIGURE 1-1. Percent of the population by race and Hispanic origin: 1990, 2000, 2025, and 2050. Reproduced from U.S. Census Bureau. (n.d.). National population projections. Retrieved December 8, 2009, from http://www.census.gov/population/www/pop-profile/natproj.html

In physical therapy, although not all physical therapists are members of the APTA, the APTA reports that approximately 93% of its membership is White (Table 1-2). A slighly greater number of people of color have recently graduated from physical therapy schools. However, as shown in Table 1-3, progress over the years has been slow. Furthermore, about 70% of APTA membership is female and this number has not changed since 1999 (APTA, 2007).

In addition to the under-representation of people of color among health professionals, the didactic and clinical educational materials used in the education of health professionals and physical therapists specifically have historically used a "Western medical model" and a Eurocentric point of view regarding disability, health, and illness. These factors contribute to a less-than-ideal delivery of care to people from other backgrounds and can result in a cultural clash and conflicting expectations between patient and therapist. Although it is best if all ethnic groups are proportionately represented within the treatment setting, it is essential to realize that it is equally important that *all* therapists, regardless of their own ethnic background, be culturally competent.

CONCLUSION

Cultural Competence: A Lifelong Journey to Cultural Proficiency provides an overview of several salient domains, the most important of which is culture. Other major topics include the influence of socioeconomic status, and race and ethnicity on one's life, health beliefs and behaviors as they relate to disability and rehabilitation, cross-cultural communication, and attitudes toward persons with disability. Baseline knowledge of these critical domains is necessary to appreciate the need to explore alternative ways to approach people from different cultures and how to develop alternative models of care. This book is intended to have theoretical and descriptive interest and value as well as practical application to physical therapists.

TABLE 1-2

PHYSICAL THERAPIST MEMBER DEMOGRAPHIC PROFILE—2008

ETHNIC ORIGIN

Hispanic or Latino	2.0
Not Hispanic or Latino	98.0

RACE

White	93.0
Asian	4.1
Native Hawaiian or Other Pacific Islander	0.3
African American or Black	1.6
American Indian or Alaskan Native	0.6

Reproduced with permission from American Physical Therapy Association. (2007). Physical therapist member demographic profile 1999–2008. Retrieved December 8, 2009, from http://www.apta.org/AM/Template.cfm?Section=Surveys_and_Stats1&Template=/MembersOnly.cfm&ContentID=46077&Token=DA435824-5557-4188-AF6A-EEFB148765AD

TABLE 1-3

ETHNICITY OF GRADUATES OF PROFESSIONAL PHYSICAL THERAPIST PROGRAMS

ETHNIC ORIGIN	2000	2001	2003	2004	2005	2007
	N=6,858	N=6,763	N=5,119	N=4,913	N=5,242	N=5,715
African American	2.9%	2.8%	4.1%	4.5%	4.8%	4.9%
American Indian/Alaskan Native	0.3%	0.3%	0.5%	0.5%	0.7%	0.5%
Asian/Pacific Islander	4.9%	5.0%	5.8%	6.5%	5.9%	5.4%
Hispanic/Latino	3.0%	3.0%	3.7%	5.0%	4.3%	4.9%
White	85.5%	85.4%	81.6%	77.9%	81.1%	81.2%
Other	1.9%	1.9%	3.6%	3.1%	1.9%	1.4%
Unknown	1.5%	1.6%	0.7%	2.5%	1.3%	1.6%

Reproduced with permission from American Physical Therapy Association. (2008). 2007-2008 fact sheet: Physical therapist education programs. Retrieved December 8, 2009, from http://www.apta.org/AM/Template.cfm?Section=Aggregate_Program_Data1&TEMPLATE=/CM/ContentDisplay.cfm&CONTENTID=51040

REFLECTION QUESTIONS

✔ Do you believe that you have a professional responsibility to move toward cultural proficiency?

✔ Where do you think you fall on the cultural competence continuum? Give some examples of why you placed yourself where you did.

✔ What is your familiarity with people of a different heritage?

✔ Can you identify an ethical dilemma related to your physical therapy practice that may be a result of two people having different value systems?

✔ How would you describe the people who live in your neighborhood? City?

✔ *Do you know any people who have recently immigrated to the United States?*

✔ *Do you enjoy being with people who are different from you?*

✔ *Did you realize the extent of the demographic transitions within the United States?*

REFERENCES

Aguirre-Molina, M., Molina, C. W., & Zambrana, R. E. (Eds.). (2001). *Health issues in the Latino community*. San Francisco, CA: Jossey-Bass Publishers.

American Physical Therapy Association. (2001). *Guidelines to physical therapy practice* (2nd ed.). Alexandria, VA: Author.

American Physical Therapy Association. (2003). Professionalism in physical therapy: Core values. Retrieved October 26, 2008, from http://www.apta.org/AM/Template.cfm?Section=Policies_and_Bylaws&TEMPLATE=/CM/ContentDisplay.cfm&CONTENTID=36073

American Physical Therapy Association. (2004). *A normative model of physical therapist professional education: Version 2004*. Alexandria, VA: Author.

American Physical Therapy Association. (2006). Code of ethics. Retrieved October 26, 2008, from http://www.apta.org/AM/Template.cfm?Section=Core_Documents1&Template=/CM/HTMLDisplay.cfm&ContentID=25854

American Physical Therapy Association. (2007). Physical therapist member demographic profile 1999-2008. Retrieved December 8, 2009, from http://www.apta.org/AM/Template.cfm?Section=Surveys_and_Stats1&Template=/MembersOnly.cfm&ContentID=46077&Token=AB6624AD-00AC-4D7C-8AD5-489B48F6CD8F

American Physical Therapy Association. (2008). 2007-2008 fact sheet: Physical therapist education programs. Retrieved December 8, 2009, from http://www.apta.org/AM/Template.cfm?Section=Aggregate_Program_Data1&TEMPLATE=/CM/ContentDisplay.cfm&CONTENTID=51040

American Physical Therapy Association. (2009). Evaluative criteria for accreditation of education programs for the preparation of physical therapists. Retrieved September 16, 2009, from http://www.apta.org/AM/Template.cfm?Section=Home&TEMPLATE=/CM/ContentDisplay.cfm&CONTENTID=62414

Cross, T. L., Bazron, B. J., Dennis, K. W., & Isaacs, M. R. (1989). *Towards a culturally competent system of care volume 1: A monograph on effective services for minority children who are severely emotionally disturbed*. Washington, DC: National Technical Assistance Center for Children's Mental Health, Georgetown University.

Frey, W. H. (2008). The Census projects minority surge. Retrieved September 11, 2009, from http://www.brookings.edu/opinions/2008/0818_census_frey.aspx

Huff, R. M., & Kline, M. V. (1999). *Promoting health in multicultural populations: A handbook for practitioners*. Thousand Oaks, CA: Sage Publications.

Jewell, D. V. (2008). *Guide to evidence-based physical therapy practice*. Sudbury, MA: Jones and Bartlett Publishers.

Leavitt, R. L. (Ed.). (1999). *Cross-cultural rehabilitation: An international perspective*. London, England: Harcourt Brace and Company.

LeMay, M. C. (2004). *U.S. immigration: A reference handbook*. Santa Barbara, CA: ABC-CLIO.

Loveland, C. (1999). The concept of culture. In R. L. Leavitt (Ed.), *Cross-cultural rehabilitation: An international perspective* (pp. 15-24). London, England: Harcourt Brace and Company.

Lynch, E. W., & Hanson, M. J. (Eds.). (1998). *Developing cross-cultural competence: A guide for working with young children and their families* (2nd ed.). Baltimore, MD: Brookes Publishing Company.

MacDorman, M. F., & Mathews, T. J. (2008). *Recent trends in infant mortality in the United States. NCHS data brief, no 9*. Hyattsville, MD: National Center for Health Statistics. Retrieved December 4, 2009, from http://www.cdc.gov/nchs/data/databriefs/db09.htm#KeyFindings

May, W. W., Morgan, B. J., Lemke, J. C., Karst, G. M., & Stone, H. L. (1995). Model for ability-based assessment in physical therapy education. *Journal of Physical Therapy Education, 9*(1), 3-6.

Miner, H. (1956). Body ritual among the Nacirema. *American Anthropologist, 58*(3), 503-507.

Morrison, E. E. (2009). Health care ethics: Critical issues for the 21st century (2nd ed.). Sudbury, MA: Jones and Bartlett Publishers.

Navarro, M. (2008). Who are we? New dialogue on mixed race. *New York Times, March 31, 2008*, A1-A15.

Purtilo, R. B. (2000). Thirty-first Mary McMillan lecture: A time to harvest, a time to sow: Ethics for a shifting landscape. *Physical Therapy, 80*(11), 1112-1119.

Siantz, M. L., & Meleis A. I. (2007). Integrating cultural competence into nursing education and practice: 21st century action steps. *Journal of Transcultural Nursing, 18*(1 Suppl), 86S-90S.

Therrien, M., & Ramirez, R. R. (2001). The Hispanic population in the United States: March 2000. Washington, DC: U.S. Census Bureau. Retrieved November 28, 2009, from http://www.census.gov/prod/2001pubs/p20-535.pdf

Tylor, E. B. (1958). *Primitive culture*. New York, NY: Harper & Row. (Original work published in 1871).

U.S. Department of Labor, Bureau of Labor Statistics. (2008). Labor force statistics from the current population survey. Retrieved August 12, 2008, from http://www.bls.gov/cps

U.S. Census Bureau. (1990). *Current population reports*. Washington, DC: Author.

U.S. Census Bureau. (1996). *Current population reports: P25-1130 population projections of the United States by age, sex, race, and Hispanic origin: 1995 to 2050*. Washington DC: Author.

U.S. Census Bureau. (2000). *Current population reports*. Washington, DC: Author.

U.S. Census Bureau. (2006). *Population estimate*. Washington, DC: Author.

U.S. Census Bureau. (2008). *Current population reports*. Washington, DC: Author.

U.S. Census Bureau. (n.d.). National population projections. Retrieved December 8, 2009, from http://www.census.gov/population/www/pop-profile/natproj.html

van Ryn, M., & Fu, S. S. (2003). Paved with good intentions: Do public health and human service providers contribute to racial/ethnic disparities in health? *American Journal of Public Health, 93*(2), 248-255.

Villa, V. M., & Torres-Gil, F. M. (2001). The later years: The health of elderly Latinos. In M. Aguirre-Molina, C. W. Molina, & R. E. Zambrana (Eds.), *Health issues in the Latino community* (pp. 157-178). San Francisco, CA: Jossey-Bass.

Wong, C. K., & Blissett, S. (2007). Assessing performance in the area of cultural competence: An analysis of reflective writing. *Journal of Physical Therapy Education, 21*(1), 40-47.

Understanding the Nature of Culture

Christine A. Loveland, PhD

CULTURE

At birth, humans must begin to adjust to a natural environment in which oxygen sustains life and to a social environment in which culture sustains life. Only when deprived of oxygen or of their usual cultural supports do people realize how crucial both are to existence. In the case of culture, this realization occurs when people leave their home and their cultural environment or when they find themselves interacting with people from different cultural backgrounds. Both types of situations are increasingly common as global travel and population movements result in frequent cross-cultural interaction. These interactions, whether as a result of necessity or choice, contain the potential for enriched communication and understanding and, paradoxically, the possibility of miscommunication and misunderstanding. One of the places where this is most evident is in all areas of clinical medicine. The rehabilitation setting provides rich opportunities for learning about another culture or for experiencing the difficulties of cross-cultural interactions. The health professional and the patient may come from different cultural backgrounds and view the presenting problem in very different ways. People in the patient's culture may see disability as something to be hidden, while the therapist's goal is to reintegrate the patient into society. The patient and her family may be very resistant to the rehabilitation professionals' efforts since they may not be able to imagine a culture in which people with disabilities (PWDs) assume a more public life. To achieve a successful therapeutic outcome, each person (patient, family members, medical personnel) involved in this situation needs to able to view the problem from another perspective.

To embark on the journey toward cultural proficiency and understand another person's perspective, it helps to understand culture, its many component parts, and examples of its influence on everyday life. This understanding begins with the notion that culture is learned, not biologically inherited. A normal human infant can learn any culture through the process of socialization (or enculturation), and by the time we are adults, our responses to any situation will be culturally based.

R. L. Leavitt (Ed.).
*Cultural Competence: A Lifelong Journey
to Cultural Proficiency* (pp. 19-30).
© 2010 SLACK Incorporated

The cultures in which we live consist of:

- The material culture, which is the tangible part of culture
- Behavior, which is based on the norms accepted in our particular culture
- The nonmaterial culture, which is the intangible part of culture, including our values, attitudes, feelings, and beliefs

Sometimes, nonmaterial culture is called our "invisible baggage" because it travels with us but is not always easily recognized. It is common for changes in the material culture to occur more quickly than changes in the nonmaterial culture. This phenomenon is called "cultural lag" and is easily seen in medical settings where the appropriate use of technology (part of the material culture) can raise extremely complex ethical issues (part of the nonmaterial culture).

Cultural universals are found in all known cultures. Examples include the presence of expressive culture; some kind of belief in the supernatural; an economic system that people use to produce, exchange, and consume goods and services; and a family and kinship system that classifies and organizes relatives. Within these categories is immense cultural variation and, because we learn about and are familiar with our own culture's religion, art, and family type, it is not always easy for us to accommodate another culture's preferences. Sometimes this discomfort can lead to strong feelings of ethnocentrism.

ETHNOCENTRISM AND CULTURAL RELATIVISM

Ethnocentrism is the belief that one's own culture is superior to others and is the standard by which other cultures should be judged. In the example of a person with a disability being set apart from mainstream society, it would be important for the health care professionals to understand why PWDs are isolated in the patient's culture. With this understanding, even though the medical staff might disagree both with the belief and the behavior, they would need to be able to consider them in any proposed rehabilitation regimen. This staff would be practicing cultural relativism, the belief that the customs and behavior of people in other cultures should not be judged on the basis of the outside observer's own culture. The concept of cultural relativism goes back to the beginning of American anthropology and continues to be an important consideration within the discipline.

There are two main approaches in the application of cultural relativism. Someone who takes the position that there is no behavior that justifies intervention in a culture is practicing absolute (or general) cultural relativism. This means that an anthropologist does not intervene even when he or she observes cross-cultural behavior, such as female genital cutting (or female genital mutilation), that can cause physical and emotional suffering.

The second approach is critical cultural relativism. Anthropologists who practice critical cultural relativism disagree with the policy of complete noninterference. In this context, "critical" does not mean that anthropologists criticize the behavior, but rather that they use critical thinking to assess the problem and possible responses to it. In addition, critical cultural relativism is based on the assumption that there are universal human rights, and that these rights cannot be denied on the basis of culture.

This discussion, in turn, leads to another contested issue: universal human rights. Who determines which rights are included? Do people in every culture in the world recognize the same moral and ethical principles? These are difficult questions and may impact how PWDs are treated within a society. A final concern is the position of someone who lives or works in a different culture and who must decide whether to become an advocate for change in that culture.

It is important to remember that cultures, like people, develop and change in response to the environment and conditions present in a particular time and place. They adapt if it is necessary and possible to do so. Cultures are not static or unchangeable, and all of the elements of a culture—the economic system, the political organization, the religion, the family structure—are interconnected. Cultural variables are woven into an intricate tapestry—pull one thread or change one color of the tapestry and the composition of the entire picture may be altered. That is why it is unrealistic to ask a person to change an aspect of his or her culture without recognizing the possibility that this may change or alter other learned values and behaviors.

The Importance of Nonmaterial Culture in Rehabilitation

In a rehabilitation context, beliefs about the cause(s) of disability and the role (appropriate behavior) of the person with a disability are part of the nonmaterial culture. The available facilities, technology, and rehabilitation equipment are part of the material culture. Sometimes similarities in the material cultures obscure profound differences in the nonmaterial cultures, and people in a cross-cultural interaction are surprised and shocked when misunderstanding develops. For example, just because a patient and therapist live in similar houses, wear similar clothing, and even speak the same language does not mean that they share the same religion, the same attitudes about disability, or the same beliefs about the appropriate behavior for men and women.

SPIRITUALITY

Spirituality provides one of the best examples of the importance of nonmaterial culture in rehabilitation. People in many cultures believe that illness, accidents, disability, and even death are supernatural punishments for the misbehavior of either the patient or a member of the patient's family. Sometimes powerful emotions such as jealousy and anger are blamed for such misfortunes; these emotions may have been unleashed in the past, even before the patient was born. If that is the case, taking a patient's history entails more than recording relevant medical information—it means an examination of the psychosocial background that can include the patient's relatives and ancestors. For some people, spiritual beliefs influence their explanation and acceptance (or lack of acceptance) of their medical condition as well as their willingness to participate in treatment and rehabilitation programs. In fact, outside of biomedicine, most medical systems consider the causes of illness and disability to lie within the souls and minds of those involved, not under a microscope or on an X-ray film. From this perspective, biomedicine treats and alleviates the symptoms, but only a truly holistic treatment that includes the emotional or psychological causes can be curative. Rehabilitation professionals should make every effort to show respect for such beliefs. When patients and families suspect that such respect isn't present, they may not discuss these beliefs with medical personnel, thereby further hampering the treatment regimen.

Johnson, Elbert-Avila, and Tulsky (2005) reviewed the literature on the importance of spiritual beliefs in the treatment preferences of African Americans, particularly as the beliefs influence decisions about care at the end of life. They found three recurrent themes: "spiritual beliefs and practices are a source of comfort, coping, and support and are the most effective way to influence healing; God is responsible for physical and spiritual health; and the doctor is God's instrument" (p. 711). These beliefs sometimes lead to clashes with medical personnel because African Americans are more likely to insist on aggressive treatment and therapies for dying patients because "limiting life-sustaining treatments may be viewed as a form of suicide" (p. 716).

In *The Scalpel and the Silver Bear* (2000), Dr. Lori Alvord, a Navajo surgeon, and Elizabeth Van Pelt describe the importance of spirituality in Navajo ideas about health and disease:

"Navajos believe in hózhó or hózhóni—'Walking in Beauty'—a worldview in which everything is connected and influences everything else. A stone thrown into a pond can influence the life of a deer in the forest, a human voice and a spoken word can influence events around the world, and all things possess spirit and power. So Navajos make every effort to live in harmony and balance with everyone and everything else. Their belief system sees sickness as a result of things falling out of balance, of losing one's way on the path of beauty. In this belief system, religion and medicine are one" (p. 14).

Although African American and Navajo spiritual beliefs are different, in both cultures these beliefs are extremely important in people's understanding of and reaction to illness. These two cultures also illustrate how very different belief systems can result in similar outcomes in a clinical setting. Alvord and Van Pelt note that "Navajos do not touch the dead. Ever. It is one of the strongest rules in our culture...When a person dies, the 'good' part of the person leaves with the spirit, while the 'evil' part stays with the body" (2000, p. 40). They go on to note the Navajos' reluctance to discuss living wills or advance directives, or to make end-of-life decisions, two of the problem areas found in the study of African American patients. Alvord and Van Pelt state that:

"...because Navajos are so uncomfortable with death and dying, speaking to them about making a decision to end life, to stop a life-support system, was nearly impossible and had to be handled very carefully. The discomfort arises partly because of the Navajo belief in the power of language, the belief that you can 'speak' something into existence. Most Navajos, for instance, would never say, 'If I fall into coma, I don't want to be kept alive.' Such verbalizing would be seen as asking for it to happen" (p. 66).

These two examples illustrate important points about the power of culture, particularly nonmaterial culture. First, with the incredible diversity of the American population, medical personnel are likely to interact with people who have widely varying spiritual beliefs, and this can be very important in a clinical setting. Second, it is possible for very different belief systems to result in very similar behavior. Both African American and Navajo patients and families may have great difficulty with end-of-life issues, resulting in similar conflicts with doctors, nurses, and therapists. For some African Americans, only God has the power to determine whether a person is healthy or sick and whether a person recovers from an illness or dies. For Navajos, fear of death and a belief in the power of speech combine to make even a discussion of end-of-life issues problematic. In both cases, hospital staff may view the families as unreasonable and unaware of the reality of the medical situation when, in fact, two very different belief systems have resulted in the same difficulties. To resolve these conflicts, it is necessary to understand enough about the culture and the relevant spiritual beliefs to work with patients and their families.

COMPARATIVE VALUE SYSTEMS

Beliefs about the supernatural and its relationship to illness are just one part of nonmaterial culture; many other values and norms are important in cross-cultural interaction. Although it can be risky to generalize about cultures because of the danger of stereotyping, many observers have identified recurrent themes and patterns in cultures (early examples include Kluckhohn & Strodtbeck, 1961; Condon & Yousef, 1975; and Hofstede, 1984). These patterns can provide overall structure to cross-cultural interaction as long as it is remembered that they are guidelines and that there will be great individual variation within each culture. Hofstede (1984, 2004; G. Hofstede & G. J. Hoftede, 2005) identified four core pairs of contrasting cultural values: individualism-collectivism (IDV), power distance index (PDI), masculinity-femininity (MAS), and the uncertainty-avoidance index (UAI). Chinese researchers later added a fifth dimension called long-term orientation (LTO). Each of these may be important in a medical setting.

According to Hofstede and Hofstede's analysis (2005, p. 78), the dominant American value is individualism. This means that social ties are relatively weak and each person's goals are important. In many other parts of the world (e.g., East Asia), the social group is more important than the individual, and social ties are stronger than they are in the U.S. In hospitals or rehabilitation facilities, this means that families or even clans might be involved in medical decisions that medical personnel interpret as more properly made by the individual patient.

American culture scores relatively low on the PDI because of its emphasis on equality and informality. Many other cultures, however, put much greater emphasis on hierarchy and formality, and people in these cultures do not like people's social status to be ambiguous or unclear. In medical settings, this has important implications for something as basic as the manner in which people are addressed. In general, people from countries like Japan and Germany expect status differences to be recognized in the use of titles and last names, and informal interaction between people of different status is not as common as it is in the U.S. It would be important for patients from countries or cultural backgrounds with a high PDI to clearly understand the medical hierarchy in a health care setting and for medical personnel to refrain from too much informal interaction (e.g., the use of first names).

Hofstede and Hofstede (2005) called the third cultural value the MAS dimension. More recently, Ferraro (2006, p. 110) called it the tough-tender dimension because of the possible gender stereotyping in the use of Hofstede's terms. In countries with an emphasis on the masculine or tough dimension, values support male behavior that is assertive and competitive, and gender roles tend to be more rigid. In a health care setting, for example, women might not be allowed to make decisions about their own health care because the men in the family have that right. In cultures and countries that are more feminine or tender, gender roles are more flexible, and people are used to seeing women in positions of responsibility.

People from cultural backgrounds with a high UAI are not very comfortable in novel or uncertain situations and prefer to have clear rules that are strictly enforced. Patients from these cultures might be uneasy when given options about their medical treatment and would do better if given clear directions on their care and rehabilitation. American culture has a low UAI and American health care professionals might be much more willing to explore an unusual treatment or to suggest multiple options for treatment than someone from a cultural background with a high UAI. A patient who dislikes uncertainty and prefers structure may not respond well to a treatment protocol that offers too many choices and puts too much reliance on the patient's decisions (G. Hofstede & G. J. Hofstede, 2005, pp. 177-178).

The lowest-ranking American cultural value is the LTO or the time dimension. This refers to a culture's emphasis on tradition and on taking a long-term approach to solving problems and maintaining relationships (e.g., business relationships). This contrasts with East Asia, in which a LTO is highly valued and emphasized (G. Hofstede & G. J. Hofstede, 2005, p. 211). In addition, American culture values the precise measurement of time (called monochronic or M-time by Hall, 1976) and the sequential ordering of tasks. People who are waiting in line expect to be helped in the order in which they lined up, and they expect (or hope) that appointments will start on time. Many other parts of the world have a much more relaxed approach to the measurement of time, and may prefer the synchronized ordering of tasks (called polychronic or P-time by Hall). Orderly lines and appointments that start when scheduled are not as important if people are used to P-time.

If health care professionals have American values, they will emphasize the autonomy and personal responsibility of their patients, expect their patients to be on time for appointments, and expect to work hard while they are there. In contrast, if their patients have a cultural value system that emphasizes the importance of the group over the individual, a casual approach to punctuality, and acceptance of fate, they may arrive after their scheduled appointment time with several family members and feel that there is little point in working too hard since much of what happens to people (including disability) is predetermined. In this situation, effective medical treatment can be derailed by cross-cultural misunderstanding and personal conflicts. In order to achieve the best possible therapeutic outcome, it therefore is imperative for rehabilitation personnel to understand not only their own culture(s), but also that of their patients. This, potentially, is just as important as their knowledge of anatomy, physiology, or manual skills.

SUBCULTURES

Subcultures (also called microcultures) are smaller units within a larger culture that have much in common with this dominant culture but are in some way(s) recognized as distinct, both by the people in the subculture and those outside it. By definition, a person who belongs to a subculture also belongs to the larger culture, and a subculture is always part of a greater cultural entity. Complex societies typically encompass many different subcultures, and people in these societies frequently engage in cross-cultural interaction without ever leaving the geographical boundaries of their home country. African Americans and Native Americans are each a subculture within the U.S. Within these subcultures, people also identify themselves as members of other subcultures. For example, a woman who considers herself to be African American may also consider herself to be Jamaican American or a "Southerner." A man who considers himself to be Native American is also proud of his tribal identity of Navajo. It may be difficult for a person who belongs to several subcultures to identify with just one of them.

Biomedicine represents another distinct subculture with its own focal vocabulary (set of specialized terms), symbols, and rules of behavior. As students complete physical therapy school, they must master not only the skills needed to become competent therapists, but also the hidden curriculum that teaches a physical therapist to be part of a medical/health care system. Members of a hospital staff are part of a system of hierarchical ranking that includes everyone from the senior attending physicians to the nursing staff to physical therapists. In this sense, hospitals and other health care facilities differ greatly from one of the primary values of American culture: egalitarianism. In many other ways, biomedicine is based on a distinct set of values that, for the most part, mirror American values (hard work, individual success, and time management).

Even within biomedicine, however, doctors do not necessarily share all of the same values. For example, Cassell (2005) contrasts the values of surgeons and intensivists (a physician who cares for critically-ill patients) and how important this is in end-of-life decisions about patient care in the surgical intensive care unit (SICU). She notes, "I repeatedly witnessed disagreement about patients' prognoses and the correct course of action. With a patient who seemed irrevocably in terminal decline, the intensivists would propose discontinuing aggressive treatment; the surgeon would insist that the patient was going to survive, refusing to endorse a shift to comfort care" (p. 72). Surgeons, who saw death as the enemy, were much less willing to support a shift to palliative or comfort care for patients than were physicians who specialized in the treatment of patients in the intensive care units. In this case, the physicians' areas of specialization were closely correlated with their attitudes toward death and end-of-life issues.

Imagine two doctors, one an intensivist and one the patient's surgeon, talking to a Navajo family about end-of-life care for their hospitalized mother. There are conflicting values, beliefs, goals, and ideas about the most basic of issues: life and death. For the best possible outcome, everyone involved should have at least some awareness of the other participants' cultural background. Since that is not always possible, everyone should at least try to respect the others' perspective; that is, they can try to practice cultural relativism.

Occupation, religion, language, and place of ancestral origin can be foundations for the development of a subculture because, in each case, the people involved differ in some way from other people in a culture. What about disability? If able-bodied people are in the majority, do PWDs belong to a distinct subculture? Do they consider themselves to be part of a (sub)culture of disability? Do other people see them in this way? As is often the case in cross-cultural inquiry, we can ask the same questions in every culture, but we will not receive the same answers.

CULTURE AND DISABILITY

The emphasis on the importance of the individual and on individual work and achievement as a measure of accomplishment and status have been important factors in the development of typical rehabilitation goals. Furthermore, social institutions in Europe gradually assumed many of the activities formerly performed by the family. This was important in the historical development and acceptance of hospitals, clinics, and other medical facilities. Sick people, and that often meant people with disabilities as well as those with short-term acute illnesses, were separated from their families and treated by professionals (Foucault, 1973). Biomedicine replaced or sometimes coexisted with traditional methods of healing (Ehrenreich & English, 1973).

This has not happened in all or even most of the world's cultures. The concept of disability is not a cultural, universal, nor means of rehabilitation. As Ingstad & Whyte (1995) point out:

> "…the concept of disability itself must not be taken for granted. In many cultures, one cannot be 'disabled' for the simple reason that 'disability' as a recognized category does not exist. There are blind people and lame people and 'slow' people, but 'the disabled' as a general term does not translate easily into many languages… The concepts of disability, handicap, and rehabilitation emerged in particular historical circumstances in Europe" (p. 7).

In many cultures, people with cognitive and physical disabilities are expected to follow the same life cycle as everyone else, including initiation (if practiced), marriage, and parenthood. They are not isolated in care facilities (which may not exist) nor are they assumed to be incapable of participation in everyday social discourse. Disability does not define their status (social position) in the culture and therefore it cannot serve as the identifying and unifying characteristic of a distinct subculture. Katherine Dettwyler's (1994) description of a Malian family's attitude toward their daughter illustrates this perfectly. While conducting fieldwork in Mali, Dettwyler noticed a little girl with unmistakable physical characteristics of a child with Down syndrome. She was particularly interested because her own son has Down syndrome. She described her conversation with the family:

> "'Do you know there's something "different" about this child?' I asked, choosing my words carefully. 'Well, she doesn't talk,' said her mother, hesitantly, looking at her husband for confirmation. 'That's right,' he said. 'She's never said a word.' 'But she's been healthy?' I asked. 'Yes,' the father replied. 'She's like the other kids, except she doesn't talk. She's always happy. She never cries. We know she can hear, because she does what we tell her to. Why are you so interested in her?'… There was no way I could explain cells and chromosomes and nondisjunction to them…would that have helped them anyway? They just accepted her as she was… Children in the United States might have the freedom to attend special programs to help them overcome their handicaps, but children in Mali have freedom from the biggest handicap of all—other people's prejudice" (Dettwyler, 1994, pp. 98-99).

In Mali, PWDs are part of the social life of their families and communities, but that certainly is not the case in all cultures. Sometimes PWDs remain isolated in their households because the disability brings shame on their families. This obviously limits their opportunities for social interaction outside of the family. Inaccessibility and lack of accommodation in the material culture (e.g., transportation, mobility aids, or suitable housing) can add to their isolation. Any or all of these conditions make it unlikely that a subculture based on disability will develop. Membership in subcultures based on ethnicity or religion also may limit social interaction. PWDs who live in societies in which residential, educational, and social segregation of subcultures exists may have little opportunity to interact with other people who have similar disabilities, unless these people already belong to the same subculture. Linguistic diversity and separation can limit cross-cultural communication also, even within the same society.

The Development of Subcultures of Disability

How does a subculture of PWD develop? People in subcultures share certain traits and life experiences, but is this true of people with different disabilities. Does a person who is blind and a person who uses a wheelchair belong to the same subculture? Or do they define themselves differently? Perhaps one is of Asian descent and considers ethnicity far more important than disability status; perhaps the other is a lawyer and considers occupation to be most important. Having a disability is a necessary but not necessarily sufficient condition for membership in a subculture of disability. Such a subculture is most likely to develop when people in a culture consider disability to be an important or even defining part of a person's identity and status.

Another important factor is the segregation of PWDs in schools, care facilities, and rehabilitation centers. Here they may have the opportunity to meet and interact with other PWDs. In addition, they are in these programs and facilities because of their disabilities and again, this implies that disability is a crucial (perhaps the most crucial) determinant of their social status. In such a situation, even if the PWDs belong to different ethnic groups or practice different religions, they may consider those experiences secondary to the shared experiences stemming from their disability.

Kohrman (2005) has traced the recent evolution of a subculture of disability and use of the concept of *canji* to refer to PWDs in China. People in some parts of China, such as Beijing, began to use this term in the 1980s and 1990s. Its use coincided with the establishment of the China Disabled Persons' Federation, a new government agency whose objectives are "to represent the common interests of all Chinese citizens with disabilities, to protect their legal rights and interests, and to mobilize social forces to serve them" (Kohrman, p. xii). The language and the definition of disability are based on those of international organizations such as the United Nations and the World Health Organization (WHO), both of which have a Western biomedical orientation. (See Edwards, 2005 for a discussion of the philosophy behind these international definitions of disability.) Recognition of disability as a separate and defining characteristic of its citizens is part of an effort by the Chinese government to bring some of its policies more in line with international attitudes and policies. Acceptance of these policies has been uneven. For example, while the term *canji* is commonly used and understood in Beijing, that is not the case in Hainan province, where Kohrman found that people were still not using it to identify PWDs as late as the mid-1990s (p. 17). There are many important conclusions in his ethnography, some of which are of particular relevance for medical personnel in rehabilitation settings. First, while the biomedical model of disability increasingly forms the basis for global definitions of disability, we should not assume that it is universal. Second, even among populations in which disability is the basis for personal identity, its use may be inconsistent and dependent on variables such as urban or rural residence.

This variation within a population can also be found in the U.S. Devlieger, Albrecht, and Hertz (2007, p. 1948) asked if "disability culture exists outside mainstream white society and if it is monolithic within and across subgroups of the larger disabled population." To answer these questions, they completed a five-year study of young African American men in the spinal cord injury unit of a rehabilitation hospital in Chicago. They concluded that disability culture in this group of people who were disabled by violent means developed because of three factors (Devlieger et al.):

> "distancing from gangs, family, friends, and community immersion in a new, safe, supportive physical and social environment; the development of personal narratives; metaphors that give meaning to their newly acquired disabilities" (p. 1957)

They also noted that "under conditions of non-violence, disability in the African American community may not be a unifying experience. For some African Americans, ethnicity, poverty, unemployment, and perhaps gang membership define their identity and culture" (p. 1956). They therefore suggest that disability as a result of a chronic or longstanding condition may not lead to a disability culture in the African American community as a whole. Thus, even if two people with disabilities share a country of origin or membership in an ethnic group, they may have very different interpretations of the meaning of disability or of their membership in a wider community of PWDs. In a rehabilitation setting, simply knowing a patient's ethnic background or country of origin is not enough because of the tremendous variation within these categories.

These ethnographic examples demonstrate the complexity of disability culture or subculture. International standards and definitions, grounded in Western biomedicine, have attained global importance. Countries such as China are developing new government agencies and bureaucracies based on Western models. However, different countries and different populations within each country have varied interpretations of the category of "disability" and the perceived needs of PWDs. In China, the recent use of *canji* to mean disability has government support, but its application and acceptance differ from province to province. In a country like Mali, where the government spent $60 per capita on health care in 2005 (WHO, 2008), none of the conditions for the development of a subculture of disability are present. This may be unfortunate, since the presence of a subculture of disability may encourage the development of disability rights organizations and improved quality of life for PWDs.

CULTURE, THE SOCIAL SCIENCES, AND CULTURAL COMPETENCE

If a physical therapist is interested in further studying culture in general, or the "culture of disability" in particular, one may need to become more familiar with some of the social sciences that emphasize these areas of study. The following introduces the physical therapist to some terminology that is not typically incorporated into physical therapy curriculums.

MEDICAL ANTHROPOLOGY

American anthropology traditionally includes four fields of study—cultural anthropology, anthropological linguistics, archaeology, and biological anthropology—and there are many subspecialties within these fields. Medical anthropology got its start as the "applied anthropology of medicine" in the years after World War II. Some of the earliest work in this field was in international development projects and public health projects in the U.S. By the 1960s, the original name was replaced by "medical anthropology," and in 1971, it gained recognition as a distinct area of specialization within American anthropology. In the years since then, medical anthropology has matured as a field of study with disparate theoretical approaches and topics of study. One of those topics has been the cross-cultural study of disability.

Some medical anthropologists take an interpretive or cultural constructivist approach to the study of disability, focusing on the symbols, values, attitudes, and reactions associated with the experience of disability. This theoretical orientation was illustrated in the study cited above of disabled African American men in Chicago. The authors included an analysis of the young men's narratives about their experiences as well as a discussion of the ways in which their families, friends, and communities reacted to their disabilities. Other medical anthropologists prefer an ecological or epidemiological approach, which stresses the origin and pattern of disease or disability. Rates of violence, particularly gun-related violence, in the U.S. and in these particular communities would be important in this type of analysis. Finally, a third theoretical approach in medical anthropology is called critical medical anthropology. This is a broad top-down approach that emphasizes political and economic forces in rates of illness and disability. In this example, important topics would include access to education, employment, and health care in these African American communities.

Medical anthropology has much to offer health care professionals who work in rehabilitation settings. It can help medical personnel understand patients' beliefs and values and place patients in a larger social and cultural context. It can also help us understand our own culture and the importance it has in our interaction with others. In summary, anthropology began as the holistic, comparative, and cross-cultural study of human beings, and this broad and inclusive approach can be seen in medical anthropology.

MEDICAL SOCIOLOGY

Medical sociology has focused on the study of human behavior in Western societies. The earliest theoretical approach to the study of illness and disability in medical sociology was based on the theories of functionalism and symbolic interactionism. Parsons (1951) elaborated on what he labeled "the sick role"—the set of expected behaviors that go along with the status of a patient or sick person—a perspective that works better with acute conditions than it does with chronic conditions. His early work led to the development of the deviance model, which has been widely used in medical sociology and in work on disability. In this model, PWDs are "deviant" because they fall outside of the boundaries of normality within a particular culture. Goffman's work (1963) is related to this because he analyzed disability as a stigmatized identity that places a person in a marginal or liminal status.

Other approaches within medical sociology take a more macro-level approach to disability and emphasize disparities in power and access to societal resources. Conflict theory has tended to view PWDs as members of a minority group because of three defining characteristics:

1. They are usually less than one-half of the population

2. They differ from the majority group in a culturally significant way

3. They lack access to economic and political power

This view of disability has been used by advocates for disability rights in the U.S. Finally, some medical sociologists have analyzed the "disability business" (the governmental and nongovernmental rehabilitation programs and policies in the U.S.).

ETHNOGRAPHY

A student of culture may employ a research methodology associated with anthropology and sociology, such as ethnography. The term *ethnography* has two meanings. It can mean the written account of a culture that is based on original research by the author, or it can refer to the research process on which this account is based. The hallmark of ethnography is its reliance on participant observation, but interviews, questionnaires, surveys, multi-sited research, team research, life histories, genealogical research, analysis of expressive culture, and problem-focused research are additional research techniques used by anthropologists and other social scientists. If the anthropologist attempts to gain a local perspective on a topic, he is taking an emic approach to ethnography. If the anthropologist takes a more academic (or scientific) approach to a topic, he is taking an etic approach to ethnography. For example, if the people of a community attribute illness to a supernatural cause, that is an emic explanation. If an epidemiologist states that the cause of this illness is a virus, that is an etic explanation. This distinction can be useful in working with PWDs whose emic explanations for their disabilities are very different from the etic (biomedical) explanations of rehabilitation staff. Understanding an ethnography of a people (or person) is typically an excellent tool to use in becoming culturally proficient.

Conclusion

Culture refers to the learned behavior, norms, and symbols that are passed from generation to generation within a society. People learn what is appropriate and acceptable within their own culture and may come to view their way of doing things as the only correct way. This attitude is called ethnocentrism, and it is common in all of the world's cultures. Successful cross-cultural communication and interaction benefit from cultural relativism, which rejects ethnocentrism, stresses the variability of culture, and emphasizes the need to try and understand other cultures in their own context. We may be better able to do this by remembering that culture has two major components: material culture and nonmaterial culture. People often are more willing to change elements of their material culture than their nonmaterial culture, contributing to cultural lag, in which the physical aspects of culture (such as styles of dress and new technology) change much more rapidly than the nonphysical aspects (such as attitudes toward new styles of dress and appropriate uses of new technology). This lag is common in biomedicine as technology (e.g., life-support systems) and research results (e.g., those in genetics) present clinicians and patients with challenging religious and ethical dilemmas. People may reject or be ambivalent toward elements of the material culture, such as a proposed medical treatment, because of the values in their nonmaterial culture. This means that rehabilitation professionals should be aware of the importance of culture (their own as well as that of their patients) and of the interconnectedness of the different parts of the material and nonmaterial culture. Such awareness is a necessity for those whose work environments include people from different cultural backgrounds. In today's world, that describes almost everyone. With an appreciation of our own and another person's culture, we can recognize not only our differences, but also our shared experiences, and perhaps establish the basis for more productive and rewarding human interaction.

Reflection Questions

✔ *What ethnic group(s) do you belong to?*

✔ *What cultural belief/behavior do you have that might impact a health care episode?*

✔ *Write one or more "fact(s)" about your culture, rituals, food, etc. that you would like others to know about.*

✔ *What specific aspect of your culture would you be most hesitant to give up?*

✔ *What quality do you think is most difficult to understand about another culture?*

✔ *What subcultures do you belong to? Which is your primary identification?*

REFERENCES

Alvord, L., & Van Pelt, E. C. (2000). *The scalpel and the silver bear.* New York, NY: Bantam.

Cassell, J. (2005). *Life and death in intensive care.* Philadelphia, PA: Temple University Press.

Condon, J. C., & Yousef, F. S. (1975). *An introduction to intercultural communication.* Indianapolis, IN: Bobbs-Merrill.

Dettwyler, K. (1994). *Dancing skeletons: Life and death in West Africa.* Long Grove, IL: Waveland Press.

Devlieger, P., Albrecht, G., & Hertz, M. (2007). The production of disability culture among young African-American men. *Social Science & Medicine, 64*(9), 1948-1959.

Edwards, S. D. (2005). Disability: Definitions, value and identity. Abingdon, UK: Radcliffe Publishing.

Ehrenreich, B., & English, D. (1973). *Witches, midwives, and nurses: A history of women healers.* New York, NY: The Feminist Press.

Ferraro, G. (2006). *The cultural dimension of international business* (5th ed.). Upper Saddle River, NJ: Prentice Hall.

Foucault, M. (1973). *The birth of the clinic: An archaeology of medicine.* New York, NY: Vintage.

Goffman, E. (1963). *Stigma: Notes on the management of spoiled identity.* Upper Saddle River, NJ: Prentice Hall.

Hall, E. T. (1976). *Beyond culture.* New York, NY: Anchor.

Hofstede, G. (1984). *Culture's consequences: International differences in work-related values.* Thousand Oaks, CA: Sage Publications.

Hofstede, G. (2004). *Cultures and organizations: Software of the mind* (2nd ed.). New York, NY: McGraw-Hill.

Hofstede, G., & Hofstede, G. J. (2005). *Cultures and organizations: Software of the mind: Intercultural cooperation and its importance for survival* (2nd ed.). New York, NY: McGraw-Hill.

Ingstad, B., Whyte, S. R. (Eds.). (1995). *Disability and culture.* Berkeley, CA: University of California Press.

Johnson, K. S., Elbert-Avila, K. I., & Tulsky, J. A. (2005). The influence of spiritual beliefs and practices on the treatment preferences of African Americans: A review of the literature. *Journal of the American Geriatric Society, 53*(4), 711-719.

Kluckhohn, F., & Strodtbeck, F. L. (1961). *Variations in value orientations.* New York, NY: Harper & Row.

Kohrman, M. (2005). *Bodies of difference: Experiences of disability and institutional advocacy in the making of modern China.* Berkeley, CA: University of California Press.

Parsons, T. (1951). *The social system.* London, England: Routledge & Kegan Paul Ltd.

World Health Organization. (2008). Mali. Retrieved November 14, 2008, from http://www.who.int/countries/mli/en

The Historical Development of Theory, Models, and Assessment Tools

Ronnie Leavitt, PhD, MPH, PT

CULTURAL COMPETENCE AND HEALTH CARE: A HISTORICAL OVERVIEW

Over time, historical events and research reports have led health professionals to become aware of the need to increase their understanding of those who may not be exactly like them. The 1960s represented a radical period in U.S. history, with increasing recognition of the "civil rights" and "feminist" movement, and the "War on Poverty." The 1968 Report of the National Advisory Commission on Civil Disorder established, beyond any doubt, the presence of health care disparity with residents of a "racial ghetto" being significantly less healthy than most other Americans. At the same time, there was increasing immigration to the U.S. by a diverse group of people from non-European countries. In the 1970s and 1980s, in response to these events, nurses and physicians began a more concentrated effort to examine ideas to encourage a more responsive health/medical community.

The idea of cultural competence can be traced to the field of medical anthropology and medical sociology. These areas of study build a bridge between anthropology or sociology and the health sciences. At their most basic, these domains attempt to see how cultural, social, and environmental factors affect health and acknowledge the alternative ways of understanding and treating disease. Anthropology recognizes that health professionals must seek the "insider's point of view" known as an emic approach. This is in contrast to the etic or outsider's point of view. An etic perspective might be to assume that everyone believes in the germ theory and the validity of penicillin. In reality, the patient may believe in supernatural causation (i.e., that they are ill because of a sin of their ancestor) or an intervention such as going to an obeah man (a healer who uses such things as parrot's beak, egg shells, or grave dirt and prayers to manipulate spiritual forces).

A review of the literature suggests that the nursing profession has the longest commitment and most experience with the topic of cultural competence. Dr. Madeline Leininger (1978), a nurse and medical anthropologist, established the theoretical foundation for the

R. L. Leavitt (Ed.).
*Cultural Competence: A Lifelong Journey
to Cultural Proficiency* (pp. 31-50).
© 2010 SLACK Incorporated

practice of transcultural nursing (study and practice of diverse cultures in the world with respect to their care, health and illness, values, beliefs, and practices) with her Theory of Culture Care Diversity and Universality. Leininger recognized that it is wrong to participate in cultural imposition (i.e., the tendency to impose one's beliefs, values, and patterns of behavior upon another culture). Formed in the early 1970s, the Transcultural Nursing Society and the *Journal of Transcultural Nursing* continue today to be at the forefront in publishing-related research, theory, and practice ideas regarding cross-cultural interactions.

Rachel Spector's *Cultural Diversity in Health and Illness* (1979) and Cecil Helman's *Culture, Health and Illness: An Introduction for Health Professionals* (1984) are two of the landmark books addressing this issue that are still published in their updated editions. The essential message from each of these has been to encourage health professionals to recognize their socialization into a biomedical/biotechnological world and to replace this perspective with one that recognizes the social-cultural environment in which one lives—to respect the world's wide-ranging cultural diversity and medical practices and to explore what people believe in and do from a traditional cultural perspective to maintain and protect their health.

Concurrently, Dr. Arthur Kleinman, both a psychiatrist and medical anthropologist, and his colleagues developed the concept of "explanatory models," or EMs, to analyze local health care systems (Kleinman, Eisenberg, & Good, 1978). This is one process of medical ethnography to explain patterns of belief about the causes of illness, the response to specific episodes of sickness, and actions taken to bring about a change in a person's health status or condition. EMs "are the notions about an episode of sickness and its treatment that are employed by all those engaged in the clinical process. The study of patient and family [explanatory models] tell us how they make sense of given episodes of illness, and how they choose and evaluate particular treatments" (Kleinman, 1980, p. 105). EMs are described in greater detail below.

Likewise, the American Medical Association (AMA) intensified its efforts in research and action (education and training) to meet the needs of culturally diverse populations. For example, in 1996, *Family Medicine* published "Recommended Core-Curriculum Guidelines on Culturally Sensitive and Competent Health Care" (Like, Steiner, & Rubel, 1996) (see Chapter 12), and in 1998, *AMA Reports* published "Efforts to Identify and Incorporate Health Needs of Culturally Diverse Populations into Broader Public Health and Community Objective" (Hedrisk, Blehert, & Scottie, 1998). Today, cultural competence is a mainstream movement within medicine (Betancourt, 2004).

Concurrent with the activities of health professionals, the U.S. government increasingly recognized the need to address the issues associated with a growing diverse population and the ability to maintain an effective and efficient health care delivery system. In the 1979 Surgeon General's Report (Public Health Service, 1979), Healthy People, and the 1990 document entitled "Healthy People 2000: National Health Promotion and Disease Prevention Objectives," (Public Health Service, 1990) the U.S. Department of Health and Human Resources (HHS) and the Department of Public Health (DPH) specified a policy agenda for a decade with particular goals and objectives to guide state and community plans. More recently, Healthy People 2010, the third set of 10-year targets for health improvements in the U.S., specifies two broad goals and 467 objectives that are grouped into 28 focus areas (HHS, n.d.). The two major goals iterated in the plan are to increase the quality and years of healthy life and to eliminate health disparities. The four enabling goals are (HHS, n.d.):

1. Promote healthy behaviors

2. Protect health

3. Provide access to quality health care

4. Strengthen community prevention

The notion of cultural competence is implicitly presumed to be embedded in the action plans. Healthy People 2020 will be released in 2010.

A significant body of work, "The Standards for Culturally and Linguistically Appropriate Service (CLAS)" was developed during the 1990s by the HHS Office of Minority Health (OMH) and finalized in 2001 (HHS, 2001) (see Chapters 9 and 12). These standards provide a blueprint for individual providers and health care organizations to develop programs and for the consumer to assess their providers in this domain. In 1994, the Joint Commission on Accreditation of Healthcare Organizations (JCAHO) mandated that in-service education concerning cultural diversity be given to all employees of health care organizations. Recently, JCAHO has promulgated more specific recommendations (see Chapter 1) (Wilson-Stronks & Galvez, 2007; Wilson-Stronks, Lee, Cordero, Kopp, & Galvez, 2008). And, in 1998, the Pew Commission listed 21 competencies for health care professionals for the 21st Century. Among these is the provision of culturally sensitive care (Beck et al., 2004).

At about the same time, the Institute of Medicine (IOM) released a report that caught the attention of government agencies and health professionals. "Unequal Treatment: Confronting Racial and Ethnic Disparities in Healthcare" (Smedley, Stith, & Nelson, 2002) became a seminal body of work that has provided momentum for those concerned with both health and human rights. The widely reported findings have led to an even greater recognition for cultural competence as a means of redressing past inequities and decreasing health and health care disparities.

Coming full circle, medical anthropology continues to play a leading role in the study of cross-cultural health care. The "newer" medical anthropology now focuses not just on descriptions of health beliefs and behaviors, but more on human rights, social justice, and structural inequality. Some medical anthropologists continue to do theoretical research, but an increasing number are involved in the application of the theory. Applied medical anthropologists apply their findings to individual health care or health promotion. They are particularly interested in primary health care or health policy both in industrialized nations and in developing countries where difference in socioeconomic status and cultural ways of life are more vivid.

To summarize, increasing numbers of health professionals, social scientists, and government agencies are pursuing the advancement of scholarly work regarding a socio-cultural perspective and health.

PHYSICAL THERAPY AND CULTURAL COMPETENCE: A HISTORICAL OVERVIEW

Physical therapy comes relatively late to recognizing the need for cultural competence. In the early 1980s, APTA created the Advisory Council (later Panel) on Minority Affairs to provide advice and counsel to the Board of Directors on issues of diversity relevant to the profession. "The Plan to Foster Minority Representation and Participation in Physical Therapy" was the basis of the initial APTA initiatives. The Office of Minority Affairs and the Minority Scholarships for Academic Excellence Award were initiated in 1988 (Meadows, 2000). Now, within the APTA, there is the Department of Minority and International Affairs.

"Concepts from Medical Anthropology for Clinicians" by Parry (1984) introduced the discipline of medical anthropology to physical therapists and suggested ways in which clinicians could restructure clinical encounters to be more culturally sensitive. In 1985, Ronnie Leavitt and Karen Schumacher founded a group now known as the Cross-Cultural and International Special Interest Group (CCISIG). CCISIG began as a networking group for PTs who wanted to share information on physical therapy internationally.

Great strides have been made since the mid 1980s in introducing cultural competence to the physical therapy profession. APTA has demonstrated a commitment to cultural competence, as reflected in its goals and policies. Within the APTA, the Department of Minority and International Affairs has a committee on cultural competence (see Chapter 1). CCISIG is stronger than ever: it is now a formally designated SIG within the health policy section of the APTA. Over time, CCISIG has broadened its goals and activities. Based on input from members, it has expanded the concept of diversity to include a range of cross-cultural issues in the U.S., including people with disabilities and the lesbian, gay, bisexual, and transgender (LGBT) community. In 1993, Leavitt and Kay facilitated the linkage between the APTA and Health Volunteers Overseas to establish Physical Therapy Overseas (PTO), which focuses specifically on physical therapy in the developing world. In 1994, *PT Magazine* had a cover story entitled "On Cultural Diversity, Anthropology, and Physical Therapy," and Parry wrote "Culture and Personal Meanings" (1994).

In addition to the APTA paying increasing attention to this topic, some of the seminal leaders of the profession began to speak about the need to think about diversity and culture. In 1995, at the World Confederation of Physical Therapy, Hislop used her keynote address to speak, in essence, about physical therapists broadening their perspectives and cultural competence, although she did not use that phrase. She stated:

> *"The value of diversity, individuality, and improvisation should be apparent to all of us. We are a group of independent clinicians, all playing the same game with the same objective, but each of us produces individual variations on the same basic theme, expressing individuality and talent that can combine to produce a unique effect, never twice the same, but powerful and beautiful… You, individually and collectively, are the only means by which a change can overtake international physical therapy and give to it the preeminence it must earn. You can force a change by acting in common cause that will result in a spurt of growth in the quality of our clinical services…that will take place in every corner of our round world"* (Hislop, 1995, p. 58).

In the 31st APTA Mary McMillan Lecture, Purtilo, using the phrase "cultural competence," called for cultural competence to be a non-negotiable skill, tested as rigorously as competence in pathokinesiology or any other field of study (2000).

In response to an editorial by Rothstein (1999) requesting input on major issues facing physical therapy as a profession during the next millennium, Bender (2000) wrote a letter entitled "Cultural Sensitivity." Bender noted that APTA's Code of Ethics first principle, "physical therapists respect the rights and dignity of all individuals," is the foundation for our decision to be more culturally sensitive in our approach to patient care (APTA, 2006; Bender, 2000). To fulfill our obligation to the Code of Ethics, Bender implored physical therapists to recognize our own biases and for the profession to actively pursue educational strategies for the student and clinician to begin the journey toward cultural competence:

> *"As physical therapists, we have known since the beginning that a patient was far more than the sum of his or her disabilities. The illness-based biomedical model was never a comfortable fit for our work because one of our profession's primary goals was to prepare patients to return to their community role in the least restrictive environment possible. We found this impossible to accomplish without accepting the patient as part of the health care team… Without a heightened awareness of the need for cultural sensitivity in our patient interactions, the patient will never really be able to participate as an equal on the team" (p. 1018).*

> *"In the past, it has sometimes been comfortable to adopt the attitude that 'it doesn't matter who my patient is because I work very hard to treat everyone in the same manner.' This attitude implies that as long as the provider feels comfortable that care is*

evenhanded and unbiased, it will be so. However, the comfort of the physical therapist is only half of the equation. The patients should also feel comfortable, and that attitude is more likely if their care takes into consideration personal beliefs, practices, and needs. One size never did fit all, and that was never more true than in the area of health care" (pp. 1018-1019).

In the mid 1990s and early 21st century, there has been much more published literature identifying and explaining the theoretical basis for cultural competence and/or providing practical examples and ways to adapt services appropriate for physical therapists. Examples include but are not limited to: *Cross-Cultural Rehabilitation: An International Perspective* (Leavitt, 1999), *Developing Cultural Competence in Physical Therapy Practice* (Lattanzi & Purnell, 2005), and *Culture in Rehabilitation: From Competency to Proficiency* (Royeen & Crabtree, 2005). The APTA published "Cultural Diversity of Older Americans," a series of six home-study booklets about different subgroups (APTA, n.d.). *PT Magazine* has had a number of articles on culture and cultural competence (Coyne, 2001; Duffy, 2001; Leavitt, 2002, 2003). The *Journal of Physical Therapy Education* has published several articles on this topic (Babyar et al., 1996; Black & Purnell, 2002; Kraemer, 2001; Romanello, 2007; Wong & Blissett, 2007). Of note is that many of these studies have pointed to a lack of adequate attention to culture and cultural competence in physical therapy education or practice. For example, Babyar et al. found that physical therapy educational programs in New York State had substantial disparity between a homogeneous student body and faculty and the diversity of the patient population and lacked material about multiculturalism. Kraemer did a qualitative study of physical therapy students' perceptions. She found that during their clinical experiences, the students lacked awareness of barriers and clinical cultural clashes, felt ill-prepared to handle such "cultural collisions," and did not know of available resources to help them.

Although scarce, there have been a few reports in the *Journal of the American Physical Therapy Association* attending to cross-cultural data and the socio-cultural aspects of physical therapy (Gannotti, Handwerker, Groce, & Crux, 2001; Kirk-Sanchez, 2004; Kolobe, 2004). Finally, there are a growing number of members of APTA who have completed their post-graduate work with an emphasis on topics related to cultural competence (Gordon, 2005; Gulas, 2005; Portee, 2007).

In the new millennium, recognition of the value for this topic continues to expand. APTA insists upon the recognition of cultural competence as a key component of high quality care. The APTA "Normative Model of Physical Therapist Education" (2004) has incorporated cultural competence notions into its document. Under performance expectations Theme 2, the graduates must demonstrate sensitivity to individual and cultural differences in all aspects of physical therapy services (APTA, 2004, 2.1). Under professional practice expectations, there is the requirement that the PT graduate will be able to identify, respect, and act with consideration for patients'/clients' differences, values, preferences, and expressed needs in all professional activities (APTA, 2004, 7.1). Embedded within the Normative Model is "Professionalism in Physical Therapy: Core Values" (APTA, 2003); the core values also imply the value of cultural competence (see Chapter 1).

The Operational Plan on Cultural Competence (APTA, 2007) is the most comprehensive document thus far. (See sidebar on page 36.)

Even so, a review of the literature, as alluded to throughout this book, indicates that the physical therapy profession (as well as the other health professions) continues to lack the means by which we adequately address cultural barriers at the personal (e.g., recognize our own biases), professional (e.g., redress the disparate numbers of students and faculty who are people of color as compared to the overall population), or institutional level (e.g., availability of departmental bi-cultural translators). The journey to cultural proficiency remains in its early stages.

THE OPERATIONAL PLAN FOR CULTURAL COMPETENCE

GOAL I:

Integrate the process of cultural competence within the physical therapy profession.

- Adopt a cultural competence model for the profession of physical therapy.
- Create an education curriculum that is consistent with the adopted cultural competence model.
- Educate stakeholders (APTA staff, PTs, PTAs, students) in the process of cultural competence.
- Facilitate ongoing assessment of the process of cultural competence within the physical therapy profession.

GOAL II:

Facilitate the development of physical therapist practices that assure physical therapy professionals are committed to serving the underserved and eliminating health disparities.

- Establish a database of effective clinical practice models that serve the underserved and eliminate health disparities.
- Promote awareness and utilization of the resources that are available to practitioners relative to the delivery of culturally competent physical therapy services.

GOAL III:

Increase the number of physical therapists and physical therapy assistants from racial/ethnic minority groups to reflect the changing demographics of U.S. society.

- Identify and communicate strategies for recruitment/retention of PTs and PTAs from racial/ethnic minority groups into PT/PTA education programs and APTA membership.
- Identify the benefits and barriers to APTA membership/governance/ participation for PTs and PTAs from racial ethnic/minority groups.
- Assess our "welcoming quotient" and develop strategies to be more inclusive for PTs and PTAs from racial/ethnic minority groups.

DEFINITIONS, THEORETICAL MODELS, AND ASSESSMENT OF CULTURAL COMPETENCE

As health care professionals from various disciplines recognize the importance of cultural competence in the delivery of culturally appropriate health care, the theoretical models and conceptual frameworks describing this domain have evolved. There are a range of associated definitions, models, assessments, and measurement tools. Some of these are described below to demonstrate the variability in approach to thinking about cultural competence and the variability of methods to attempt to measure cultural competence for an individual or organization. A review of the literature reveals that the definitions/phrases and models share many similarities, especially in the theoretical underpinnings, although some differences exist as well. As you read the following, it can be useful to determine which of the selected ideas and methods are really the most useful and practical for you. It is also appropriate to recognize that it takes time and practice for the PT to feel comfortable with any kind of assessment. As with other capabilities, one must work toward the goal of competence, and hopefully excellence at completing the task at hand. Whether your primary physical therapy identity is student, educator, clinician, manager, or researcher, you can ponder the information presented and choose to use that which meets your personal and professional goals of improved functional outcome for the patient and greater professional satisfaction derived from better interactions with the patient.

DEFINITIONS OF KEY CONCEPTS
ASSOCIATED WITH CULTURAL COMPETENCE

A fuller understanding of cultural competence requires more analysis and parsing of the terms associated with it. Some of the more commonly used terms are described here, although the evolutionary nature of the concept requires that definitions and meanings will continue to develop. Many terms associated with cultural competence are often used interchangeably. For example, *cross-cultural*, *trans-cultural*, and *intercultural*, are often used interchangeably. Nursing tends to use the latter two terms more than physical therapists.

Cultural diversity alludes to the fact that people are different. This phrase has been used to simplify the presence of human variation within the health care system. There has been a history of providing "cultural diversity" education, generally focusing on cultural awareness and cultural knowledge by giving information about specific groups of people. Recognizing diversity, although a first step, does nothing to meet the varying needs of diverse peoples. Likewise, increasing cultural knowledge about particular ethnic groups may be of interest, but knowledge alone does not necessarily translate into action. The concept of cultural diversity also applies to the idea that there are diverse ways to receive health care.

The term *multicultural* reflects the idea that a culture is heterogeneous with regard to age, color, ethnicity, gender, national origin, political ideology, race, religion, and sexual orientation, and it includes the presence and participation of people with disabilities and those from different socioeconomic backgrounds. In the context of this book, the concept of multiculturalism is considered something to accept and even strive for. Typically, we are talking about today's reality of "living in a multicultural world" or supporting the concept of a "multicultural environment." The concept must utilize the sensitivity, knowledge and skill development, and adaptation components of cultural competence to effect meaningful changes in a multicultural world made of individuals with diverse ideas, perspectives, and backgrounds.

Medical pluralism suggests that in every society, although there may be a predominant system for delivering health care, alternative systems exist simultaneously. It may also indicate that a single entity (person or family) may pick and choose elements of a range of systems. For example, in 1993, Eisenberg et al. published the first national survey describing the use of complementary and alternative medical therapies (CAM) (i.e., defined as those health care and medical practices that are not currently an integral part of conventional medicine). At that time, approximately one-third of adults in the U.S. had used at least one CAM during the last year. A follow-up survey in 1997 concluded that 42% of the population used CAM (Eisenberg et al., 1993).

Culturally congruent care is a term initiated by Leininger (1991). This occurs when health professionals think and act in ways that fit with a person or group's beliefs and lifeways. Culturally congruent care can occur only if one knows, and uses in a meaningful and appropriate way, the values, expressions, patterns, and practices of culturally diverse groups and individuals. This term is used more often in nursing literature.

New terms continue to enter the cultural competence lexicon. *Cultural humility* (Tervalon & Murray-Garcia, 1998) has been defined as a commitment to make the lifelong journey toward cultural proficiency through self-critique and action toward changing the power imbalances in the client-health care professional relationship. Nuñez (2000) has suggested the term *cross-cultural efficacy* to represent the ability of a caregiver to be effective in interactions that involve individuals of different cultures by ensuring that neither the caregivers' nor patients' culture is the preferred or the more accurate view.

Fisher, Burnet, Huang, Chin, and Cagney (2007) have coined the term *cultural leverage* when designing and implementing culturally congruent interventions. That is "a focused strategy for improving the health of racial and ethnic communities by using their cultural practices, products, philosophies, or environments as vehicles that facilitate behavior change of patients and practitioners" (Fisher et al., p. 245S).

Still and all, the term *cultural competence* has taken hold most often as advocates for a better approach to care realize its more encompassing nature. Cross, Bazron, Dennis, and Isaacs (1989) have developed the most widely utilized definition and framework for understanding the meaning of cultural competence (see Chapter 1). Cultural competence is a set of behaviors, attitudes, and policies that come together in a continuum to enable a health care system, agency, or individual rehabilitation practitioner to function effectively in transcultural interactions. In practice, cultural competence acknowledges and incorporates—at all levels—the importance of culture, the assessment of cross-cultural relations, the need to be aware of the dynamics resulting from cultural differences, the expansion of cultural knowledge, and the adaptation of services to meet culturally unique needs. The goal of moving toward cultural proficiency, the last stage of cultural competence on Cross et al.'s continuum, is the purpose of this book.

Models of Cultural Competence

Theorists and health practitioners have developed numerous models and/or approaches to foster the goal of cultural proficiency. Some of the more widely accepted and utilized are described here. My goal in reviewing these models (and assessment tools below) is to allow the reader to more fully understand the robust nature of cultural competence. All of the models imply that cultural competence is a never-ending, always evolving, non-linear process that will continue to challenge us throughout our lifetime. All of these are similar yet distinct enough to warrant recognition.

Cross et al. (1989) developed a model of cultural competence whereby one moves along a continuum from cultural destructiveness to cultural proficiency. (This, the most widely used and this author's preference, has been described in Chapter 1.)

Arguably, in today's health system environment, the model described by Campinha-Bacote (2002) is used most often after Cross et al. (1989). Campinha-Bacote defines *cultural competence* as "the process in which the healthcare provider continuously strives to achieve the ability to effectively work within the cultural context of a client, individual, family, or community" (p. 54). Her model has five essential constructs that are interdependent and necessary to reach cultural competence:

1. *Having cultural desire*: "The motivation of the health care professional to 'want to' engage in the process of becoming culturally competent; not the 'have to'" (p. 15). Because this is viewed as the pivotal element in one's journey to cultural competence, it is described first. Cultural desire presumes the ability to sacrifice one's prejudice and biases toward those who are different and "includes a passion and commitment to be open and flexible with others; a respect for differences, yet a commitment to build upon similarities; a willingness to learn from clients and others as cultural informants; and a sense of humility" (p. 16).

2. *Having cultural awareness* (*cultural sensitivity* is often the term used): Requires considerable self-examination regarding one's own biases and the recognition of one's own cultural beliefs, values, and behaviors. Becoming culturally aware requires cultural openness both cognitively and emotionally, learning about others, and integrating a range of approaches and world views as necessary.

3. *Increasing cultural knowledge*: Requires learning to seek information about different groups in order to understand the theoretical and conceptual frameworks for the worldviews of other people. This can cover a range of domains (see Chapter 4), but general worldview and value system, health-related beliefs and behaviors, disease

incidence and prevalence, and treatment efficacy are especially important. Embedded in this construct are ideas such as what is the highest cultural value for a group/individual (axiology) or how does a cultural group come to know truth or knowledge (epistemology).

4. *Developing cultural skills*: The ability to collect culturally relevant data in a culturally appropriate way so that a culturally relevant treatment plan can be developed.

5. *Having a cultural encounter*: The exposure to people from different cultures with an opportunity to help them achieve shared goals.

Similar to Cross et al. (1989), Campinha-Bacote (2002) has described a cultural competence continuum. That is, one can move from unconscious incompetence (having a "cultural blind spot syndrome" or assuming there are no differences in culture between the professional and client) to conscious incompetence (recognizing one's lack of knowledge) to conscious competence (learning about other peoples' cultures, verifying generalizations, and adapting interventions to be culturally appropriate) to unconscious competence (spontaneously providing culturally relevant care for diverse patients). At this later stage, the process is natural and comfortable (Campinha-Bacote).

Yet another framework is Borkan and Neher's Developmental Model of Ethnosensitivity (1991). This model assesses the health care workers' ability to grasp cultural issues by describing a continuum from ethnocentrism to ethnorelativity. One can move from fear (mistrust) to denial (cultural blindness, overgeneralization) to superiority (negative stereotyping) to minimization (reductionism) to relativism (acceptance) to empathy (pluralism) to a final stage of being ethnosensitive whereby one has the ability to appreciate values and behaviors within the context of specific cultural norms and apply this ability to one's health care practice.

Anthropologist Milton Bennett (1993) has suggested a continuum of cultural competence that begins with avoidance and progresses to integration as a final stage. The first three stages are considered ethnocentric and the last three ethnorelative:

1. *Denial/avoidance*: A person denies cultural differences or is unaware that others do not share a similar world view.

2. *Defense/protection*: Although a person acknowledges the existence of differences, these are considered threatening to one's sense of self. Thus, defense mechanisms must be employed such as denigration of others and believing in one's own superiority.

3. *Minimization*: An individual trivializes the cultural differences that exist and focuses on presumed similarities (i.e., Person X is just like me) in an effort to emphasize humanity as a unified group.

4. *Acceptance*: Cultural worldviews are recognized and accepted but the individual is more focused on behaviors as opposed to values.

5. *Adaptation*: Individuals improve skills to interact and communicate with people from other cultures.

6. *Integration*: People value a range of cultures and work toward conscious evaluation of alternative behavior and values. These individuals try to integrate aspects of their own culture and those from other cultures into clinical practice.

Most recently, Schim, Doorenbos, Benkert, and Miller (2007) applied a puzzle metaphor to understand culturally congruent care. The puzzle represents a nonlinear and interconnected visual tying the constructs together. The model is still evolving, but the four basic constructs of the puzzle for the health care provider are cultural diversity (a fact of life), cultural awareness (the cognitive construct), cultural sensitivity (the affective or attitudinal construct), and cultural competence (the behavioral construct). The client layer of the model is equally important. It recognizes individuals, families, and communities.

ELICITING CULTURAL INFORMATION USING PATIENT-CENTERED MODELS

In contrast to the above theoretical models defining cultural competence and/or focusing on the process by which health professionals can become culturally competent, some models are more patient-centered. That is, the models are means by which to gain knowledge about what people think, feel, want, and need. Models generally recognize the necessity of including an affective, cognitive, behavioral, and environmental domain. The physical therapist should explore these regarding their patient to the degree that is appropriate and practical.

The Purnell Model for Cultural Competence is an organizing framework to assess cultural values, beliefs, behaviors, and health care practices of individuals. It is a holistic model that may be applicable for a range of providers, but not all of the components are directly applicable to physical therapist practice. Nevertheless, recognition of the global society (e.g., world politics/conflicts, natural disasters, business practices, and more), community (a group of people having a common interest or identity through physical or social connections), family (e.g., physically or socially connected individuals), and person (a biological, psychological, sociological, cultural being) as well as the broad range of interconnected domains enumerated assist the PT to think broadly and can assist one in working toward cultural proficiency. The dark circle in the middle represents unknown phenomena, a concept that I find appealing since I cannot imagine that we know everything about ourselves, let alone others. The jagged line under the circle represents the nonlinear concept of a cultural competence continuum.

Purnell and Palunka (2003) define cultural competence as an act whereby a health professional develops an awareness of one's existence, sensations, thoughts, and environment without letting these factors have an undue influence on those for whom care is provided and being able to adapt the care in a manner that is congruent with the client's culture (Figure 3-1).

Leininger (2002) uses a "sunrise" graphic to describe her Theory of Culture Care Diversity and Universality (Figure 3-2). She identifies the influence of seven cultural and social structure dimensions on a person's well-being. These are:

1. Cultural values and life ways
2. Religious, philosophical, and spiritual beliefs
3. Economic factors
4. Educational factors
5. Technological factors
6. Kinship and social ties
7. Political and legal factors

Leininger (2002) suggests that information gleaned about the above domains be used by the provider to guide their determination of approach(es). This guidance can occur through cultural care preservation, cultural care accommodation, and cultural care restructuring if a cultural practice is deemed detrimental to health (Leininger).

Giger and Davidhizar (2002) posit that cultural competence is a dynamic, fluid, continuous process whereby an individual, system, or agency finds useful and meaningful strategies to deliver care based on knowledge of the cultural heritage, attitudes, and behaviors of those to whom care is delivered. Their Transcultural Assessment Model focuses on how six factors can influence health beliefs and practices of each culturally unique person. An understanding of these can assist health care professionals in assessing patients from diverse cultures. The six cultural phenomena to be considered are:

1. *Communication*: Verbal and nonverbal style
2. *Space*: Personal boundaries

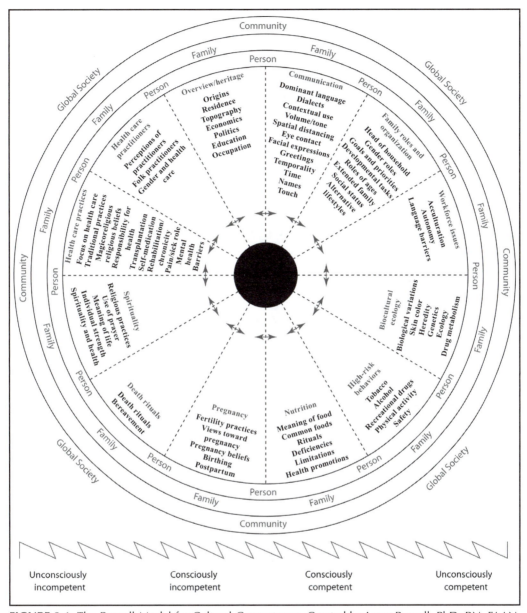

FIGURE 3-1. The Purnell Model for Cultural Competence. Created by Larry Purnell, PhD, RN, FAAN. Reprinted with permission.

3. *Social organization*: Family structure and religious values

4. *Time*: Time reckoning and consideration of past, present and future

5. *Environmental control*: Health practices

6. *Biological variation*: Physical attributes, nutritional preferences, and diseases specific to their cultural group

Related to the patient-centered models that explore specific domains of culture, others are focused on a more general approach regarding what questions the provider should ask and how to ask them. The following are some of the more commonly used guides to elicit socio-cultural information from a patient.

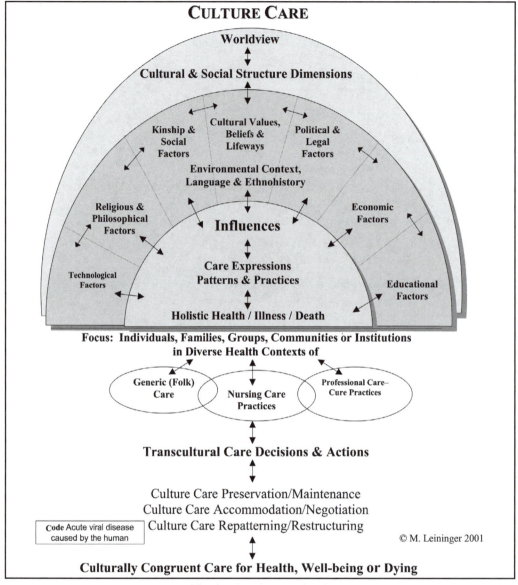

FIGURE 3-2. Leininger's Sunrise Enabler for the Theory of Culture Care Diversity and Universality. Leininger, M. M. Culture care theory: A major contribution to advance transcultural nursing knowledge and practices. *Journal of Transcultural Nursing, 13*(3), pp. 189-192, copyright © 2002 by SAGE Publications. Reprinted by permission of SAGE Publications.

Arguably, the most well-known is that of the Explanatory Model (EM), defined by Kleinman (1980) as mentioned previously. Open-ended questions are used to allow patients to discuss their health based on their perceptions of a particular illness or condition. The physical therapist can ask the patient questions such as:

- What do you call your problem?
- What do you think caused your problem?
- What are the greatest problems your illness has caused for you?
- What do you fear most about the consequences of this illness?
- What kind of treatment do you think you should receive?
- What are the most important results you hope to get from your treatment?

Kleinman reminds health care professionals that although we need to focus on the patient's explanatory model, it is essential to understand that clinicians also have an explanatory model and operate within their own distinct culture. The patient and his or her family cannot be expected to always and completely comply with the practitioner's explanatory model, and the health care professional cannot be expected to "buy into" the patient's explanatory model. (An example of the use of EMs is given in Chapter 9.)

Additionally, there are a range of useful mnemonics that have been suggested for assessing a client's culture or when trying to skillfully gather information from the patient. These mnemonics are generally intended to foster respect for client centrality, avoid stereotyping, and allow for adoption of mutually acceptable ways to encourage success. No one is the best for all situations.

Berlin and Fowkes (1983) have suggested using the mnemonic LEARN when assessing your patient's culture (see Chapter 9):

- *Listen* to the client's perception of the problem.

- *Explain* your perception of the problem from a health professional point of view.

- *Acknowledge* the similarities and differences between the two perceptions.

- *Recommend* a plan of care that takes into account the patient's perceptions and builds upon similarity of ideas as much as possible.

- *Negotiate* a treatment plan that can work for both parties and realistically be carried out.

Alternatively, Stuart and Lieberman (1993) suggest the mnemonic BATHE for eliciting the patient's psychological context with regard to their visit to the health professional. The following are the suggested questions:

- *Background*: What is going on in your life?

- *Affect*: How do you feel about what is going on?

- *Trouble*: What about the situation troubles you the most?

- *Handling*: What are you doing about the problem?

- *Empathy*: The provider should offer psychological support.

MEASURING CULTURAL COMPETENCE: A CHALLENGE

The actual quantifiable measurement of cultural competence can focus on a number of factors. For example, does the organization want to focus on consumer and community perceptions, management policies or skill levels, workers' personal attitudes, or disparities of outcome? Do educators want to assess their students' likelihood of being open to this field of study or the actual knowledge that a student has gained about a particular group of people? Do you as a physical therapist want to do a self-analysis of your awareness and sensitivity toward people who are different than you? Do you want to learn about your style of communication? Is it of interest to delve deeper into whether your personal value system is more aligned with an individualistic or collectivistic culture?

There are many challenges to measuring the elements of cultural competence. The concept of culture is so complex, fluid, and multi-faceted that it is difficult to use concrete measurement tools that can capture the relationship of culture to an individual, organization, health care delivery system, and society. Furthermore, as is noted throughout this book, the multiplicity of factors influencing health-related outcomes makes it rather difficult to isolate the contribution of cultural competence. A full description of organizational and individual assessment and evaluation concepts is outside the scope of this book. Nevertheless, some review of the literature and particular assessment tools are reviewed here so the reader can become familiar with some of the available options.

It is wise to realize that multi-method and multi-domain assessment strategies can lead to a richer understanding of cultural competence, in addition to patient-centered care and quality improvement. Some specific suggestions for physical therapists, physical therapy departments/clinics, and hospitals are provided in Chapter 12.

Perhaps the most comprehensive review of this topic was completed by the HHS, OMH (Fortier & Bishop, 2004). The project is a stepping stone for the advancement and practical understanding of how to measure cultural competence. Recognizing that cultural competence is essential for accessible, responsive, high-quality care, Fortier and Bishop embarked on a literature review to understand how the complex construct of cultural competence can be measured. The material was organized according to the well-established framework for determining quality of health care systems developed by Avedis Donabedian (1966). Donabedian uses three constructs to measure quality of care:

1. *Capacity/structure*: Staffing, facilities, equipment, governance and administrative systems

2. *Process*: Method of delivery

3. *Outcome*: Results

In addition to using the traditional levels of analysis in health services research, that is, the individual, organizational, and societal level, they also analyzed measurements for the health care delivery system as a whole. From this, Fortier and Bishop further identified nine domains for potential measurement (2004):

1. Values and attitudes

2. Cultural sensitivity

3. Communication

4. Policies and procedures

5. Training and staff development

6. Facility characteristics, capacity, and infrastructure

7. Intervention and treatment model features

8. Family and community participation

9. Monitoring, evaluation, and research

For example, a process indicator of the percentage of clients with limited English proficiency who have access to bilingual staff or interpretation services can measure the domain of communication. From an organizational viewpoint, an indicator can be based on a checklist from the National Center for Cultural Competence (NCCC) on communication style indicating behaviors that a provider may do (i.e., "I attempt to determine familial colloquialisms that may impact assessment": never, rarely, occasionally, or frequently). A measure of capacity or structure is the number of trained translators and interpreters available. An outcome measure for quality of communication can be the decrease in misdiagnosis and inadequate treatment plans resulting from failure to communicate effectively with consumers from different ethnic groups.

Fortier and Bishop (2004) concluded that, thus far, outcome measures represent the least prevalent type of measure and process measures the most common.

Under the auspices of the HHS Agency for Healthcare Research and Quality, Brach and Fraser (2000) identified nine cultural competency techniques that could theoretically improve outcome measures (and decrease disparities) for diverse populations. These are: interpreter services, recruitment and retention policies, training, coordinating with traditional healers, use of community health workers, culturally competent health promotion, including family/community members, immersion into another culture, and administrative and organizational accommodations.

In 2004, a final report was prepared (Fortier & Bishop, 2004), concluding the Brach and Fraser project. Although limited in scope and mostly descriptive in nature, existing studies suggest that the proposed interventions noted above do have the potential to affect health care delivery and health outcomes. Unfortunately, due to variations in definitions and study design, findings are inconsistent and cannot be easily generalized, and further research is strongly advised. The difficulty linking specific interventions to specific outcomes is recognized. Nevertheless, recommendations were made for priority research agendas: topics generating the most interest included language assistance interventions; cultural competence education and training; and racial, ethnic, and linguistic concordance between patients and providers.

Similarly, based on an extensive review of the medical and public health literature, Schim et al. (2007) conclude that measurement of culturally competent behaviors and interventions cluster into three areas:

1. Organizational (e.g., workforce diversity)

2. Structural (e.g., addressing processes, barriers, and facilitators)

3. Clinical (e.g., transcultural communication and adaptation of care)

In summary, more research to assess the affect of cultural competence is essential. Some stakeholders appear willing to undertake interventions without "proof of value," possibly secondary to consumer demand. Others insist upon more solid outcomes research.

SELF-ASSESSMENT OF CULTURAL COMPETENCE BY HEALTH PROFESSIONALS

There are many self-assessment tools to help individuals and agencies examine their cultural and linguistic competence. Self-assessments have inherent limitations, yet they are also beneficial for gathering information to begin a lifelong process of developing more awareness, knowledge, and skills. A large number of instruments have been used in the nursing, mental health, and social work professions to measure one or more constructs of cultural competence, although many do not have data supporting their reliability and validity (Roizner, 1996). New materials are being generated as cultural competence takes to center stage in efforts to improve functional health outcomes and diminish health disparities. Selected tools are listed here.

A review of the literature indicates that most titles associated with cultural competence assessment are actually recommended check-off lists of personal, departmental, or organizational characteristics and activities that one can consider in determining the degree of cultural competence. Rather than list these here, Chapter 12 provides summarizing examples. Your personal style and work place requirements will influence your decisions regarding which of these you use.

The Cultural Competence Health Practitioner Assessment (CCHPA), modifying the work of Cross et al. (1989), is a self-assessment tool developed by the NCCC (n.d.) at the request of the Health Resources and Services Administration (HRSA), HHS, and the Bureau of Primary Health Care (BPHC) to promote better delivery of health care services to culturally and linguistically diverse people and underserved communities. The CCHPA measures data in six subscales (NCCC):

1. Values and belief systems

2. Cultural aspects of epidemiology

3. Clinical decision making

4. Life cycle events

5. Cross-cultural communication

6. Empowerment/health management

It takes approximately 20 minutes to complete and it is suggested that practitioners consider completing the CCHPA for a distinct ethnic group. The NCCC continues to develop innovative self-assessments for individuals and health service organizations.

Schim, Doorenbos, Miller, and Benkert (2003) and Doorenbos, Schim, Benkert, and Borse (2005) have developed a cultural competence assessment (CCA) instrument for use by health care providers. The CCA has an internal consistency reliability of 0.89 overall, with 0.91 and 0.75 for the two subscales. Construct validity was supported and mean scores were significantly higher for providers who reported previous diversity training compared to those who had not.

Arguably, the most used instrument to measure cultural competence of physical therapists is that developed by Campinha-Bacote (2002). The Inventory for Assessing the Process of Cultural Competence Among Healthcare Professionals—Revised (IAPCC-R) measures the level of cultural competence among health professionals. It is a self-administered tool consisting of 25 items that measure the five cultural constructs enumerated in her model of desire, awareness, knowledge, skill, and encounters. Scores are based on a 4-point Likert scale, with higher scores indicating greater competence. Content validity has been established by national experts and reliability has been calculated by coefficient Cronbach alpha scores of 0.85 and 0.90 for two groups of nurses.

Physical therapist Charles Gulas (2005) did a study using the IAPCC-R specifically with physical therapy students. His findings support the idea that this assessment is reliable for measuring cultural competence with physical therapy students (Cronbach alpha of 0.78 and Guttman Split-half coefficient of 0.77). Interestingly, the student sample scored the highest on the constructs of cultural desire and cultural awareness. Given that cultural desire may be the most important construct to motivate students or health care practitioners, this may be a good sign.

However, based on an item analysis of the work by Gulas (2005), Kraemer and Beckstead (2003), Shore and Steinbroner (2004), and Woehrle (2004) suggesting that the IAPCC- R tool is not totally appropriate for physical therapy students or sensitive enough to measure change over time (e.g., after an intervention), Campinha-Bacote has followed up with revision.

The newest version of the IAPCC is the IAPCC-SV to measure the level of cultural competence among students in health professions (Campinha-Bacote, 2007). It consists of 20 items measuring the five cultural constructs on a 4-point Likert scale. Content validity was established by national expert review and reliability testing demonstrated a Cronbach's alpha of 0.783 (Fitzgerald, Cronin, & Campinha-Bacote, in press).

Other self-assessment scales measuring different aspects of cultural competence that have demonstrated moderate or better internal consistency and reliability (Cronbach's alpha coefficients of > 0.70) include the Cross Cultural Adaptability Inventory (CCAI) (Kelley & Meyers, 1995), the Multicultural Awareness, Knowledge, and Skills Assessment (MAKSS) developed by D'Andrea, Daniels, and Heck (1991), the Multicultural Counseling Inventory (MCI) (Sodowsky, Taffe, Gutkin, & Wise, 1994), the Cultural Self-Efficacy Scale (CSES) (Smith, 2001), and the Self-Assessment Questionnaire (CCSAQ) (Mason, 1995).

The critical question, to what degree can an individual move toward cultural competence and cultural proficiency, remains murky. D. B. Pope-Davis, Prieto, Whitaker, and S. A. Pope-Davis (1993) measured cultural competency among occupational therapists and found higher scores for those with higher levels of education, work experience with diverse populations, or who had taken courses related to multiculturalism. Similarly, D. B. Pope-Davis and Ottavi (1994) found that nursing students who had worked with a diverse population scored higher on a multicultural sensitivity and knowledge scale compared to students without such experience.

In "Assessing the Impact of Cultural Competency Training Using Participatory Quality Improvement Methods," Like, Fulcomer, Kairys, Wathington, and Crosson (2004) note that physicians' self-perceived cultural competence knowledge, skill, and comfort levels improved significantly over time, but the lack of experimental design or control did not allow the authors to conclude that it was the training intervention per se that caused the changes. The authors did suggest that quality improvement teams may improve the provision of culturally responsive care in clinical settings.

The Association of American Medical Colleges (AAMC) has developed a Tool for Assessing Cultural Competence Training (TACCT) as part of a comprehensive curricular needs assessments for medical schools. The TACCT consists of 67 items measuring knowledge, skill, or attitude with regard to cultural competence (Lie, Boker, & Cleveland, 2006).

In brief, it is generally believed that increased cultural knowledge without concurrent changes in attitudes and behavior is of limited value, and may even prove harmful if stereotypes are merely reinforced (Tervalon & Murray-Garcia, 1998). As noted earlier, Tervalon and Murray-Garcia encourage cultural humility, that is, a lifelong commitment to self-evaluation and critique in order to develop mutually beneficial health care partnerships. Or, as Cross et al. (1989) suggest, a lifelong commitment to highly value the role of culture in our and our patients' lives, that is, cultural proficiency, the penultimate step of cultural competence.

In summary, the conclusion of Brach and Fraser (2000) still seems most accurate. Rigorous research on cultural competency techniques and outcomes is lacking. That is, "...while there is substantial research evidence to suggest that cultural competency should in fact work, heath systems have little evidence about which cultural competency techniques are effective and less evidence on when and how to implement them properly" (Brach & Fraser, p. 181). This author hopes that *Cultural Competency: A Lifelong Journey to Cultural Proficiency* is one means by which physical therapists will be encouraged to answer the questions implied above.

REFLECTION QUESTIONS

✔ *What do you think are the strengths and weaknesses of the cultural competence models described?*

✔ *Which models do you think you can practically use in your clinical setting?*

✔ *Which model would you ideally use in your clinical setting?*

✔ *What is your "explanatory model" when you have the flu?*

✔ *Do you believe cultural desire is a required component of cultural competence?*

✔ *How do you define excellence in your personal and professional life?*

REFERENCES

American Physical Therapy Association. (2003). Professionalism in physical therapy: Core values. Retrieved October 26, 2008, from http://www.apta.org/AM/Template.cfm?Section=Policies_and_Bylaws&TEMPLATE=/CM/ContentDisplay.cfm&CONTENTID=36073

American Physical Therapy Association. (2004). *A normative model of physical therapist professional education: Version 2004.* Alexandria, VA: Author.

American Physical Therapy Association. (2006). Code of Ethics. Retrieved October 26, 2008, from http://www.apta.org/AM/Template.cfm?Section=Core_Documents1&Template=/CM/HTMLDisplay.cfm&ContentID=25854

American Physical Therapy Association. (2007). Strategic plan for cultural competence. Retrieved September 18, 2009, from http://www.apta.org/AM/Template.cfm?Section=Home&TEMPLATE=/CM/ContentDisplay.cfm&CONTENTID=54391

American Physical Therapy Association, Section on Geriatrics. (n.d.). Continuing education home study module. Retrieved September 18, 2009, from http://www.geriatricspt.org/members/homestudy.cfm

Babyar, S., Sliwinski, M., Krasilovsky, G., Rosen, E., Thornby, M., & Masefield, J. R. (1996). Survey of inclusion of cultural and gender issues in entry-level physical therapy curricula in New York State. *Journal of Physical Therapy Education, 10*(2), 53-62.

Beck, B., Wolff, M., Bates, T., Beversdorf, S., Young, S., & Ahmed, S. (2004). Development, implementation and evaluation of a M3 community health curriculum. *Med Educ Online, 9*(5). Retrieved December 8, 2009, from http://www.med-ed-online.org

Bender, D. G. (2000). Cultural sensitivity. *Physical Therapy, 80*(10), 1018-1019.

Bennett, M. J. (1993). Towards ethnorelativism: A developmental model of intercultural sensitivity. In R. M. Paige (Ed.), *Education for the intercultural experience* (2nd ed.). Boston, MA: Intercultural Press.

Berlin, E. A., & Fowkes, W. C., Jr. (1983). A teaching framework for cross-cultural care: Application in family practice. *Western Journal of Medicine, 139*(6), 934-938.

Betancourt, J. R. (2004). Cultural competence—marginal or mainstream movement? *New England Journal of Medicine, 351*(10), 953-955.

Black, J. D., & Purnell, L. D. (2002). Cultural competence for the physical therapy professional. *Journal of Physical Therapy Education, 16*(1), 3-9.

Borkan, J. M., & Neher, J. O. (1991). A developmental model of ethnicity in family practice training. *Family Medicine, 23*(3), 212-217.

Brach, C., & Fraser, I. (2000). Can cultural competency reduce racial and ethnic health disparities? A review and conceptual model. *Medical Care Research and Review, 57*(Suppl 1), 181-217.

Campinha-Bacote, J. (2002). The process of cultural competence in the delivery of healthcare services: A model of care. *Journal of Transcultural Nursing, 13*(3), 181-184.

Campinha-Bacote, J. (2007). *The process of cultural competence in the delivery of healthcare services: The journey continues* (5th ed.). Cincinnati, OH: Transcultural C.A.R.E Associates.

Coyne, C. (2001). Cultural competency: Reaching out to all populations. *PT Magazine, 9*(10), 44-50.

Cross, T. L., Bazron, B. J., Dennis, K. W., & Isaacs, M. R. (1989). *Towards a culturally competent system of care: A monograph on effective services for minority children who are severely emotionally disturbed.* Washington, DC: CASSP Technical Assistance Center, Georgetown University Child Development Center.

D'Andrea, M., Daniels, J., & Heck, R. (1991). Evaluating the impact of multicultural counseling training. *Journal of Counseling and Development, 70*, 143-150.

Donabedian, A. (1966.) Evaluating the quality of medical care. *Milbank Memorial Fund Quarterly, 44*(3 Suppl), 166-206.

Doorenbos, A. Z., Schim, S. M., Benkert, R., & Borse, N. N. (2005). Psychometric evaluation of the cultural competence assessment instrument among health care providers. *Nursing Research, 54*(5), 324-331.

Duffy, P. (2001). Cultural competence strengthens our profession. *PT Magazine, 9*, 24-25.

Eisenberg, D. M., Kessler, R. C., Foster, C., Norlock, F. E., Calkins, D. R., & Delbanco, T. L. (1993). Unconventional medicine in the United States: Prevalence, costs, and patterns of use. *New England Journal of Medicine, 328*(4), 246-252.

Fisher, T. L., Burnet, D. L., Huang, E. S., Chin, M. H., & Cagney, K. A. (2007). Cultural leverage: Interventions using culture to narrow racial disparities in health care. *Medical Care Research and Review, 64*(5 Suppl), 243S-82S.

Fitzgerald, L., Cronin, S., & Campinha-Bacote, J. (in press). Psychometric testing of the inventory for assessing the process of cultural competence among healthcare professionals—Student version (IAPCC-SV). *Journal of Theory Construction & Testing.*

Fortier, J. P., & Bishop, D. (2004). *Setting the agenda for research on cultural competence in health care: Final report.* Edited by C. Brach. Rockville, MD: U.S. Department of Health and Human Services, Office of Minority Health, and Agency for Healthcare Research and Quality.

Gannotti, M. E., Handwerker, W. P., Groce, N. E., & Crux, C. (2001). Sociocultural influences on disability status in Puerto Rican children. *Physical Therapy, 81*(9), 1512-1523.

Giger, J. N. & Davidhizar, R. (2002).The Giger and Davidhizar transcultural assessment model. *Journal of Transcultural Nursing, 13*(3), 185-188.

Gordon, S. (2005). *An exploration of educators' perceptions concerning the multicultural education of students in New England physical therapist programs.* Unpublished Doctoral dissertation. Orono, ME: University of Maine.

Gulas, C. (2005). *Establishing the reliability of using the inventory for assessing the process of cultural competence among healthcare professionals with physical therapy students.* Unpublished dissertation. Saint Louis, MO: Saint Louis University.

Hedrisk, H., Blehart, B., & Scotti, M. (1998). Efforts to identify and incorporate health needs of culturally diverse populations into broader public health and community objective. *AMA Reports, Section X*, 374-382.

Helman, C. G. (1984). *Culture, health and illness.* London, England: John Wright and Sons.

Hislop, H. (1995). In common cause. *PT Magazine, 3*(9), 56-61.

Kelley, C., & Meyers, J. (1995). *Cross-cultural adaptability inventory manual*. Minneapolis, MN: National Computer Systems.

Kirk-Sanchez, N. J. (2004). Factors related to activity limitations in a group of Cuban Americans before and after hip fracture. *Physical Therapy, 84*(5), 408-418.

Kleinman, A. (1980). *Patients and healers in the context of culture: An exploration of the borderland between anthropology, medicine, and psychiatry*. Berkeley, CA: University of California Press.

Kleinman, A., Eisenberg, L., & Good, B. (1978). Culture, illness, and care: Clinical lessons from anthropologic and cross-cultural research. *Annals of Internal Medicine, 88*(2), 251-258.

Kolobe, T. H. A. (2004). Childrearing practices and developmental expectations for Mexican-American mothers and the developmental status of their infants. *Physical Therapy, 84*(5), 439-453.

Kraemer, T. J. (2001). Physical therapist students' perceptions regarding preparation for providing clinical cultural congruent cross-cultural care: A qualitative case study. *Journal of Physical Therapy Education, 15*(1), 36-51.

Kraemer, T. J., & Beckstead, J. (2003). Establishing the reliability of using the Cross Cultural Adaptability Inventory with physical therapist students. *Journal of Physical Therapy Education, 17*(1), 27-32.

Lattanzi, J. B., & Purnell, L. D. (2005). *Developing cultural competence in physical therapy practice*. Philadelphia, PA: F.A. Davis.

Leavitt, R. L. (Ed.). (1999). *Cross-cultural rehabilitation: An international perspective*. London, England: Harcourt Brace and Company.

Leavitt, R. L. (2002). Developing cultural competence in a multicultural world: Part I. *PT Magazine, 10*(12), 36-48.

Leavitt, R. L. (2003). Developing cultural competence in a multicultural world: Part II. *PT Magazine, 11*(1), 56-70.

Leavitt, R. L., & Kay, E. D. (1993). PTs seek coordination of overseas volunteer work. *PT Bulletin*, June 16.

Leininger, M. M. (1978). *Transcultural nursing: Concepts, theories and practices*. Hoboken, NJ: John Wiley & Sons.

Leininger, M. M. (1991). *Culture care diversity and universality: A theory of nursing*. Sudbury, MA: Jones and Bartlett Publishers.

Leininger, M. M. (2002). Culture care theory: A major contribution to advance transcultural nursing knowledge and practices. *Journal of Transcultural Nursing, 13*(3), 189-192.

Lie, D., Boker, J., & Cleveland, E. (2006). Using the tool for assessing cultural competence training (TACCT) to measure faculty and medical student perceptions of cultural competence instruction in the first three years of the curriculum. *Academic Medicine, 81*(6), 557-564.

Like, R. C., Fulcomer, M., Kairys, J., Wathington, K., & Crosson, J. (2004). *Assessing the impact of cultural competency training using participatory quality improvement methods*. Hartford, CT: Aetna Foundation.

Like, R. C., Steiner, R. P., & Rubel, A. J. (1996). Recommended core curriculum guidelines on culturally sensitive and competent health care. *Family Medicine, 28*(4), 291-297.

Mason, J. L. (1995). *Cultural competence self-assessment questionnaire: A manual for users*. Portland, OR: Portland State University.

Meadows, J. (2000). Cultural diversity in physical therapy: The APTA's perspective. *GeriNotes, Newsletter of the Section on Geriatrics, 7*(6), 10-13.

National Center for Cultural Competence. (n.d.). Cultural competence health practitioner assessment (CCHPA). Retrieved November 19, 2008, from http://www11.georgetown.edu/research/gucchd/nccc/features/CCHPA.html

Nuñez, A. E. (2000). Transforming cultural competence into cross-cultural efficacy in women's health education. *Academic Medicine, 75*(11), 1071-1079.

Parry, K. (1984). Concepts from medical anthropology for clinicians. *Journal of Physical Therapy, 64*(6), 929-933.

Parry, K. (1994). Culture and personal meanings. *PT Magazine, 2*(10), 39-45.

Pope-Davis, D. B., Prieto, L. R., Whitaker, C. M., & Pope-Davis, S. A. (1993). Exploring multicultural competencies of occupational therapists: Implications for education and training. *American Journal of Occupational Therapy, 47*(9), 838-844.

Pope-Davis, D. B., & Ottavi, T. M. (1994). Examining the association between self-reported multicultural counseling competencies and demographic variables among counselors. *Journal of Counseling & Development, 72*, 651-654.

Portee, C. (2007). *An exploration of cultural competency pedagogical strategies and assessment methods in entry-level physical therapist educational programs*. Unpublished Doctoral dissertation. Fort Lauderdale, FL: Nova Southeastern University.

Public Health Service. (1979). Healthy people: The Surgeon General's report on health promotion and disease prevention. Washington, DC: U.S. Department of Health, Education, and Welfare.

Public Health Service. (1990). Healthy people 2000: National health promotion and disease prevention objectives. Washington, DC: U.S. Department of Health and Human Services.

Purnell, L. D., & Palunka, B. J. (Eds.). (2003). *Transcultural health care: A culturally competent approach* (2nd ed.). Philadelphia, PA: F.A. Davis.

Purtilo, R. B. (2000). Thirty-first Mary McMillan lecture: A time to harvest, a time to sow: Ethics for a shifting landscape. *Physical Therapy, 80*(11), 1112-1119.

Roizner, M. A. (1996). *A practical guide for the assessment of cultural competence in children's mental health organizations.* Boston, MA: Technical Assistance Center for the Evaluation of Children's Mental Health Systems, Judge Baker Children's Center.

Romanello, M. L. (2007). Integration of cultural competence in physical therapist education. *Journal of Physical Therapy Education, 21*(1), 33-39.

Rothstein, J. (1999). The curmudgeon finds good news. *Physical Therapy, 79*(12), 1120-1121.

Royeen, M., & Crabtree, J. L. (2005). *Culture in rehabilitation: From competence to proficiency.* Upper Saddle River, NJ: Prentice Hall.

Schim, S. M., Doorenbos, A. Z., Benkert, R., & Miller, J. (2007). Culturally congruent care: Putting the puzzle together. *Journal of Transcultural Nursing, 18*(2), 103-110.

Schim S. M., Doorenbos, A. Z., Miller, J., & Benkert, R. (2003). Development of a cultural competence assessment instrument. *Journal of Nursing Measurement, 11*(1), 29-40.

Shore, S., & Steinbroner, A. E. (2004). *Curricular initiatives toward the development of cultural sensitivity: A practical model.* Nashville, TN: Paper presented at the APTA Combined Sections Meeting.

Smedley, B. D., Stith, A. Y., & Nelson, A. R. (Eds.). (2002). *Unequal treatment: Confronting racial and ethnic disparities in health care.* Washington, DC: National Academies Press.

Smith, L. S. (2001). Evaluation of an educational intervention to increase cultural competence among registered nurses. *Journal of Cultural Diversity, 8*(2), 50-63.

Sodowsky, G. R., Taffe, R. C., Gutkin, T. B., & Wise, S. (1994). Development of the multicultural counseling inventory (MCI): A self-report measure of multicultural competencies. *Journal of Counseling Psychology, 41,* 137-148.

Spector, R. E. (1979). *Cultural diversity in health and illness.* Upper Saddle River, NJ: Prentice Hall.

Stuart, M. R., & Lieberman, J. A., 3rd. (Eds.). (1993). *The fifteen minute hour: Applied psychotherapy for the primary care physician* (2nd ed.). Westport, CT: Praeger Publishers.

Tervalon, M., & Murray-Garcia, J. (1998). Cultural humility versus cultural competence: A critical distinction in defining physician training outcomes in multicultural education. *Journal of Health Care for the Poor and Underserved, 9*(2), 117-125.

U.S. Department of Health and Human Services, Office of Disease Prevention and Health Promotion. (n.d.). Healthy People 2010. Retrieved September 21, 2009, from http://www.healthypeople.gov

U.S. Department of Health and Human Services, Office of Minority Health. (2001). *National standards on culturally and linguistically appropriate services in health care: Final report.* Washington, DC: Author.

Wilson-Stronks, A., & Galvez, E. (2007). *Hospitals, language, and culture: A snapshot of the nation.* Oakbrook Terrace, IL: The Joint Commission.

Wilson-Stronks, A., Lee, K. K., Cordero, C. L., Kopp, A. L., & Galvez, E. (2008). *One size does not fit all: Meeting the health care needs of diverse populations.* Oakbrook Terrace, IL: The Joint Commission.

Woehrle, J. (2004). *Measuring cultural competency of physical therapy learners: A time-series analysis.* Unpublished dissertation. Minneapolis, MN: Capella University.

Wong, C. K., & Blissett, S. (2007). Assessing performance in the area of cultural competence: An analysis of reflective writing. *Journal of Physical Therapy Education, 21*(1), 40-47.

4

Exploring Cultural Diversity

ELICITING A CLIENT'S ETHNOGRAPHY

Ronnie Leavitt, PhD, MPH, PT

No matter which particular model of cultural competence or assessment tool you prefer (and each therapist will likely use a combination of those previously described), a less structured review of a range of socio-cultural and biological variables may provide the best overview of a patient's worldview and way of life. In an effort to learn about the material realities and beliefs and behaviors of patients and clients and to facilitate the process of becoming culturally competent in the practice of physical therapy, clinicians must, in essence, do a health care ethnography. An *ethnography* is a description of a culture. It is an attempt to understand another way of life from the point of view of the people of that culture. The ethnographer seeks to learn from people, to observe and be taught by them, and to discover the insider's emic (rather than the outsider's etic) point of view (Spradley, 1979). This process requires that ethnocentrism be minimized. Ethnographic exploration of patients' lives is closely linked to medical anthropology, in which the responses to impairments and disease (disturbances in body processes) and illness and disability (culturally mediated responses) are compared across cultures.

Many variables—including degree of acculturation, socioeconomic status, the effects of racism, incidence and prevalence of disease and disability, comparative value orientations, methods of communication, and health beliefs and behaviors—must be considered during the process of ethnography. Each of these variables must be assessed so that the examination and the interventions may be appropriately modified based on a person's culture. The variables explored below never exist alone; they are complex and intertwined with each other. Furthermore, greater emphasis needs to be on the difficult task of sorting out the relative influence of these variables (e.g., separating biological/genetic factors from socioeconomic factors from cultural lifestyle habits). In other words, what is the relative influence of family structure, diet, exercise, alcohol consumption, income, community, and other variables? We need to sense patterns and variations without over-generalizing.

In this chapter, an overview of the salient special considerations that a physical therapist should know about and some recent data about these variables with regard to specific populations are given. The importance of asking the right questions to elicit this

R. L. Leavitt (Ed.).
*Cultural Competence: A Lifelong Journey
to Cultural Proficiency* (pp. 51-76).
© 2010 SLACK Incorporated

information cannot be overemphasized. See Chapter 9 for examples from Masin's experiences in an early intervention program in Florida where miscommunication and cultural mal-alignments were altered after efforts to elicit her patients' emic perspective. Some of these topics are covered in greater depth and from a different perspective in other chapters. Paying attention to these factors (recognizing our own perspectives and our patients' potentially different world views) is one way in which we can contribute to the process of gaining improved outcomes for our patients and greater personal and professional satisfaction secondary to knowing that we have done our best.

DEGREE OF ACCULTURATION

Acculturation is the process by which people from one culture adopt the traits of the mainstream culture. A term associated with acculturation is *heritage consistency*, that is, the degree to which one's lifestyle reflects his or her respective tribal culture. Many of the variables discussed below are more or less significant, depending on the person's level of acculturation. Generally, a person can be the following:

- *Highly assimilated*: The person has largely adopted the new culture (e.g., Italian American, Greek American, Irish American)

- *Bicultural*: The person functions comfortably in two cultures (e.g., Hispanic/Latino, Jewish, people from South Asia [India, Pakistan, Bangladesh])

- *Highly traditional*: The person's values and behaviors are similar to those found in the country of origin (e.g., Hmong, Bantu)

In the U.S., the degree to which people acculturate to the mainstream culture (what has been referred to as the "White, Anglo-Saxon, Protestant" culture) is influenced by factors such as age, level of education, number of years in this country, and socioeconomic status. Acculturation may affect people's health status, their perspective on health, and their interaction with the health care system and the clinician (Mainous, Diaz, & Geesey, 2008). If an individual appears to be highly acculturated or bicultural and somewhat comfortable in a clinic setting, a PT might have a misperception about one's "true" cultural life ways.

Migration history is one means to assess the degree of acculturation. Physical therapists should be aware of when, why, and how migration occurred. Immigration often does not occur under ideal conditions; therefore, many patients and clients are not seen under ideal circumstances. For example, Mexicans came to the U.S. in large numbers in 1848 and 1910 during postwar periods. Their decision to emigrate was influenced by both the need for a labor force in the U.S. to build railroads and by the extreme poverty and the religious persecution of Christians in their home country. Since the 1940s, large numbers of Mexicans came to perform agricultural labor, and this immigrant group remains relatively poor and politically powerless (S. Santana & F. O. Santana, 2001).

From the beginning, there has apparently been a divide between Mexicans based on whether they are "documented." Most recently, there has been less migration into the U.S., but as noted in Chapter 1, Mexicans remain the largest immigration group (S. Santana & F. O. Santana, 2001).

Puerto Rican people have been coming to the mainland in significant numbers since the Spanish American War in 1898. After World War II, many came to join the manufacturing and service industries—industries that are now diminishing in the U.S.—and thus there is more unemployment for people who are not otherwise trained. In 1953, Puerto Rico became a Commonwealth, and Puerto Ricans have U.S. citizenship (Huff & Kline, 1999).

For both of the above groups, the continuous migration back and forth to the country of origin increases the likelihood of maintaining bicultural status. In contrast, Cuban

Americans have mostly come to the U.S. during periods of large-scale migration as a result of political circumstances, and they cannot go back and forth to Cuba. In 1959, many upper- and middle-class people emigrated. In 1980, the Mariel boatlift brought more working class exiles to the U.S. Overall, although there is a distinction between the first and second wave of immigrants, this population has achieved parity (or better) with White Americans regarding health statistics and socioeconomic status (Huff & Kline, 1999).

The Hispanic population, more than a third of whom have been born outside of the U.S., is typically considered to be bicultural with strong ties to their homeland. Descriptions of these three Hispanic/Latino subgroups remind us of how important it is to consider intercultural and intra-cultural variation.

Other immigrant groups also show distinct intra-ethnic differences depending on the time of immigration. Vietnamese who arrived in the U.S. during the mid-1970s were primarily well-educated, upper class, and Christian, and were escaping a repressive political regime. In contrast, Vietnamese immigrants during the 1980s were more likely to be escaping economic as well as political deprivation, and they arrived with fewer economic resources, different and more considerable health problems, and a more marginalized social support system.

Most recently, forced migration for immigrants groups from war-torn nations such as Iraq or Somalia also demonstrates a range of diversity. In 2007, approximately 7000 Somalians and 1600 Iraqis arrived in the U.S. (U.S. Department of Health and Human Services [HHS], 2007). For the most part, the people from Somali, the largest African refugee group in the U.S., are coming directly from refugee camps where they have lived for a decade or more due to political turmoil in their native land. They arrive extremely disadvantaged with no economic or educational resources, some not even knowing how to sign their name ("A Profile of Somali Refugees, n.d."). Refugees from Iraq are more likely to be familiar with Euro-American ways of life. The potential for members from these two groups to assimilate to the U.S. way of life, at least to some degree, is vastly different for each group.

In general, a number of factors predict the presence of more traditional beliefs and behaviors, including emigration from a rural area, frequent returns to the country of origin, limited formal education, little or no ability to speak or read English, low socioeconomic status, recent immigration to the U.S., immigration at an older age, and housing segregation. Typical ways to measure the degree of acculturation are based on the language used within the home (for example, 78% of Hispanics speak Spanish at home), the language of preferred media sources, and the people who are part of the person's primary support system (Huff & Kline, 1999).

Although physical therapists might not formally measure their patients' level of acculturation, they can ask questions about these subjects that will help them better understand their patients' degree of assimilation. For example, immigration status is a significant determinant of living arrangements (Choi, 1999). Mexican Americans who immigrate after the age of 50 and become ill are more likely to move in with other people than have someone move in with them (J. L. Angel, R. J. Angel, & Markides, 2000). One who immigrates after the age of 60 years is more likely to live in extended family arrangements (Wilmoth, DeJong, & Himes, 1997).

SOCIOECONOMIC STATUS (SES)

Socioeconomic status, which includes level of income, education, and occupation, is arguably the most relevant variable affecting one's worldview and health status. There is a direct linear correlation between class (primarily evaluated through SES) and health. See Chapter 7 for more in depth information on the relationship of poverty to health. The relationship of education to health status is especially important—even more than income.

Yet, there is considerable intra-ethnic diversity when reviewing these data. For example, physical therapists should be aware that high school graduation rates have reached new highs—89% of non-Hispanic Whites, 80% of Blacks, and about 57% of Hispanics have graduated high school (U.S. Department of Commerce, 2004). Among Hispanics, the rates were 46% of Mexican Americans, 60% of Puerto Ricans, and 62% of Cuban Americans (Huff & Kline, 1999). Clinicians should also consider that people with lower educational levels may use "traditional medicine" to a greater extent than people with higher levels of education. More educated Hispanics have fewer health impairments, especially Cubans (Tran & Williams, 1998). Lack of education, more common among older Hispanics, is an obstacle when trying to promote health and prevent disease and disability.

Although most poverty in this country is categorized as relative (i.e., people are able to afford some basic necessities but are unable to maintain an average standard of living), it is commonly known that people who live in poverty have more health problems than people with higher incomes, and that the effects of socioeconomic status tend to be stronger for the poorest populations. Poverty is not randomly distributed through the population. Rather, it is strongly related to such variables as race or ethnicity, gender, age, and disability status. Although socioeconomic advancement continues for most, conservative estimates are that 13% of families in the U.S. are below the poverty line. Data from 2007 shows that for adults in the U.S., about 25% of African-American families and 21% of Hispanic families live in poverty, compared with about 10% of Asian and Pacific Islanders and 8% of White families (U.S. Census Bureau, 2008). For children under 18 years of age, the data are worse. The rate for Whites is about 14%, African Americans is 33%, Hispanic Americans is 27%, and Asian Americans is 12% (U.S. Census Bureau, 2008). The median income also varies—for Hispanics, it is $24,000 versus $41,000 for non-Hispanics. Intra-cultural diversity is again apparent in that Puerto Ricans as a group are the most impoverished Hispanics, whereas Cuban Americans are the least. Mexican Americans fall in between (Huff & Kline, 1999). Some of the small but growing Hispanic population subgroups are especially poor. For instance, Dominicans in the U.S. have mean earnings below $8000, and more than one-third live in poverty (López-De Fede & Haeussler-Fiore, 2002). Female-headed households are associated with poverty, and over 40% of Puerto Rican households are headed by a female (with the figure being about 19% for Mexican and Cuban Americans) (Huff & Kline, 1999; Tran, Dhooper, & McInnis-Dittrich, 1997).

These data have tremendous implications. There is a direct correlation between poverty and access to comprehensive, effective, and efficient medical care (Collins et al., 2002; Mansfield, Wilson, Kobrinski, & Mitchell, 1999; McDonough, Duncan, Williams, & House, 1997; Reviere & Hylton, 1999; Smedley, Stith, & Nelson, 2002). More than one-fourth of U.S. Hispanics do not have a usual health care provider (about twice as likely as blacks and three times as likely as Whites) (Livingston, Minushkin, & Cohn, 2008). Being among the working poor or being undocumented often leads to lack of health insurance. About one-third, and the largest subgroup among the approximately 46 million people in the U.S. that do not have insurance, is the Hispanic population (U.S. Census Bureau, 2008). There is wide intra-cultural diversity: about 41% of Mexican Americans do not have health insurance, the highest percent of all subcultures (S. Santana & F. O. Santana, 2001). Almost 90% of the uninsured are working, but there is no employer-based coverage. Recent immigrants, including the great majority who are legal residents, are also less likely to be insured (Brown, Ojeda, Wyn, & Levan, 2000). Furthermore, the changing economic and political landscape of the early 21st Century (e.g., welfare reform, immigration reform, tighter eligibility requirements and reduced benefits for Medicare and Medicaid, a weakening economy) may significantly impact low income and less acculturated older patients due to their considerable reliance on Medicare and Medicaid. One-third of the Puerto Rican people in the U.S. are on Medicaid (associated with high numbers living in female-headed households in New York).

Additional frequently cited obstacles to maintaining health are associated with poverty. Poor housing (or even homelessness) and unsafe environmental conditions, inadequate food sources and nutrition, harmful lifestyle habits, and lack of access to transportation are all prevalent. Being poor is also associated with stress and a sense of alienation, hopelessness, powerlessness, and isolation. All of these feelings can lead to further estrangement (with a concomitant loss of social support systems) and marginal participation in society, including the health care system. Poverty at a young age has multiple effects on health as a person ages, notwithstanding the availability of Medicare. Poverty among people who are not elderly and who are expected to care for their older family members adds to their personal economic challenge and limits the amount of assistance they can provide to their older relatives (Power, Manor, & Matthews, 1999).

Although not just a problem among low-income people, physical, emotional, and sexual abuse is nevertheless often associated with the stress of poverty. Physical therapists need to be familiar with signs and symptoms of abuse and available resources. PTs might be the ones to first notice indications that abuse is present. Sensitivity to this issue can be tricky. Asking the right questions in the most comfortable way is something that is learned over time. How does one inquire without being insulting or taking away one's pride? This is one area where level of skill development can be especially important.

RACISM

Physical therapists must be cognizant of the marked effect of racism on health status and health care interactions (Collins et al., 2002; Schneider, Zaslavsky, & Epstein, 2002; Smedley et al., 2002). Although more typically associated with African Americans in this nation, Hispanic people (especially those of darker skin), Native Americans, Asians, and Middle Easterners are likely to have felt the effects of prejudice and racism as well (Berger, 1998; Facione & Katapodi, 2000; Lefebvre & Lattanzi, 2007).

According to Schneider et al. (2002), after adjustment for potential confounding factors, there were disparities in the quality of health care for African Americans who were Medicare beneficiaries and enrolled in managed care plans. They were less likely than Whites to receive eye examinations, beta blocker medication after myocardial infarction, and follow-up after hospitalization for mental illness (Schneider et al.). Moreover, the collective historical health care experience of African Americans, including the Tuskegee syphilis study, sterilization initiatives, and sickle cell screening abuses, have led to a distrust of the medical profession by many African Americans (Berger, 1998). See Chapter 6 for a more detailed discussion of the effects of racism on health.

INCIDENCE AND PREVALENCE OF DISEASE AND DISABILITY

Disease and disability are not randomly distributed. Many factors, including race, ethnicity, age distribution, socioeconomic status, sexuality, geography, and migration history, play a role in determining the incidence and prevalence of disease and disability. Discovering the determinants of disease (i.e., those risk factors related to the development and cause of the condition) is a major aspect of epidemiological work. Sometimes, a single variable is associated with a pathology (such as with vector-borne diseases), but often several risk factors are associated with a disease. Broadly speaking, risk factors can be related to inherited characteristics (e.g., genetic make-up), environmental factors (e.g., pollution), or personal behavior and lifestyle (e.g., diet) (Braithwaite & Taylor, 2001; Knutsen, Leavitt, & Sarton, 1995; Paul & Thorburn, 1999).

In the U.S., there are substantial health disparities between ethnic and racial groups—people of color have many more health problems than the White population (Aguirre-Molina, Molina, & Zambrana, 2001; Berger, 1998; Chu, Miller, & Springfield, 2007; Collins et al., 2002; HHS, n.d.; National Center for Health Statistics, 2007; Reviere & Hylton, 1999;

Smedley et al., 2002) (see Chapters 6 and 7). They are also more likely to report poor health and more restricted activity (Berkman & Gurland, 1998; Dunlop, Song, Manheim, Daviglus, & Chang, 2007; Feinglass, Rucker-Whitaker, Lindquist, McCarthy, & Pierce, 2005; Tran & Williams, 1998). Latinos have significantly more functional impairments than Blacks or Whites, which may result from lower income and education levels and from their residential environment (Berkman & Gurland, 1998). Puerto Ricans have more health problems than any other group (Tran & Williams, 1998). Women from all ethnic groups are especially disadvantaged and report greater limitation in activities of daily living (Villa & Torres-Gil, 2001). People of color have a lower life expectancy, higher infant mortality rates, and higher morbidity and mortality rates for a wide range of diseases. The elimination of health care disparities between people of color and Whites is one of the two major goals of Healthy People 2010, a guiding document for the U.S. Public Health Service (HHS, 2000).

However, some surprises do exist. For example, although cardiovascular disease is the number one cause of death for older people overall in the U.S., Hispanic/Latinos have the same level of heart disease mortality or lower than Whites, despite their high rates of diabetes and obesity and high blood lipid levels. Intra-ethnic diversity is once again a factor because this advantage is present for Mexican American men, but not women. Paradoxically, Mexican American men have twice the rate of angina pectoris compared with White men. It is believed that their genetic makeup leaves them vulnerable to some diseases (such as angina and diabetes) but less prone to having a fatal outcome (Angel et al., 2000; Huff & Kline, 1999; Villa & Torres-Gil, 2001).

Another paradox is that Hispanic/Latinos historically have lower rates of some of the most common kinds of cancer (e.g., lung, breast, colorectal, and prostate cancers), yet have higher rates for other cancers (e.g., stomach, gall bladder, liver, and cervical cancers) (Huff & Kline, 1999; McDougal, Medeleine, Daling, & Li, 2007; Tran & Williams, 1998). Once cancer is diagnosed, however, the higher-than-expected death rates from cancer among the Hispanic/Latino population are thought to be related to culturally motivated resistance to screening tests and early treatment because of language and communication barriers and the cultural belief in fatalism (Berger, 1998; Flores, 2000; Hubbell, Chavez, Mishra, & Valdez, 1996; Mickley & Soeken, 1993; Perez-Stable, Sabogal, Otero-Sabogal, Hiatt, & McPhee, 1992; Saurez, Roche, Nichols, & Simpson, 1997).

Non–insulin-dependent diabetes mellitus (type II) is the most significant medical concern for Hispanic/Latino and Native American people (and a disease common among African Americans as well) (Black, 2002; Huff & Kline, 1999; Nakamura, 1998; Peek, Cargill, & Huang, 2007). It deserves special attention because of its excessive prevalence and the severity of its complications and consequences. Family history, genetics, obesity, and age are key risk factors. The so-called "thrifty" gene theory related to Mexican Americans and Native Americans with diabetes is an example of the interaction of both genetic and lifestyle variables. When particular tribes were semi-nomadic, they frequently subsisted on a feast-or-famine diet. The tribes genetically developed an ability to metabolize their food efficiently. Today, when people exercise less and food is more abundant and likely to be high in fats and calories, there is a higher rate of obesity and diabetes. People with more Native American heritage are more resistant to insulin and unable to break down glucose in the blood. On the positive side, some Native Americans have the benefit of a gene that causes their blood sugar levels to respond to moderate exercise more quickly than other groups (Huff & Kline, 1999; Pember, 2002; Wasson, 1999).

Black people are disproportionately affected by cardiovascular disease, hypertension, and strokes (Davis, Vinci, Okwusa, Chase, & Huang, 2007; Nakamura, 1998). AIDS is increasingly a disease affecting African Americans: the HIV infection rates are seven times higher than for Whites (the rates for Hispanics are three times higher than for Whites) (Krisberg, 2008). Obesity, a health problem unto itself and a risk factor highly associated with disease and disability, is increasingly a problem in the U.S., and especially so for people of color. African American women have the highest rates of obesity, followed by Mexican American women (Huff & Kline, 1999; Urgo, 1998). Several factors contribute to obesity, such as genetic admixture, limited ability to metabolize carbohydrates, low socioeconomic status, decreased exercise, and cultural attitudes toward food and weight. A greater degree of acculturation is associated with decreased rates of obesity (Huff & Kline, 1999).

Regarding access to the health care system, people of color, once ill, are more likely to receive episodic, crisis-oriented care that occurs later and less frequently than for White people (Collins et al., 2002; Lurie & Dubowitz, 2007; Rowley, Jenkins, & Frazier, 2007). Recent immigrants are typically unfamiliar with how the American health care system works. They will commonly use the emergency room for primary care, which wastes resources and is not conducive to comprehensive care (Collins et al., 2002). Tran et al. (1997) report that community-based social and health services are underutilized by Hispanics. Strong social networks predict more regular use of the health care system to address medical needs (Friedenberg & Hammer, 1998). Some of the barriers to formal assistance include lack of knowledge about availability, accessibility, and eligibility for services and discomfort with bureaucracy (Dietz, 1996). In addition, there are few health promotion and disease and disability prevention programs. Hispanics and Asian Americans receive fewer preventive screening tests (e.g., mammograms) than African Americans and Whites (Collins et al., 2002). Under these conditions, greater complications and higher morbidity rates are inevitable.

An additional line of inquiry and data are related to the variation between and among ethnic groups and their level of health-related behaviors (D'Alonzo & Fischetti, 2008; McArthur & Raedeke, 2009). For example, Neighbors, Marquez, and Marcus (2008) have compared leisure-time activities between Hispanic and non-Hispanic White persons. All Hispanic subgroups were less active than their non-Hispanic White counterparts, but there was significant variation among Hispanic subgroups. Cuban and Dominican subgroups were the least active, particularly among women. Mexican Americans were the most active. Socioeconomic covariates had an impact on reducing the disparity among men, but had a much smaller effect on leisure-time activity disparities among women.

Although the focus here has been on disparities between people of color and those who are White, it is also necessary to recognize that disparities exist based on other variables such as sexuality. For example, women who are lesbians are more likely to smoke cigarettes, abuse alcohol, be overweight, and participate in vigorous physical activity and are less likely to have had a Papanicolaou or mammogram exam during the previous two years as compared to women in opposite-sex relationships (Aaron et al., 2001). Lesbians are also less likely than women in opposite-sex relationships to have health insurance coverage, to have seen a medical provider in the previous 12 months, or to have a regular source of health care (Heck, Sell, & Gorin, 2006). In contrast, men in same-sex relationships were as likely or more likely to report adequate health care access as compared to men in opposite-sex relationships (Heck et al., 2006).

Physical therapists need to be knowledgeable about the variables affecting the incidence and prevalence of medical conditions so they can be better prepared to treat these conditions, answer patient and family questions concerning the condition, and develop special preventive and educational programs targeted to those in need.

COMPARATIVE VALUE ORIENTATIONS

In contrast to material culture (the more easily observed and understood parts of culture, such as clothing, food, music, forms of greeting, ceremonial rites of passage), a person's nonmaterial culture (which includes values and morals) is more difficult to assess. Sometimes similarities in the material cultures of the patient and the physical therapist obscure profound differences in their nonmaterial cultures that are very relevant to the therapist-patient interaction. In fact, comparative value orientations and world view may provide important clues that can help the physical therapist and the patient to better understand each other.

Table 4-1 lists recurrent themes and patterns in cultures that many observers have identified (Leavitt, 2003; Loveland, 1999; Lynch & Hanson, 1998). These cultural elements may be the core of a person's worldview, or they may be the values that a person lives by. People from groups that have been most heavily influenced by European culture typically will have the values listed in the left-hand column, whereas people from those groups influenced by Hispanic/Latino, Asian, Middle Eastern, or African cultures typically will have the values listed in the right-hand column. However, a person's worldview also can be heavily influenced by personality traits, socioeconomic status, level of acculturation, and other factors. Moreover, a person does not necessarily fit into a rigid category; he or she may fall at the far end of one dichotomous scale, in the middle of a second, or at the other end of a third.

The defining element represented in Table 4-1 may be the comparison between types of social organization and relationships—individualism/privacy versus collectivism/group welfare. There are innumerable ways in which these two "value orientations" can influence the therapeutic encounter. For example, European values emphasize the importance of the individual and the ability of each person to affect his or her future through hard work (Lynch & Hanson, 1998). In this type of cultural orientation, both time and nature are commodities to be used profitably, and the success (or lack of success) of each person is credited to that person. A patient with an individualistic worldview may prefer to use assistive technology in order to live independently. Health care professionals with this type of worldview might emphasize the autonomy and personal responsibility of their patients and expect them to work hard at therapy.

What if patients have a cultural value system that emphasizes the importance of the group over the individual? In these societies, conformity is prized and behavior is constrained by social roles. Family roles (e.g., head of household, gender roles, attitudes toward the young and the old) are likely impacted by these cultural value systems. To illustrate, in the Hispanic/Latino culture, many cultural characteristics reflect the values of a collectivist society. One of the most significant values is *familismo*, or family commitment and responsibility. The welfare and honor of the family are preeminent concerns. Traditional gender roles within the family—known as *machismo* for men and *marianismo* for women—are related to *familismo*. The oldest man or the father is typically the authority figure and the final arbiter. The mother is central within the household and is responsible for child rearing and the cultural and social stability of the family. She is often described as having a sacrificing nature. Women are considered to be morally and spiritually superior to men; however, men typically make the final decisions within the household (S. Santana & F. O. Santana, 2001).

In collectivist cultures, kinship bonds across generations are common. Thus, a patient may arrive at the clinic with several family members. The patient may feel there is little point to working too hard because the family will provide care and because the patient believes that much of what happens to people—including disease and disability—is predetermined by fate (fatalism). In order for both the patient and the clinician to "save face," the patient might act very polite and accommodating when, in fact, he or she may not understand the clinician's instructions. Patients also might recognize that their goals and the clinician's goals are not the same. For instance, the patient may not want to use assistive technology because independence is not the goal.

Related collectivist cultural values associated with the Hispanic/Latino culture may include, but are not limited to, *respeto* (respect toward individuals based on age, gender, and social position or authority), *personalismo* (friendliness and individualized attention

TABLE 4-1	
COMPARATIVE VALUE SYSTEMS	
EURO-AMERICAN	**CROSS-CULTURAL COMPARISON**
Individualism/privacy	Collectivism/group welfare
Personal control over environment	Fate
Time dominates	Human interaction dominates
Precise time reckoning	Loose time reckoning
Future orientation	Past orientation
Doing (working, achieving)	Being (personal qualities)
Human equality	Hierarchy/rank/status
Self-help	Birthright inheritance
Competition	Cooperation
Informality	Formality
Directness/openness/honesty	Indirectness/ritual/"face"
Practicality/efficiency	Idealism/theory
Materialism	Spiritualism
Values youth	Values elders
Relative equality of sexes	Relative inequality of sexes

Adapted from Ferraro, G. (2002). *The cultural dimensions of international business* (4th ed.). Upper Saddle River, NJ: Prentice Hall. and Hanson, M. J. (1998). Families with Anglo-European roots. In E. W. Lynch and M. J. Hanson (Eds.), *Developing cross-cultural competence: A guide for working with young children and their families* (2nd ed., p. 121). Baltimore, MD: Paul Brooks Publishing Co.

and responsiveness to interpersonal interactions), *simpatia* (kindness, being nice), and fatalism (belief that events are predetermined) (Flores, 2000; Zungia, 1998). Generally speaking, these cultural values may be viewed as cultural strengths to be worked with (and not against) to foster more positive health outcomes.

The cultural beliefs and values of Native American people are also collectivistic. Sanchez, J. A. Plawecki, and H. M. Plawecki (1996) identify generosity and sharing, respect for elders, respect for nature, choice, freedom, and courage as the most important values.

In a rehabilitation setting, even the development of group exercise programs may be influenced by comparative value systems. For example, does the patient value competition or cooperation? Would a patient rather work hard and increase the number of repetitions, or would the patient not want to "show off" to others? Is the patient comfortable exercising among both men and women?

The patient's opinion on the role and status of medical personnel may be different depending on his or her culture. On one hand, an older patient from Cuba may expect the health care provider to demonstrate respect by addressing them first, by using the proper titles, and by asking about the family. On the other hand, a patient from a Middle Eastern subculture might tend to defer to the health care professional, who is considered to be an authority figure worthy of high esteem. The patient may be especially reluctant to express negative feelings and may be unlikely to share concerns about taking medication ordered by a physician or to ask questions that may be perceived as "stupid." An interactive conversation about health care options is less likely to occur (Salimbene, 2000).

PACE OF LIFE AND THE NOTION OF TIME

Perhaps the most difficult cultural differences to overcome, especially for those with a European cultural viewpoint, relate to pace of life and the notion of time (Brice & Campbell, 1999; Hall, 1984). *Monochronism* is the belief that time is an important concept, that events happen in chronological order, that there is a separation of work tasks and socializing, and that adherence to schedules is important. Many Whites are monochronistic—they are action-oriented and value punctuality. *Polychronism*, on the other hand, is the belief that events can happen concurrently and that fixed schedules are insignificant. The focus is on a more personal interaction, with less concern about completion of the task at hand (i.e., the value of personalism). Work orientation and the acquisition of material goods may not be present among people who value a relaxed, relationship-oriented lifestyle more highly.

Imagine the potential for misunderstanding if a Hispanic/Latino man, for example, arrives late for an appointment and expects the therapist to chat for a few minutes about non-therapeutic issues—such as the well-being of his family—and the therapist, already annoyed about her schedule being interrupted, immediately launches into a discussion about how to do exercises. These differences can also have an economic impact—late patients can disrupt a therapist's schedule and decrease his or her efficiency.

VALUES ACROSS THE LIFE SPAN

Comparative value systems may affect the behaviors of patients of a particular age group. For instance, expectations for the behavior of Asian American adolescents may be different from those for the behavior of a typical White adolescent. Older Asian American children are expected to be well disciplined and to take on some adult roles. An older adolescent sibling may be expected to accept personal sacrifice and to care for young children in the extended family while simultaneously working hard to maintain a strong academic record. A sense of duty or obligation to the family may be pronounced and is learned through role modeling. If the older sibling misbehaves, he or she might be rebuked for not setting a good example for the younger ones. High expectations may be a source of stress. Adolescents are likely to be recipients of a parenting style that is somewhat controlling, restrictive, and protective. This may lead to distancing behaviors or a distrust of outsiders. Discussions about sensitive topics such as sexuality may need to be avoided, and the patient's willingness to discuss personal issues related to treatment might be minimal (Chan, 1998).

Similarly, there may be special considerations when working with older people. Respect for older people is a value prevalent among many ethnic groups. Signs of respect may include using terms of address such as "Ma'am" or "Sir" or asking for tales of wisdom. In many cultures, it is expected that adult children will provide an economic and social base for their older parents. Older Asian and Hispanic/Latino people are more likely to live with other family members or friends and are less likely to be segregated, to live alone or in a nursing home or other institution, or to use professional home nursing services. Mutual assistance, especially in times of illness, is counted on both because of cultural preferences and because of strategic adjustments to American society (Baxter, Bryant, Scarbro, & Shetterly, 2001; S. Santana & F. O. Santana, 2001; Wilmoth et al., 1997).

Comparative value systems may have an impact on gift-giving from a patient to a therapist. In some cultures, gift-giving is the norm rather than the exception. APTA's Guide for Professional Conduct (2004) states that the physical therapist should at all times ensure that his or her professional judgment is not affected by a patient's gift. The physical therapist should also ensure that the gift has not created an obligation for either the therapist or the patient. The physical therapist, however, needs to consider the patient's value system when deciding whether accepting a modest gift from the patient or the patient's family is ethically appropriate. In many cultures, it would typically be a great insult to refuse a gift—a person's pride may be at stake. On a personal note, I have been given the gift of a few crackers or a couple of fresh eggs from a farm. These kinds of gifts have been the most meaningful to me.

THE ROLE OF RELIGION

The role that religion plays in a person's explanatory model can be closely aligned to their general health beliefs and behaviors and their comparative value systems. Religious beliefs and customs may affect the acceptance and the administration of more standard medical and rehabilitation practices (Mickley & Soeken, 1993).

Religious beliefs may be an area in which health care professionals have difficulty accepting someone else's moral and ethical viewpoint and actions. One well-known point of conflict is the refusal of a person who is a Jehovah's Witness to allow a medical intervention if it requires a blood transfusion. Conflicts also may occur when patients have a strong faith that a supreme spiritual being (e.g., God, Allah, Brahma) will cure them, and they, therefore, avoid treatment. A Lubavitcher orthodox Jew may turn to a *rebbe* for healing prayers or an African American may turn to a "tent meeting." People from Southeast Asia may adhere to *karma*, a belief that one's present life is based on a previous existence, and they thus accept a misfortune as predestined.

Religious beliefs can also affect care delivery. A traditional Muslim woman is forbidden to expose her skin (except for the hands and face) to a man other than her husband, and, therefore, she would require a woman for a physical therapist. The "Sabbath" days mean different things in different religions, and how these religions celebrate the Sabbath may affect patient care. For example, the Jewish Sabbath begins at sundown on Friday and extends to sundown on Saturday, which would affect the times that therapists can provide care, especially in the home.

COMMUNICATION STYLES

Communication and language are intertwined with and are inseparable from culture. The ability to communicate effectively, therefore, is an exceptionally important variable when working cross-culturally or seeking to understand a patient's cultural value system and "explanatory model" (see Chapter 9).

English is the primary language in the U.S. Spanish is the second most commonly used language, followed by French, which lags far behind (Johnson, 1999). However, there are dozens of other languages that are used by large numbers of people in the U.S. About 55 million people in the U.S. speak a language other than English in their homes, and 24 million of those speak English "less than very well" (Limited English Proficiency, n.d.; U.S. Census Bureau, 2007). Ideally, the physical therapist and patient would speak the same language. More realistically, physical therapists should learn a few key words in the primary language of their patients. Translators are often a necessity, and typically family (often children) or friends are called upon to act as translators. Although this may be the only available alternative, it is fraught with problems. The HHS Office of Minority Health (2001) strongly advises that children should not be used as interpreters, especially for adults. When a family member or friend is the translator, physical therapists should be aware that they are dealing with an untrained third party who may be "interpreting" the information before passing it on to them and that some topics may be inappropriate to discuss with the translator because they are of a more personal or sensitive nature (e.g., family planning, spousal abuse, terminal illness).

If possible, a professional translator should be used. Translation requires knowledge of medical terminology, a good memory, the ability to concentrate, and the ability to know how and when to edit messages so that the true meaning can be accurately transmitted. The ideal professional interpreter is bicultural and has a good grasp of both medical and cultural nuances (HHS, 2001; Ross, 2001).

Limited proficiency in English is one of the most important variables associated with poor health status and is a barrier to accessing the health care system (Collins et al., 2002; Flores, 2000; Smedley et al., 2002). Because a language barrier is so common and such a significant obstacle to good health care, the Office of Civil Rights in the HHS has developed policies to better serve people with limited English proficiency, including language assistance appropriate to the needs of each facility (Ross, 2001).

INTERACTIVE STYLES

In addition to the spoken word, there are obvious and subtle differences in the interactive styles. For example, verbal communication in individualistic societies is associated with direct, "low-context" communication. Patients with this cultural background may expect that the physical therapist will get right to the point and may assume that they do not have to rely on the surrounding context for interpretation. They would expect that what is found in the verbal message is what is being communicated. The notion of privacy is important, and questions of a more personal nature might be considered off-limits (Brice & Cambell, 1999; Hall, 1984; Lynch, 1998). In contrast, a person from a collectivist culture may speak indirectly, in a more circular fashion, always keeping in mind the need for everyone to "save face." Communication is more "high-context" and listener-focused (i.e., sensitive to situational and contextual features). There may be more "spiral" (or indirect) logic, more indirect verbal negotiation, and subtle nonverbal nuances. The notion of privacy is less pervasive, but no party should be embarrassed or "lose face." The focus is more on human relationships (e.g., *personalismo*). It may take a long time to establish a solid, trusting relationship, but once it exists, it is likely to be strong and lasting (Brice & Cambell, 1999; Chan, 1998; Johnson, 1999).

Another difference in verbal communication is the amount of "wait time" or time gaps that occur during conversation. Native Americans typically have a longer wait time than Whites because the pace of conversation is slower. Physical therapists should wait until the person has finished speaking before interrupting or asking questions. European Americans typically are uncomfortable with silence. Wait time is also increased when patients need to translate the words into their own language before responding. In some cultures, many people may speak at once (Ladyshewsky, 1999).

Different cultural groups also may have many nonverbal, observable differences in communication style. In fact, Mehrabian (1980) suggests that as much as 93% of the total meaning of an encounter is communicated by nonverbal factors such as body language (55%) and tone of voice (38%). Differences in interpretation occur with regard to eye contact, facial expression, body movement, personal space, and overall formality. The physical therapist may believe a patient is acting disinterested if eye contact is not direct, when in reality, the patient may believe it is impolite to look directly at someone who is perceived as the authority figure. A physical therapist may always give a firm handshake upon introduction to a patient and may presume that this is an appropriate, friendly, and polite gesture. Native American or traditional Asian American patients, however, may consider this aggressive or hostile, because a subtle, "soft," nonthreatening handshake is the norm in their cultures.

What is the patient's preferred requirement for personal space? How close does the patient like to stand when speaking with health care providers? Physical therapists should observe their patient's response when they stand closer or further away during a general conversation. During a treatment session, does a person of the opposite sex seem more uncomfortable than might be expected? How do people from different cultures stand with each other as compared with how they stand with the therapist? Touch can provide reassurance and kindness, or it can be a discomfort and annoyance.

Gender and age are important variables influencing personal space. For example, people from Hispanic/Latino and Middle Eastern subcultures tend to prefer standing close and are comfortable with physical contact between members of the same sex (Lynch, 1998). People who are members of the orthodox branches of Islam or Judaism, meanwhile, might not be comfortable being touched by someone of the opposite sex.

LEARNING STYLES

The physical therapist who is educating a patient about a diagnosis or a home program must recognize, in addition to education and literacy rates, that many cultures have different methods of teaching and learning. The existence of different learning methods becomes an especially important consideration when the physical therapist is working with a patient who was educated outside of the U.S. or who is a recent immigrant. People of European ancestry, for example, often rely on note taking and studying written texts as well as intense discussions with a great deal of interaction between the physical therapist and the patient. People of other cultures, in contrast, may rely more on a lecture format with few questions and little discussion. Members of other cultural groups, such as Blacks and African Americans, may rely almost entirely on oral training and demonstration. A written list of exercises, even with diagrams, may not be as effective as "hearing and feeling" these exercises. When possible, physical therapists should include family members in discussions about home programs and other aspects of patient care; inclusion of the family is especially important for patients from cultures that have collectivist values (Levitt, 1999).

If the patient has limited proficiency in English, it is wise to speak slowly (not loudly) and to avoid colloquialisms and idioms. Statements should be rephrased often, and physical therapists should check to be sure that their patient or client understands their meaning.

Written patient instructions should be translated into grammatically correct, simple language using appropriate, meaningful vocabulary to help ensure that these materials are used as intended and are culturally relevant to the patient. The material should be translated back into the original language to see if something does not make sense.

Rapport is also likely to be enhanced if the clinic environment has been adapted to make someone from a different cultural background feel more welcome. Therapists should consider the types of magazines that are placed in public meeting spaces or in the waiting area. Are these publications and the signs around the workplace in more than one language? Do pictures in the literature look like the people who frequent the facility? What images decorate the space? A consideration of these questions, an understanding of a range of communication styles (both verbal and nonverbal) and learning styles, and the ability to properly interpret an interaction will undoubtedly minimize barriers that may otherwise exist.

WHEN DIFFERENCES IN CULTURAL VALUES AND COMMUNICATION ARE NOT CONSIDERED

If the physical therapist does not consider differences in cultural values and does not act on them appropriately, miscommunication and misunderstanding between the patient and the clinician may be more likely (The Provider's Guide, n.d.). Based on reports in the medical literature regarding the impact of language and cultural differences on the patient-provider relationship, it could be inferred that problems in communicating might result in the following (Carrasquillo, Orav, Brennan, & Burstin, 1999; David & Rhee, 1998; Doescher, Saver, Franks, & Fiscella, 2000; Flores et al., 2003; Morales, Cunningham, Brown, Liu, & Hays, 1999):

1. The physical therapist could make errors in the examination and diagnostic process.
2. The patient might not fully participate in the therapy program.
3. The patient may report overall dissatisfaction with the physical therapy service.

HEALTH BELIEFS AND BEHAVIORS

Historically, models for the provision of care in the U.S. generally have relied on the values and belief systems of the "majority" (i.e., the White middle-class). These models are culturally insensitive because they deny the existence of "non-Western" systems of thinking, sometimes referred to as "folk," "indigenous," or "tradiational" systems. At the most basic level for physical therapists, we need to understand the meaning of disability for our patients. The World Health Organization (WHO) defines disability as "an umbrella term for impairments, activity limitations and participation restrictions. It denotes the negative aspects of the interaction between an individual (with a health condition) and that individual's contextual factors (environmental and personal factors)" (WHO, 2001, p. 190). The *Guidelines to Physical Therapist Practice* (APTA, 2001) defines disability as "the inability or restricted ability to perform actions, tasks, and activities related to required self-care, home management, work, community, and leisure roles in the individual's sociocultural context and physical environment" (see Chapter 5).

Although many health care professions have embraced these or similar definitions of disability, the concept of disability is not a cultural universal. As Ingstad and Whyte (1995) state, "In many cultures, one cannot be 'disabled' for the simple reason that 'disability' as a recognized category does not exist. There are blind people and lame people and 'slow' people, but 'the disabled' as a general term does not translate easily into many languages" (p. 7). In cultures in which disability does not define who a person is, people with a disability are expected to follow the same life cycle as everyone else.

It is not necessary to catalog every known variation in disability beliefs, but it is appropriate for practitioners to understand how other people conceptualize disability and rehabilitation. This understanding can have a positive effect on the manner in which rehabilitation professionals are received and regarded and on their ability to serve their patients (Groce, 1999).

CAUSES OF DISABILITY AND DISEASE

Although there are general similarities among folk beliefs about the causes of illness and disability—including psychological states such as fear, envy, and family turmoil; environmental or natural conditions such as bad air and excess cold or heat; and supernatural causes such as witchcraft or bad spirits—these beliefs also vary (Pachter, 1994). Physical and mental illnesses are sometimes intertwined, and emotional, spiritual, social, and physical factors can be major contributing forces to illnesses. Overall, however, physical disabilities are more accepted by the community and the family than mental disabilities (Foster, 1976; Galanti, 1991; Groce & Zola, 1993).

Although many people hold folk health care beliefs and Western health care beliefs simultaneously, traditional beliefs from a patient's cultural background may be brought to the forefront during times of stress or uncertainty, especially in patients with lower levels of education. In an ethnographic study conducted in rural Jamaica, Leavitt (1992) recorded that one mother explained that her child's disability originated from jaundice because the hospital did not have the ability to "burn" the jaundice out when her child was born. Another mother stated that, because she did not eat more nutritious food while she was pregnant, her daughter was born with a disability, when in fact her daughter had Down syndrome. Physical therapists need to recognize that patients express beliefs based on their personal worldview.

In some cultures, people may believe that illness and disability are forms of divine punishment. A person may have sinned or violated a taboo, either in this life or a previous life, thereby causing the wrath of God, which may take the form of an illness or disability visited on the offender or a family member. Many people throughout the world believe in the "evil eye." The evil eye typically is a spell, usually motivated by envy, which is believed to cause the victim to fall ill. In an article about disability by Mardiros (1989), one Mexican American woman claimed that one of her husband's previous lovers asked a *bruja* (a sorcerer or witch) to put a hex on them, which the woman blamed for all of their "bad luck."

In any culture, there may be people who believe that an imbalance of elements is responsible for an ailment. This "elemental" system resembles the ancient Greek concept of an imbalance of the four humors, and it includes a system of classification for diseases, body organs, herbal remedies, and foods. All four of these mutually complementary forces are required for a person to be in harmony with nature, and a belief in this concept might affect the patient's decision regarding what medicines to use and foods to eat. In India, the Ayurvedic system equates health with balance. Traditional Chinese medicine requires a balance of yin and yang. The Navajo believe that their health depends on harmony with family, community, self, and nature, and they do not have a concept of communicable disease. Their language, for example, does not have a word for *germ* (Berger, 1998).

In some communities, harmony between the physical and spiritual world requires a balance of "hot" and "cold." Examples of diseases considered to be "hot" by the Hispanic/Latino culture are hypertension, diabetes, acid indigestion, and other diseases characterized by vasodilation and a high metabolic rate. "Cool" remedies such as bananas, passion flowers, and lemon juice are used for a "hot" illness. "Cold" diseases include menstrual cramps, pneumonia and other respiratory diseases, colic, and anemia. If a person is anemic, he or she might eat more "hot" foods, such as organ meats with a lot of blood products. Blood is "hot" and is associated with strength, virility, and *machismo*. For a cold, orange juice (vitamin C) might be recommended by a physician, but the Hispanic/Latino folk tradition is to treat a "cold" with a "hot" remedy such as red chili peppers (which, by the way, also have vitamin C) (Nakamura, 1998; Rubel & Moore, 2001; Spector, 2000).

SELECTION OF INTERVENTIONS

Decision making about health behaviors can be complex. In some cultures, when a person is sick, the family and a hierarchy of lay healers are often the first line of defense. Next, people seek out either a Western biomedical health care professional or a folk healer who practices traditional medicine. Sometimes, health care professionals and traditional healers are seen simultaneously. Typically, people are more likely to partake in indigenous health care practices if they are less acculturated, poorer, and live in rural areas (Young & Garro, 1982). Practical matters such as cost, severity of illness, and availability of practitioners often determine the utilization of traditional health care practices (Young & Garro, 1982).

Treatment for a disease or disability is also culturally specific, although intra-ethnic variation abounds. Indigenous folk healers, or practitioners of traditional medicine, are prevalent in every society. The *curanderos* may be preferred by Mexican Americans, the singer by the Navajo, the voodoo priest by Haitians, the *santeria* by Cubans, the herbalist by the Chinese, and so on. For the Laotian Hmong, the shaman may use herbal concoctions and animal sacrifice (Fadiman, 1997). In Jamaica, the *obeah* may use materials such as blood, feathers, parrots' beak, grave dirt, egg shell, and medicinal herbs to treat a person with a disability (Leavitt, 1992). In Puerto Rico, an *espirtista* (usually a female medium), helps people with physical or emotional problems by connecting them with good spirits and exorcising evil spirits (Nakamura, 1998). For many Native American tribes, "talking circles"—where stories are shared—are used to demonstrate the interconnectedness of life, the cycle of life and death, and the balance in the natural world required for good health. In fact, health care professionals may use "talking circles" to educate people about preventive and treatment measures so that the notion of fatalism can be replaced with the idea of control over one's health (Pember, 2002). Over 400 herbal remedies have been identified for use among Native Americans (Sanchez et al., 1996).

In the U.S., the medical establishment considers many of the interventions cited above as complementary and alternative medicine (CAM). These include mind-body interventions (hypnosis or prayer), biological-based interventions (herbal therapies and dietary supplements), manipulative and body-based interventions (massage, manipulation) and energy therapies (focusing on the role of energy sources within the body). Yet, for people with non-Western belief systems, these types of intervention are the norm, and it is the Western bio-medical model that can be complementary and alternative.

Today, there is increased knowledge that many people in the U.S., of all ethnic backgrounds, are using CAM. As noted above, Eisenberg et al. (1993) and Eisenberg et al. (1998) did seminal work in this area. More recently, the U.S. National Health Interview Survey (NHIS) (Barnes, Powell-Griner, McFann, & Nahin, 2004), concluded that greater than one-third of adults used CAM during the preceding year. When the definition of CAM was expanded to include prayer, the percent rose to 62%. Other than prayer, some of the most common CAM therapies used were herbal therapies, meditation, chiropractic care, yoga, and massage. Consistent with earlier reports, gender (women), education (higher educational attainment), and recent medical history (hospitalized within the past year) was associated with higher CAM usage. There is a growing amount of research on the use of CAM by people of color to explore its use and to discover whether use of CAM results from health disparities or causes them. In general, Whites used CAM most (36%) with Hispanics next (27%), closely followed by Blacks (26%) (Graham et al., 2005).

Two theoretical explanations for why ritual healing practices may be successful are based on neurobiology or psychology. The first explanation is neurobiological. Endorphins may play a role in diminishing pain (Oyama, Jin, Yamaya, Ling, & Guillemin, 1980). The release of these neurochemicals, produced by the brain, may be influenced by psychological experiences (e.g., transcendental meditation) (Infante et al., 1998). The second explanation is the placebo effect, which may help the body to heal itself (Kaptchuk, 2002). A placebo may be a word or an action, not just a pharmaceutical substance. By engaging the patient's mind and emotions, the healer may aid physiological repair (Nakamura, 1998).

Traditional practices may also influence the responses of a patient or client to a Western medical protocol. Many Vietnamese believe that Western medicine is designed to suit the body size of people in Western cultures. Thus, the quantity of drugs prescribed may be seen as inappropriate for the Vietnamese person, who is typically much smaller than the average White American (Ladinsky, Volk, & Robinson, 1987). Likewise, the physical therapist working in the area of women's health might want to know that there may be special considerations associated with childbirth. Different Asian subcultures, for example, prepare special dishes to assist with the involution of the uterus, chase the "bad blood" away, and regulate menstrual flow (Chan, 1998).

Often, the use of an alternative treatment is the source of misunderstanding and conflict. A practitioner of Western medicine may perceive that Asian practices used to draw "evil" from the body—such as coin rubbing, in which a coin is rubbed on the skin until a raised red mark appears, or cupping, in which a heated glass is placed on the body to create a vacuum that causes the skin to rise and become red—are harmful (Chan, 1998). On the other hand, a traditional Hmong person may have superstitions about health care practitioners in the U.S. Some Hmong believe that U.S. surgeons cut out body parts of the deceased to eat them or to sell them as food (Fadiman, 1997).

Many texts and studies detail patients' beliefs in folk illnesses and their use of herbal and other home remedies and alternative healers for conditions as diverse as asthma, diabetes, AIDS, and depression. Yet, most patients do not report the use of CAM to their health provider (Berger, 1998).

Sometimes, home remedies are harmful. One remedy, known as *greta* or *azarcon*, which is used for gastroenteritis, has a very high lead content and is considered dangerous. (Huff & Kline, 1999; Spector, 2000). Lead, mercury, and arsenic have been detected in a some Indian-manufactured traditional Ayurvedic medicines. Metals may be present due to the practice of *rasa shastra* (combining herbs with metals, minerals, and gems) (Saper et al., 2008).

When using typical Western medical and physical therapy interventions, it is necessary to consider whether they are appropriate in the context of the patient's culture. For example, people from many Asian subcultures usually squat rather than sit on chairs and thus require greater range of motion in the hip, knee, and ankle, even at the expense of stability. It is much less likely for someone to receive a total hip replacement in Asia than in the U.S. because it does not allow for flexion beyond 90 degrees. Also, eating with hands or chopsticks may require different movement patterns and range of motion than are typically used by people from European-influenced subcultures.

CULTURE-BOUND SYNDROMES

Culture-bound syndromes, sometimes referred to as folk illnesses, exist in most cultures. They are associated with unique beliefs about the cause of an illness and may require specific culturally prescribed treatments. *Susto* is perhaps the most studied culture-bound, psychosomatic illness within Hispanic/Latino subcultures. *Susto*, or "shock," occurs when a frightening event causes the soul to leave the body. Symptoms of *susto* include sleepiness, loss of appetite, insomnia, and generalized depression. Psychiatrists consider these symptoms to be body metaphors for psychological distress (Rubel & Moore, 2001). Other culture-bound syndromes within the Hispanic community include *emphacho* (stomach aches, diarrhea, vomiting, and fever are symptoms of having eaten an inappropriate food, which is said to "stick" to the stomach lining), *envidia* (set off when a person is envious of another), and *mal aire* (bad air caused by an evil wind, with symptoms similar to those of a cold or flu) (Nakamura, 1998; Rebhun, 1994).

A culture-bound syndrome from the Haitian culture is "arrested pregnancy syndrome," in which a woman who expects to be carrying a child and feels as though she is pregnant is not actually pregnant. It is often associated with infertility in a culture that highly values the ability to have children (Coreil, Barnes-Jasiah, Augustin, & Cayemittes, 1996). Anorexia nervosa, a psychological disorder with which most U.S. physical therapists are familiar, is considered a culture-bound syndrome of White North Americans (Basch, 1999).

In summary, although one cannot say with certainty how many individuals have non-Western health care belief systems, physical therapists must consider that these belief systems are more prevalent than they expect. Variables such as the patient's level of acculturation and place of origin can influence a belief system. It is wise to expect that traditional beliefs are somewhere in a person's cultural background and may be brought to the forefront during times of stress or uncertainty. Researchers often have a difficult time uncovering a respondent's belief system because they do not ask the right questions or the respondent may fear looking "ignorant" or "backward." This author believes that physical therapists need to become comfortable talking about these beliefs and behaviors with patients. Greater and appropriate communication should lead to greater understanding and movement toward cultural proficiency.

DIETARY PRACTICES ACROSS CULTURES

Physical therapists serving patients from a wide range of cultures would also benefit from knowledge about their patients' dietary practices. For many cultural groups, there is profound social and cultural meaning, as well as nutritional value, in food. For example, specific foods for the African American community are identified as "soul food." These may be unhealthy from a nutritional perspective (high salt and high fat content) but significant to an individual, representing a rich cultural history and memories.

To use a second example, for people of Jewish ancestry, traditional Jewish foods are associated with religious celebrations and are a unifying component of ethnic identity. Foods commonly associated with Jewish living are chicken soup (sometimes referred to as "Jewish penicillin"), bagels and lox (smoked salmon), *knaidle* (matzah heal dumplings served in soup at Passover or on the Sabbath), chopped liver, *kugel* (noodle pudding), gefilte fist (ground freshwater fish served in oblong pieces with horseradish), blintzes (crepes filled with fruit or cheese), and more (Leavitt, 2006). No matter what the eating patterns of an individual are, it is generally unlikely that a person will completely alter their eating habits on your suggestion to eat more healthily. Finding a compromise is likely the best solution.

Jewish people who are more observant may obey the Jewish dietary laws of *kashrut*. When one maintains these specific dietary laws with regard to food and utensils, one is considered *kosher*. In brief, certain foods are restricted such as pork and shellfish. Meat and chicken need to be slaughtered in a way that minimizes the animal's pain in order to be considered *kosher*. Meat and dairy foods are separated in preparation, serving, and eating (Leavitt, 2006). People of the Islamic faith have some of the same dietary practices.

PAIN ACROSS CULTURES

Physical therapists often have patients in pain, and thus, must recognize that people respond to pain quite differently from each other. The way people react to and feel about pain is not just based on a physiologic response to tissue damage, but rather typically guided by cultural rules. Researchers on the psychosocial and behavioral aspects of pain have found significant relationships among ethnic variation, perception of pain intensity, and the responses to pain (Bates & Edwards, 1998; Weissman, Gordon, & Bidar-Sielaff, n.d.; Zborowski, 1952).

In a seminal study, Zborowski (1952) compared different White populations—including Jewish, Italian, Irish, and "old" or "Yankee" Americans—and determined that some cultural groups, such as Italian Americans, allowed their members to complain about pain, whereas other groups, such as "old" Americans, expected their members to "report" pain in a dispassionate manner. Zborowski also found that members of some groups, including Italian Americans, wanted immediate relief of pain from painkillers, whereas others, including Jewish Americans, worried more about the long-term implications of pain and did not want to use medications for fear that they would mask a more serious problem. Societal rules regarding pain tolerance also promote gender or age differences, but these are not cultural universals.

During the late 1980s, Bates and Edwards (1998) investigated patients' meanings and explanations associated with pain. U.S.-born "old" American (mostly Protestants), Hispanic, Irish, Italian, French Canadian, and Polish people, all of whom were outpatients in a Massachusetts pain treatment facility, were studied. Variation in ethnic identity and locus-of-control style were consistently associated with differences in pain intensity and response. The Hispanic group demonstrated (presumed to be primarily Puerto Ricans since the study was in Massachusetts) the highest pain expressiveness, the greatest interference with work and social activities, and the highest degree of emotional and psychological stress. The Italian group was second in each of these categories, and either the Polish or "old" American group was the lowest in each category. According to the authors, the results of the study supported the idea of interethnic group variation in the response to pain.

In addition, Bates and Edwards (1998), reinforcing the notion of intracultural diversity, reported that intragroup variation analysis demonstrated within group differences in the response to pain based on both generation and degree of heritage consistency (i.e., the degree to which a person's lifestyle reflects his or her traditional culture). More recent immigrants or people who are the first generation born in the U.S., people who have high degrees of heritage consistency, and people who believe that they have a strong support system report less severe responses to pain.

Looking more closely at one particular group, S. Santana and F. O. Santana (2001) cite a 1995 study by Villarruel, who identified the ways in which Mexican Americans experience pain. Beliefs about pain include the following:

- Pain is an accepted and expected part of life
- Pain does not negate one's responsibilities and duties
- Pain is predetermined by the gods
- Pain is a consequence of immoral behavior
- Pain should be endured with a stoic attitude
- Pain may best be alleviated by maintaining balance

PTs need to contemplate the meaning of pain for an individual patient.

A study comparing normative pain responses among college students in the U.S. and India found that students in India were less accepting of overt pain expression than those in the U.S. Females believed that overt pain expression was more appropriate than males. Thus, Indian males had the highest pain tolerance. Reported pain intensity predicted 28% of the variance in pain tolerance and beliefs predicted another 5% (Nayak, Shiflett, Eshun, & Levine, 2000). Refer to Helman's text, *Culture, Health and Illness* (1984) for more information on pain and culture.

It also should be noted that physiological or biological differences can result in different responses to and side effects from drugs. Chinese patients, for instance, appear to metabolize drugs differently than White patients and require lower dosages of some pain medications (Matthews, 1995; Preble, Quveryn, & Sinatra, 1992; Zhou & Liu, 2000; Zhou, Koshakji, Silberstein, Wilkinson, & Wood, 1989).

END-OF-LIFE BELIEFS AND BEHAVIORS

Health beliefs and behaviors associated with end-of-life decisions deserve special attention by physical therapists specializing in geriatrics. Although physical therapists do not typically deal with end-of-life decisions, it is, nevertheless, a possible topic of conversation, especially with family members. Because of language and cultural barriers, people of color may not have adequate knowledge of the purpose and availability of hospice services.

In Asian and Hispanic/Latino subcultures that have a belief in fatalism, disclosure of a terminal disease may take away any hope that the patient may have. The family, especially the eldest son, has a very strong obligation to protect loved ones from emotional distress. In actuality, it is not common for elderly Chinese people to discuss the likelihood of death at all because it is believed to be a bad omen. The Navajo feel similarly—negative thoughts would be in conflict with the concept of *hozho*, which involves goodness, harmony, and a positive attitude.

Older adults are likely to have varied attitudes toward advance directives. For example, elderly Chinese people may be less likely to write something down, because they honor the spoken word. Elderly Japanese people tend to place great faith in family and professional relationships, and it is less likely that decisions would be made by the individual alone. For the Navajo as well, major decisions are collaborative, and the family and the tribe would have input into any advance directives (Berger, 1998).

Hispanic/Latino people generally are less knowledgeable about, and less likely to write, living wills than other ethnic groups. According to Berger (1998), Mexican Americans have a more negative attitude toward advance directives than Whites or African Americans, although there is a correlation to the degree of acculturation. In general, it is less likely that the Hispanic/Latino person would make these decisions alone. As with many other cultural groups, major decisions are collaborative, and the family would have input into any advance health directives.

Once death occurs, some cultural groups (e.g., Orthodox Jews, Christian Scientists) are less likely to consent to an autopsy because they believe a mutilated body may cause suffering in the afterlife (Berger, 1998). With regard to bereavement, grief responses also depend on personal characteristics and culture. In contrast to the European American culture, in which people are encouraged to grieve and "move on," many non-Western cultures encourage people to continue their relationship with the deceased, possibly through a specific altar dedicated to the loved one where they can pray or bring food and other offerings (Craig & Baucum, 2001).

CONCLUSION

The concept of cultural competence is complex, multi-dimensional, and still evolving. Health professionals and health policy experts have recognized its potential impact on improving health outcomes for individual clients and larger populations, decreasing cost for the health care system (long term if not immediately), and improving professional job satisfaction for health professionals. Physical therapists need to understand various models of cultural competence and possible methods to assess their own beliefs and behaviors regarding culture and diversity, as well as their ability to adapt to culturally diverse patient needs within their place of employment. Cultural competence needs to be a non-negotiable skill, valued and tested as rigorously as competence in any clinical science or other field of study.

REFLECTION QUESTIONS

✔ *How long has your family been in the United States?*

✔ *Why did your ancestors come to America?*

✔ *Do members of your family display different degrees of acculturation to the "normative" American culture?*

✔ *What values do you hold most dear? Are these related to your cultural heritage?*

✔ *Where do you fall on the cultural value continuum (i.e., if you drew a line across each of the paired cultural values, where do you place yourself on that line)? Are you happy with that placement?*

✔ *How do you feel when people do not speak English well?*

✔ *Do you know anyone who does not speak English at home?*

✔ *Do you enjoy going to restaurants that serve food that is different than what you typically eat?*

✔ *How often do you make an effort to learn about people of a different ethnic group or faith?*

✔ *How often do you go to a cultural event or partake in a holiday related to another ethnic or religious group?*

✔ *What stereotypes do you hold about people from a different religion?*

✔ *What biases do you hold toward individuals from a different religion?*

✔ *What do you believe are the values of people who are of _____ heritage?*

✔ *How do you feel about complementary and alternative medicine?*

REFERENCES

A profile of Somali refugees in the United States. (n.d.). Retrieved November 6, 2009, from http://paa2006.princeton.edu/download.aspx?submissionId=61036

Aaron, D. J., Markovic, N., Danielson, M. E., Honnold, J. A., Janosky, J. E., & Schmidt, N. J. (2001). Behavioral risk factors for disease and preventive health practices among lesbians. *American Journal of Public Health, 91*(6), 972-975.

Aguirre-Molina, M., Molina, C. W., & Zambrana, R. E. (Eds.). (2001). *Health issues in the Latino community.* San Francisco, CA: Jossey-Bass.

American Physical Therapy Association. (2001). *Guidelines to physical therapy practice* (2nd ed.). Alexandria, VA: Author.

American Physical Therapy Association. (2004). APTA guide for professional conduct. Retrieved October 26, 2008, from http://www.apta.org/AM/Template.cfm?Section=Core_Documents1&Template=/CM/HTMLDisplay.cfm&ContentID=24781

Angel, J. L., Angel, R. J., & Markides, K. S. (2000). Late-life immigration: Changes in living arrangements, and headship status among older Mexican-origin individuals. *Social Science Quarterly, 81*(1), 389-403.

Barnes, P. M., Powell-Griner, E., McFann, K., & Nahin, R. L. (2004). Complementary and alternative medicine use among adults: United States, 2002. *Advance Data, 27*(343), 1-19.

Basch, P. F. (1999). *Textbook of international health* (2nd ed.). New York, NY: Oxford University Press.

Bates, M., & Edwards, W. T. (1998). Ethnic variations in the chronic pain experience. In P. J. Brown (Ed.), *Understanding and applying medical anthropology* (pp. 267-278). New York, NY: McGraw-Hill.

Baxter, J., Bryant, L. L., Scarbro, S., & Shetterly, S. M. (2001). Patterns of rural Hispanic and non-Hispanic white health care use. *Research on Aging, 23*(1), 37-60.

Berger, J. T. (1998). Culture and ethnicity in clinical care. *Archives of Internal Medicine, 158*(19), 2085-2090.

Berkman, C. S., & Gurland, B. J. (1998). The relationship between ethnoracial group and functional level in older persons. *Ethnicity & Health, 3*(3), 175-188.

Black, S. A. (2002). Diabetes, diversity, and disparity: What do we do with the evidence? *American Journal of Public Health, 92*(4), 543-548.

Braithwaite, R. L., & Taylor, S. E. (Eds.). (2001). *Health issues in the black community* (2nd ed.). San Francisco, CA: Jossey-Bass.

Brice, A., & Campbell, L. (1999). Cross-cultural communication. In R. L. Leavitt (Ed.), *Cross-cultural rehabilitation: An international perspective* (pp. 83-94). London, England: Harcourt Brace and Company.

Brown, E. R., Ojeda, V. D., Wyn, R., & Levan, R. (2000). *Racial and ethnic disparities in access to health insurance and health care.* Los Angeles, CA: UCLA Center for Health Policy Research and the Henry J. Kaiser Family Foundation.

Carrasquillo, O., Orav, E. J., Brennan, T. A., & Burstin, H. R. (1999). Impact of language barriers on patient satisfaction in an emergency department. *Journal of General Internal Medicine, 14*(2), 82-87.

Chan, S. (1998). Families with Asian roots. In E. W. Lynch, & M. J. Hanson (Eds.), *Developing cross-cultural competence: A guide for working with young children and their families* (2nd ed., pp. 251-344). Baltimore, MD: Brookes Publishing Company.

Choi, N. G. (1999). Living arrangements and household compositions of elderly couples and singles: A comparison of Hispanics and blacks. *Journal of Gerontological Social Work, 31*(1-2), 41-61.

Chu, K. C., Miller, B. A., & Springfield, S. A. (2007). Measures of racial/ethnic health disparities in cancer mortality rates and the influence of socioeconomic status. *Journal of the National Medical Association, 99*(10), 1092-1100, 1102-1104.

Collins, K. S., Hughes, D. L., Doty, M. M., Ives, B. L., Edwards, J. N., & Tenney, K. (2002). *Diverse communities, common concerns: Assessing health care quality for minority Americans.* New York, NY: The Commonwealth Fund.

Coreil, J., Barnes-Josiah, D. L., Augustin, A., & Cayemittes, M. (1996). Arrested pregnancy syndrome in Haiti: Findings from a national survey. *Medical Anthropology Quarterly, 10*(3), 424-436.

Craig, G. J., & Baucum, D. (2001). *Human development* (9th ed.). Upper Saddle River, NJ: Prentice Hall.

D'Alonzo, K. T., & Fischetti, N. (2008). Cultural beliefs and attitudes of Black and Hispanic college-age women toward exercise. *Journal of Transcultural Nursing, 19*(2), 175-183.

David, R. A., & Rhee, M. (1998). The impact of language as a barrier to effective health care in an underserved urban Hispanic community. *Mount Sinai Journal of Medicine, 65*(5-6), 393-397.

Davis, A. M., Vinci, L. M., Okwusa, T. M., Chase, A. R., & Huang, E. S. (2007). Cardiovascular health disparities: A systematic review of health care interventions. *Medical Care Research and Review, 64*(5 Suppl), 29S-100S.

Dietz, T. (1996). *Bureaucracy and the Mexican American elderly: Policy and programming issues* [association paper]. Knoxville, TN: Society for the Study of Social Problems.

Doescher, M. P., Saver, B. G., Franks, P., & Fiscella, K. (2000). Racial and ethnic disparities in perceptions of physician style and trust. *Archives of Family Medicine, 9*(10), 1156-1163.

Dunlop, D. D., Song, J., Manheim, L. M., Daviglus, M. L., & Chang, R. W. (2007). Racial/ethnic differences in the development of disability among older adults. *American Journal of Public Health, 97*(12), 2209-2215.

Eisenberg, D. M., Davis, R. B., Ettner, S. L., Appel, S., Wilkey, S., Van Rompay, M., et al. (1998). Trends in alternative medicine use in the United States, 1990-1997. *Journal of the American Medical Association, 280*(18), 1569-1575.

Eisenberg, D. M., Kessler, R. C., Foster, C., Norlock, F. E., Calkins, D. R., & Delbanco, T. L. (1993). Unconventional medicine in the United States. *New England Journal of Medicine, 328*(4), 246-252.

Facione, N. C., & Katapodi, M. (2000). Culture as an influence on breast cancer screening and early detection. *Seminars in Oncology Nursing, 16*(3), 238-247.

Fadiman, A. (1997). *The spirit catches you and you fall down: A Hmong Child, her american doctors, and the collision of two cultures.* New York, NY: Farrar, Straus, and Giroux.

Feinglass, J., Rucker-Whitaker, C., Lindquist, L., McCarthy, W. J., & Pearce, W. H. (2005). Racial differences in primary and repeat lower extremity amputation: results from a multihospital study. *Journal of Vascular Surgery, 41*(5), 823-829.

Ferraro, G. (2002). *The cultural dimensions of international business* (4th ed.). Upper Saddle River, NJ: Prentice Hall.

Flores, G. (2000). Culture and the patient-physician relationship: Achieving cultural competency in health care. *Journal of Pediatrics, 136*(1), 14-23.

Flores, G., Laws, M. B., Mayo, S. J., Zuckerman, B., Abreu, M., Medina, L., et al. (2003). Errors in medical interpretation and their potential clinical consequences in pediatric encounters. *Pediatrics, 111*(1), 6-14.

Foster, G. (1976). Disease etiologies in non-Western medical systems. *American Anthropologist, 78*(4), 773-782.

Freidenberg, J., & Hammer, M. (1998). Social networks and health care: The case of elderly Latino in East Harlem. *Urban Anthropology, 27*(1), 49-85.

Galanti, G. (1991). *Caring for patients from different cultures: Case studies from american hospitals.* Philadelphia PA: University of Pennsylvania Press.

Graham, R. E., Ahn, A. C., Davis, R. B., O'Connor, B. B., Eisenberg, D. M., & Phillips, R. S. (2005). Use of complementary and alternative medical therapies among racial and ethnic minority adults: Results from the 2002 National Health Interview Survey. *Journal of the National Medical Association, 97*(4), 535-545.

Groce, N. (1999). Health beliefs and behavior towards individuals with disability cross-culturally. In R. L. Leavitt (Ed.), *Cross-cultural rehabilitation: An international perspective* (pp. 37-47). London, England: Harcourt Brace and Company.

Groce, N. E., & Zola, I. K. (1993). Multiculturalism, chronic illness, and disability. *Pediatrics, 91*(5 Pt 2), 1048-1055.

Hall, E. T. (1984). *The dance of life: The other dimension of time.* Garden City, NY: Anchor Press/Doubleday.

Hanson, M. J. (1998). Families with Anglo-European roots. In E. W. Lynch and M. J. Hanson (Eds.), *Developing cross-cultural competence: A guide for working with young children and their families* (2nd ed., p. 121). Baltimore, MD: Paul Brooks Publishing Co.

Heck, J. E., Sell, R. L., & Gorin, S. S. (2006). Health care access among individuals involved in same-sex relationships. *American Journal of Public Health, 96*(6), 1111-1118.

Helman, C. G. (1984). *Culture, health and illness.* London, England: John Wright and Sons.

Hubbell, F. A., Chavez, L. R., Mishra, S. I., & Valdez, R. B. (1996). Differing beliefs about breast cancer among Latinas and Anglo women. *Western Journal of Medicine, 164*(5), 405-409.

Huff, R. M., & Kline, M. V. (1999). *Promoting health in multicultural populations: A handbook for practitioners.* Thousand Oaks, CA: Sage Publications.

Infante, J. R., Peran, F., Martinez, M., Roldan, A., Poyatos, R., Ruiz, C., et al. (1998). ACTH and beta-endorphin in transcendental meditation. *Physiology & Behavior, 64*(3), 311-315.

Ingstad, B., & Whyte, S. R. (Eds.). (1995). *Disability and culture.* Berkeley, CA: University of California Press.

Johnson, F. L. (1999). *Speaking culturally: Language diversity in the United States.* Thousand Oaks, CA: Sage Publications.

Kaptchuk, T. J. (2002). The placebo effect in alternative medicine: Can the performance of a healing ritual have clinical significance? *Annals of Internal Medicine, 136*(11), 817-825.

Krisberg, K. (2008). New CDC training reveals higher U.S. HIV infection rate. *The Nation's Health, 38*(8), 8.

Knutson, L. M., Leavitt, R. L., & Sarton, K. R. (1995). Race, ethnicity and other factors influencing children's health and disability: Implications for pediatric physical therapists. *Pediatric Physical Therapy, 7*(4), 175-183.

Ladinsky, J. L., Volk, N. D., & Robinson, M. (1987). The influence of traditional medicine in shaping medical care practices in Vietnam today. *Social Science & Medicine, 25*(10), 1105-1110.

Ladyshewsky, R. (1999). Cross-cultural supervision of students. In R. L. Leavitt (Ed.), *Cross-cultural rehabilitation: An international perspective* (pp. 163-172). London, England: Harcourt Brace and Company.

Leavitt, R. L. (1992). *Disability and rehabilitation in rural Jamaica: An ethnographic study.* Madison, NJ: Fairleigh Dickinson University Press.

Leavitt, R. L. (2003). Developing cultural competence in a multicultural world: Part II. *PT Magazine, 11*(1), 56-70.

Leavitt, R. L. (2006). Cultural considerations for Jewish clients. In J. B. Lattanzi & L. D. Purnell. *Developing cultural competence in physical therapy practice.* Philadelphia, PA: F.A. Davis.

Lefebvre, K., & Lattanzi, J. B. (2007). Health disparities and physical therapy: A literature review and recommendations. *HPA Resource/HPA Journal, 7*(1), J1-J10.

Levitt, S. (1999). The collaborative learning approach in community based rehabilitation. In R. L. Leavitt (Ed.), *Cross-cultural rehabilitation: An international perspective* (pp. 151-161). London, England: Harcourt Brace and Company.

Limited English Proficiency. (n.d.). Questions and answers. Retrieved December 1, 2008, from www.lep.gov/faqs/faq.html

Livingston, G., Minushkin, S., & Cohn, D. (2008). Hispanics and health care in the United States: Access, information and knowledge. Retrieved October 20, 2008, from http://pewhispanic.org/reports/report.php?ReportID=91

López-De Fede, A., & Haeussler-Fiore, D. (2002). *An introduction to the culture of the Dominican Republic for rehabilitation service providers.* Buffalo, NY: Center for International Rehabilitation Research Information and Exchange (CIRRIE). CIRRIE Monograph Series.

Loveland, C. (1999). The concept of culture. In R. L. Leavitt (Ed.), *Cross-cultural rehabilitation: An international perspective* (pp. 15-24). London, England: Harcourt Brace and Company.

Lurie, N., & Dubowitz, T. (2007). Health disparities and access to health. *Journal of the American Medical Association, 297*(10), 1118-1121.

Lynch, E. W. (1998). Developing cross-cultural competence. In E. W. Lynch, & M. J. Hanson (Eds.), *Developing cross-cultural competence: A guide for working with young children and their families* (2nd ed., pp. 47-89). Baltimore, MD: Brookes Publishing Company.

Lynch, E. W., & Hanson, M. J. (Eds.). (1998). *Developing cross-cultural competence: A guide for working with young children and their families* (2nd ed.). Baltimore, MD: Brookes Publishing Company.

Mainous, A. G., Diaz, V. A., & Geesey, M. E. (2008). Acculturation and healthy lifestyle among Latinos with diabetes. *Annals of Family Medicine, 6*(2), 131-137.

Mansfield, C. J., Wilson, J. L., Kobrinski, E. J., & Mitchell, J. (1999). Premature mortality in the United States: The roles of geographic area, socioeconomic status, household type, and availability of medical care. *American Journal of Public Health, 89*(6), 893-898.

Mardiros, M. (1989). Conception of childhood disability among Mexican-American parents. *Medical Anthropology, 12*(1), 55-68.

Matthews, H. W. (1995). Racial, ethnic, and gender differences in response to medicines. *Drug Metabolism and Drug Interaction, 12*(2), 77-91.

McArthur, L. H., & Raedeke, T. D. (2009). Race and sex differences in college student physical activity correlates. *American Journal of Health Behavior, 33*(1), 80-90.

McDonough, P., Duncan, G. J., Williams, D., & House, J. (1997). Income dynamics and adult mortality in the United States, 1972 through 1989. *American Journal of Public Health, 87*(9), 1476-1483.

McDougall, J. A., Medeleine, M. M., Daling, J. R., & Li, C. I. (2007). Racial and ethnic disparities in cervical cancer incidence rates in the United States, 1992-2003. *Cancer Causes & Control, 18*(10), 1175-1186.

Mehrabian, A. (1980). *Silent messages: Implicit communication of emotions and attitudes* (2nd ed.). Belmont, CA: Wadsworth Publishing.

Mickley, J., & Soeken, K. (1993). Religiousness and hope in Hispanic- and Anglo-American women with breast cancer. *Oncology Nursing Forum, 20*(8), 1171-1177.

Morales, L. S., Cunningham, W. E., Brown, J. A., Liu, H., & Hays, R. D. (1999). Are Latinos less satisfied with communication by health care providers? *Journal of General Internal Medicine, 14*(7), 409-417.

Nakamura, R. M. (1998). *Health in America: A multicultural perspective.* San Francisco, CA: Benjamin-Cummings Publishing Company.

National Center for Health Statistics. (2007). Table 27. In *Health, United States, 2007 with chart book on trends in the health of Americans.* Hyattsville, MD. Retrieved September 22, 2009, from http://www.cdc.gov/nchs/data/hus/hus07.pdf#027

Nayak, S., Shiflett, S. C., Eshun, S., & Levine, F. M. (2000). Culture and gender effects in pain beliefs and the predication of pain tolerance. *Cross-Cultural Research, 34*(2), 135-151.

Neighbors, C. J., Marquez, D. X., & Marcus, B. H. (2008). Leisure-time physical activity disparities among Hispanic subgroups in the United States. *American Journal of Public Health, 98*(8), 1460-1464.

Oyama, T., Jin, T., Yamaya, R., Ling, N., & Guillemin, R. (1980). Profound analgesic effects of beta-endorphin in man. *Lancet, 1*(8160), 122-124.

Pachter, L. M. (1994). Culture and clinical care: Folk illness beliefs and behaviors and their implications for health care delivery. *Journal of the American Medical Association, 271*(9), 690-694.

Paul, T., & Thorburn, M. (1999). Epidemiological considerations in the assessment of disability. In R. L. Leavitt (Ed.), *Cross-cultural rehabilitation: An international perspective* (pp. 137-150). London, England: Harcourt Brace and Company.

Peek, M. E., Cargill, A., & Huang, E. S. (2007). Diabetes health disparities: A systematic review of health care interventions. *Medical Care Research and Review, 64*(5 Suppl), 101S-156S.

Pember, M. (2002). The Ho-Chunk way. *Washington Post.* Health section: F1, 6–7.

Perez-Stable, E. J., Sabogal, F., Otero-Sabogal, R., Hiatt, R. A., & McPhee, S. J. (1992). Misconceptions about cancer among Latinos and Anglos. *Journal of the American Medical Association, 268*(22), 3219-3223.

Power, C., Manor, O., & Matthews, S. (1999). The duration and timing of exposure: Effects of socioeconomic environment on adult health. *American Journal of Public Health, 89*(7), 1059-1065.

Preble, L., Quveryn, J., & Sinatra, R. (1992). Patient characteristics influenceing postoperative pain management. In R. Sinatra, A. Hord, B. Ginsburg, & L. Preble (Eds.), *Acute pain: Mechanisms and management* (10th ed., pp. 140-150). St Louis, MO: Mosby-Year Book.

Rebhun, L. A. (1994). Swallowing frogs: Anger and illness in Northeast Brazil. *Medical Anthropology Quarterly, 8*(4), 360-382.

Reviere, R., & Hylton, K. (1999). Poverty and health: An international overview. In R. L. Leavitt (Ed.), *Cross-cultural rehabilitation: An international perspective* (pp. 59-69). London, England: Harcourt Brace and Company.

Ross, H. (2001). HHS' Office of Civil Rights focuses on Title VI policy, provides guidance for ensuring linguistic access. *Closing the Gap, Cultural Competency Part II,* February/March, 4-7.

Rowley, D. L., Jenkins, B. C., & Frazier, E. (2007). Utilization of joint arthroplasty: Racial and ethnic disparities in the Veterans Affairs Health Care System. *Journal of the American Academy of Orthopedic Surgeons, 15*(Suppl 1), S43-S48.

Rubel, A. J., & Moore, C. C. (2001). The contribution of medical anthropology to a comparative study of culture: Susto and tuberculosis. *Medical Anthropology Quarterly, 15*(4), 440-454.

Salimbene, S. (2000). *What language does your patient hurt in? A practical guide to culturally competent care.* Amherst, MA: Diversity Resources.

Sanchez, T. R., Plawecki, J. A., & Plawecki, H. M. (1996). The delivery of culturally sensitive health care to Native Americans. *Journal of Holistic Nursing, 14*(4), 295-307.

Santana, S., & Santana, F. O. (2001). *An introduction to Mexican culture for rehabilitation service providers.* Buffalo, NY: Center for International Rehabilitation Research Information and Exchange (CIRRIE). CIRRIE Monograph Series.

Saper, R. B., Phillips, R. S., Sehgal, A., Khouri, N., Davis, R. B., Paquin, J., et al. (2008). Lead, mercury, and arsenic in U.S.- and Indian-manufactured Ayurvedic medicines sold via the Internet. *Journal of the American Medical Association, 300*(8), 915-923.

Schneider, E. C., Zaslavsky, A. M., & Epstein, A. M. (2002). Racial disparities in the quality of care for enrollees in Medicare managed care. *Journal of the American Medical Association, 287*(10), 1288-1294.

Smedley, B. D., Stith, A. Y., & Nelson, A. R. (Eds.). (2002). *Unequal treatment: Confronting racial and ethnic disparities in health care.* Washington, DC: National Academies Press.

Spector, R. E. (2000). *Cultural diversity in health and illness* (5th ed.). Upper Saddle River, NJ: Prentice Hall.

Spradley, J. P. (1979). *The ethnographic interview.* New York, NY: Harcourt, Brace, Jovanovich.

Suarez, L., Roche, R. A., Nichols, D., & Simpson, D. M. (1997). Knowledge, behavior, and fears concerning breast and cervical cancer among older low-income Mexican-American women. *American Journal of Preventative Medicine, 13*(2), 137-142.

The Provider's Guide to Quality and Culture. (n.d.). The impact of cultural competence on clinical outcomes. Retrieved November 6, 2002, from http://erc.msh.org/mainpage.cfm?file=7.1.0.htm&module=provider&language=English

Tran, T. V., Dhooper, S. S., & McInnis-Dittrich, K. (1997). Utilization of community based social and health services among foreign born Hispanic American elderly. *Journal of Gerontological Social Work, 28*(4), 23-43.

Tran, T. V., & Williams, L. F. (1998). Poverty and impairment in activities of living among elderly Hispanics. *Social Work in Health Care, 26*(4), 59-78.

Urgo, M. (1998). New obesity guidelines: Minority women at risk. *Closing the Gap. Minority Women's Health Initiative,* June/July, 6-7.

U.S. Census Bureau. (2007). Selected social characteristics in the United States: 2007. Retrieved December 8, 2009, from http://factfinder.census.gov/servlet/ADPTable?_bm=y&-qr_name=ACS_2007_1YR_G00_DP2&-geo_id=01000US&-ds_name=ACS_2007_1YR_G00_&-_lang=en

U.S. Census Bureau. (2008). Income, poverty and health insurance coverage in the United States: 2007. Retrieved September 22, 2009, from http://www.census.gov/prod/2008pubs/p60-235.pdf

U.S. Department of Commerce. (2004). High school graduation rates reach all-time high: Non-Hispanic White and Black graduates at record levels. *U.S. Census Bureau News*. Retrieved December 2, 2009, from http://www.census.gov/Press-Release/www/releases/archives/education/001863.html

U.S. Department of Health and Human Services, Administration for Children and Families. (2007). Fiscal year 2007 refugee arrivals. Retrieved September 22, 2009, from http://www.acf.hhs.gov/programs/orr/data/fy2007RA.htm

U.S. Department of Health and Human Services, Office of Disease Prevention and Health Promotion. (2000). Healthy People 2010. Retrieved September 21, 2009, from http://www.healthypeople.gov

U.S. Department of Health and Human Services, Office of Minority Health. (2001). *National standards on culturally and linguistically appropriate services in health care: Final report*. Washington, DC: Author.

Villa, V. M., & Torres-Gil, F. M. (2001). The later years: The health of elderly Latinos. In M. Aguirre-Molina, C. W. Molina, & R. E. Zambrana (Eds.), *Health issues in the Latino community* (pp. 157-178). San Francisco, CA: Jossey-Bass.

Wasson, S. (1999). Treatment of the Native American population. *Orthopedic Physical Therapy Clinics of North America, 8*(2), 215-223.

Weissman, D. E., Gordon, D., & Bidar-Sielaff, S. (n.d.). Fast fact and concept #78: Cultural aspects of pain management. Retrieved December 1, 2008, from http://www.mywhatever.com/cifwriter/library/eperc/fastfact/ff78.html

Wilmoth, J. M., DeJong, G. F., & Himes, C. L. (1997). Immigrant and non-immigrant living arrangements among America's White, Hispanic, and Asian elderly population. *International Journal of Sociology and Social Policy, 17*(9-10), 57-82.

World Health Organization. (2001). *ICF: International classification of functioning, disability, and health*. Geneva, Switzerland: Author.

Young, J. C., & Garro, L. Y. (1982). Variation in the choice of treatment in two Mexican communities. *Social Science & Medicine, 16*(16), 1453-1465.

Zborowski, M. (1952). Cultural components in responses to pain. *Journal of Social Issues, 8*, 16-30.

Zhou, H. H., Koshakji, R. P., Silberstein, D. J., Wilkinson, G. R., & Wood, A. J. (1989). Altered sensitivity to and clearance of propranolol in men of Chinese descent as compared with American whites. *New England Journal of Medicine, 320*(9), 565-570.

Zhou, H. H., & Liu, Z. Q. (2000). Ethnic differences in drug metabolism. *Clinical Chemistry and Laboratory Medicine, 38*(9), 899-903.

Zuniga, M. E. (1998). Families with Latino roots. In E. W. Lynch & M. J. Hanson (Eds.). *Developing cross-cultural competence: A guide for working with young children and their families* (2nd ed., pp. 209-250). Baltimore, MD: Brookes Publishing Company.

5

Disability Across Cultures

Ronnie Leavitt, PhD, MPH, PT and
Susan E. Roush, PhD, PT

Disability exists in all societies, yet how much does the casual observer (or even reha-bilitation professionals) understand about the meaning of disability? How does one ever understand the lived experiences of persons with disabilities (PWD)? While physical ther-apists, of course, have disability-related expertise, that expertise encompasses a relatively limited perspective. Broader appreciation of the reality of living with a disability is rare among any health care professionals, including therapists who may consider themselves disability advocates.

Greater rates of disability are inevitable. Patterns of health and disease determinants and consequences are continuing to change as we enter the new millennium. The major health problems in the world are shifting from acute infectious diseases and peri-natal problems to chronic, degenerative conditions and injury resulting from violence, war-fare, and traffic accidents (Brundtland, 2002). This process, known as the epidemiologic transition, is associated with a demographic transition characterized by an increase in raw numbers and the aging world population. At the same time, there is a major para-digm shift occurring in social institutions, communications, technology, and world cul-tures that will affect how disability is defined, encountered, and interpreted (Albrecht, Selman, & Bury, 2001).

In essence, this chapter is an introduction to the emerging field of disability studies, a specialty area that focuses on sociocultural perspectives rather than exclusively focusing on biomedical factors to appreciate the lives of PWD. Although the study of the meaning of disability is relatively new and research has been limited, disability studies and the culture of disability are fast becoming recognized as key bodies of knowledge for reha-bilitation professionals (Eddey & Robey, 2005). Disability studies has its roots in the social sciences, humanities, and rehabilitation sciences. The melding of these disciplines has not occurred without tension for rehabilitation sciences as disability studies specifically "seek to reframe rehabilitation's understanding and responses to disability" by exploring the concept that rehabilitation is not an objective practice, but rather one that "reflect[s] particular historical and ideological forces" (Kielhofner, 2005, p. 487).

R. L. Leavitt (Ed.).
*Cultural Competence: A Lifelong Journey
to Cultural Proficiency* (pp. 77-98).
© 2010 SLACK Incorporated

THE SUBCULTURE OF DISABILITY

In reality, the concept of disability is not a cultural universal. That is, disability as we know it is not a concept found in all known cultures. In some cultures, PWDs are expected to follow the same life cycle as everyone else. Disability does not define their status in the culture and thus does not serve as the identifying and unifying characteristic of a subculture. As Ingstad and Whyte (1995) state:

> *"In many cultures, one cannot be 'disabled' for the simple reason that 'disability' as a recognized category does not exist. There are blind people and lame people and 'slow' people, but 'the disabled' as a general term does not translate easily into many languages…The concepts of disability, handicap, and rehabilitation emerged in particular historical circumstances in Europe" (p. 7).*

If disability does exist in a society as a recognized category, there is variation in its meaning. Its significance for the individual and their family depends upon each society's values. Attitudes toward individuals with a disability; concepts of rehabilitation; the sociocultural, biological, and economic implications of disability; and policy affecting individuals with a disability also vary.

For individuals from a Euro-American culture, it is more likely that a subculture (a smaller group within a larger culture that is in some way distinct) based on disability can be found. That is, the following conditions are more likely to be present and contribute to a subculture of disability (Loveland, 1999):

- Medical treatment makes survival with disabilities common
- Culture-wide concepts of normality and disability exist
- Cultural values stress individualism and achievement, and PWD are likely to strive for independence and autonomy
- Disability is an overriding determinant of status and identity
- PWD have opportunities to meet and interact with one another
- PWD have access to education and technology that facilitate their interaction with others
- PWD have access to a modern infrastructure such as transportation and communication systems

In the past 20 years, much scholarly effort has been directed at explaining the experience of disability in Euro-American culture. From this work, several models have emerged. Although features of the multiple models overlap, they can be conceptualized on a continuum that has a medical (or bio-medical) paradigm at one end and a social justice paradigm at the other. A brief review of these models will illustrate the context in which the phenomena of disability as a subculture emerged.

The medical paradigm is the traditional model that still carries significant weight; this approach views disability as a deviation from normal that needs to be "fixed" (See Hughes, 2002; Linton, 1998; or Smart, 2001 for examples). Historically, as the name implies, medical and medical-related education and practice have been grounded in this approach. This includes the preparation of rehabilitation professionals. For those with disabilities, the limitations of the medical model are obvious—individuals with conditions that can't be "fixed" are devalued because they inherently represent failure. It is believed that many of the stereotypes and negative stigma associated with disability are consequent to this perspective. It may also contribute to the paucity of resources for persons with disabilities and the low priority typically associated with their needs when compared against others (Oliver, 2004).

A more complex and moderately more positive conceptualization of disability emerged from the harsh negative interpretation of these conditions offered by the medical model. These new models offer theoretical definitions of disability and parse disability into a number of components (see Altman, 2001 for a comprehensive treatment of this topic). Nagi (1965, 1969, 1991), the first to introduce these ideas, defined four components: pathology, impairment, functional limitation, and disability. Considering tendonitis of the rotator cuff as an example, the pathology would be inflammation of the tendons of the rotator cuff muscles, the impairment is loss of active range of motion at the shoulder, the functional limitation is the inability to reach overhead, and the associated disability might be dependence in combing or washing one's hair.

Other Nagi-inspired models of disability exist, including models put forth by the World Health Organization (WHO) (1980, 2000, 2001), and the Institute of Medicine (Brandt & Pope, 1997; Pope & Tarlov, 1991), the latter of which incorporates prevention. Another model comes from Verbrugge and Jette (1994). Using language from the 1980 WHO model as an illustration, disability is conceptualized as having three components: impairment, disability and handicap. An impairment in these models is similar to Nagi's impairment (e.g., cerebral palsy). The disability relates to activities that cannot be performed (e.g., verbal communication) and the handicap relates to how the disability impacts a particular role (e.g., limitations in employment or the work role).

Interestingly, these models all define disability differently, variously including terms such as *roles, activities, patterns of behavior, life activities, domains of human activity, demands of the environment,* and others. The exclusion of the subjective experience of the person and factors such as self-determination and autonomy has been criticized (Hemmingsson & Jonsson, 2005). Indeed, the focus in these models of disability remains the perceived deficit, although later models begin to address the role of the environment and serve as a bridge to the next major category on the disability continuum.

This next major category of models used to understand the experience of disability shifts the perspective from the individual and what is "wrong" with him or her to the environment and its role in defining, amplifying, and/or ameliorating the effects of disability. The environmental, functional, and minority rights models (Michalko, 2002) are examples. Assistive technology, classroom accommodations, and some civil rights-inspired laws are tools that have grown out of these models. Unlike the medical and medical-inspired models, this approach acknowledges prejudice and discrimination as significant contributors to the disability experience. The focus, however, in some of these models is still at the level of the individual. Emphasis on the societal factors is most prominent in the minority group model (Michalko), which emphasizes the shared subjugated experiences of persons with disabilities, who as a group have been oppressed by the dominant (i.e., non-disabled) population. The Disability Rights Movement is founded on this model, and this is where disability as a subculture begins to emerge on the continuum. It also connects this middle aspect of the disability continuum with the social justice end.

The social justice perspective of understanding disability builds upon the Disability Rights model but fully shifts the focus from individuals and their collective experience to society (Abberley, 1987; Oliver, 1990). This perspective introduces the term *ableism*, which is defined as "a pervasive system of discrimination and exclusion that oppresses people who have mental, emotional, and physical disabilities" (Rauscher & McClintock, 1997, p. 198) or, alternatively in a lay publication, "discrimination in favor of the able-bodied" (Tullock, 1993). It is conceptually analogous to racism and sexism. Universal Design and its application in educational settings, Universal Instructional Design (Evans, 2008), are practical tools that are consistent with the social justice model. Key principles of both of these tools are that environments should be usable by the greatest number of people to the greatest extent possible and that designing for inclusion in advance is preferable to after-the-fact accommodations. Although implementation of these principles eliminates many barriers, its primary strength may be that it also addresses the recalcitrant prejudice and negative stigma associated with disability. The social justice model eliminates, as much as possible, any exceptional treatment directed at persons with disabilities and the associated potential for that treatment to be patronizing, condescending, exploitive, or repressive. Instead, it promotes the view that disability is part of the human experience, something most, if not all of us, experience in some way or at some time in our lives. Disability from this perspective is to be appreciated as another aspect of the rich diversity that defines who we are and is something to be valued and perhaps even celebrated.

While there are many parallels between a social justice approach to understanding the experience of disability and understanding the experience of other minority groups, there are important differences as well. Disability is the only group in which everyone has the potential to become a member. The fear of acquiring a disability has been referred to as "the existential angst of disability," (Smart, 2001, p. 115) a phrase that captures the dread associated with unexpected danger. Also, it is much less common for persons with disabilities to have family members sharing their minority status than it is for most other minority groups. While some disabling conditions are inherited with multiple people in the same family affected, many persons with disabilities are the only one in their family with this minority status. The gay, lesbian, bisexual, and transsexual community may be the closest to sharing this common isolated experience with persons with disabilities.

A final difference to be considered is the one that has the potential to have the greatest impact on those who work in rehabilitation. Disability is the only minority group seeking social justice to have a billion dollar industry (health care) devoted to preventing, eliminating, or ameliorating its existence. Asking health care professionals to simultaneously fully engage in changing or at least minimizing disability and celebrate its existence is paradoxical. Many professionals (e.g., physical therapists) are specifically trained to detect the most nuanced, subtle signs of disability and alter them to improve function. This approach necessarily implies that disability is not just different, but less—otherwise, why change it? Health care professionals, particularly those who work with patients with disabilities, are asked to integrate the opposite ends of the disability continuum: the medical model and the social justice model. Block and her colleagues (2005) provide an interesting look at this attempted integration by way of content analysis of the language occupational therapy students use in describing a visit to an independent living center. Moving beyond description, Oliver (2004) provides guidance in this paradoxical task of integrating the two extreme models. This work offers the perspective that individual interventions (e.g., rehabilitation) do not necessarily conflict with the social model of disability, it should just not be the predominant paradigm that defines disability. Research, however, tells us that health care professionals have not done a satisfactory job of integrating the medical model and the social justice model. For example, professionals have consistently been shown to underestimate the quality of life and self-esteem of their patients with disabilities (summarized in Basnett, 2001). Basnett further explores the negative consequences that arise because of the limiting stereotypes facilitated by the medical model—consequences that are potentially monumental in the lives of persons with disabilities because of the prominent role these professionals play.

In addition to the conceptual models that have developed to understand the experience of PWD, it is important to consider that the subculture of disability may be, more or less, salient for an individual or group. For example, people with hearing impairments often primarily identify with "the deaf community" (culture), and deafness may be one's major identifying factor. Deafness is not viewed as a limitation, but rather a biological characteristic that has given rise to a specific culture and the slogans of "deaf pride" and "disability pride" (Groce, 1999; Ravaud & Stiker, 2001).

In contrast, much of the world does not have the above named conditions, models, or concepts associated with the subculture of disability, and the disability rights/social justice understanding of disability are absent or in the early stages of development. This may influence the interaction between the therapist and the client. For example, the client may not understand their rights or those rights do not exist in their culture. They may not conceptualize their disability as compatible with the pursuit of multiple life options, or they may not understand a complex medical response to what they view as a spiritual or sacred phenomenon (Fadiman, 1998).

A Complex Picture

To get a better understanding of a client's "worldview" when assessing disability and associated beliefs and behaviors, an assessment of many specific variables is essential. Key variables such as ethnicity or socioeconomic status may be the most important determinants in helping to define an individual. These highly influence other variables such as acculturation status, that is, the degree to which an individual has taken on the characteristics of the normative culture. Level of acculturation is particularly relevant to health status and how one interacts with the health care delivery system.

Another critical variable to understand is one's worldview and/or value system. The core values of a Euro-American physical therapist are likely to include individualism and a value for youthfulness. In contrast, core values held by people of Asian descent (and others) emphasize collectivism (placing family first), and great respect for elders. Children must remain ever loyal for the sacrifices their parents made, and they are expected to provide financial, emotional, and practical support for their parents. The PT must consider how these core values will affect one's disability status and/or interaction with the therapist. Patient independence, valued so highly by American health care professionals, may not be the goal for some patients. Religion is also relevant and closely allied to one's worldview. Most physical therapists in the U.S. will be Christian, yet many Asian clients will be Buddhist. Buddhism views pain and suffering as a part of life and not to be complained about, and thus the patient may not report discomfort to the therapist (Leavitt, 2003; Ling, 2003).

A person's disability status may also impact their verbal and nonverbal communication style, which itself may be closely tied to ethnicity and other broader cultural factors. In addition to the potential expected style differences between and within cultural groups, such as those affecting spatial distancing, touch, and more, there are further considerations due to the presence of a disability. For example, a PWD should be greeted with the same respect as someone without a disability. If an individual has difficulty greeting someone with a typical handshake, it is appropriate for the PT to reach out to the patient's right hand or shake the left hand. Or, if someone is in a wheelchair, it is important for the therapist to sit, thus facilitating "eye to eye" contact. Furthermore, if the PWD is unable to communicate easily, one cannot make an assumption about the intelligence of the client. Accommodation through alternative means of communication (writing, sign language) may be in order.

As health professionals, a range of factors such as those mentioned above need to be considered during all points within the rehabilitation process—assessment, examination, plan of care, and intervention. One must recognize the complexity of the situation and consider both intercultural diversity and intra-cultural diversity related to the presence of subgroups and individuality. The assumption should be made that a client with a disability will, in addition, have many other primary and secondary cultural characteristics that are also relevant in defining who that person is. One cannot simply put people in groups and generalize to an individual based on a population. Each client is unique.

Cultural Response to the Presence of Disability at the Societal Level: An Historical Perspective

PWD have always been part of human society, although documentation of their life experiences is limited. Ancient art and early legends from Greece, Rome, India, China, and the Americas all show evidence of the existence of PWD (Braddock & Parish, 2001; Groce, 1999). In Iraq, there is evidence of a skeleton of an elderly Neanderthal with a withered arm and blindness in one eye. The gravesite, covered with flowers, gives an indication that he was a valued member of society.

What were the prevailing attitudes toward PWD in earlier times? The data point to a mixed picture. For example, the Old Testament commanded "Thou shall not curse the deaf nor put a stumbling block before the blind, nor maketh the blind to wander out of the path" (Leviticus 19:14), while at the same time also warning "if you do not follow His commands and decrees...all these curses will come upon you and overtake you: the Lord will afflict you with madness, blindness, and confusion of mind" (Deuteronomy 28:15, 28-29) (Braddock & Parish, 2001).

Although there is evidence of negative attitudes toward people with disabilities in all three of the monotheistic religions (Judaism, Christianity, and Islam), in early times, these religious groups found ways to modify the burdens imposed on PWD (Miles, 1999). For example, Jewish priests had the task of examining sacrificed animals to ensure that they were offered without blemish. Thus, good eyesight was a requirement. Conversely, blind people could memorize sacred texts and speak them on special occasions. Over time, this "work" became an honored occupation for blind men, especially within Islam. Today, for many, much of the Koran is recited from memory.

The classical literature of Buddhism and Hinduism also point to a mixed picture. Some historical documents point to the exclusion of PWD and others to exhortations for charity. As an example, in the Indian epic of Mahabharata, there are several references to the rulers' duties to cherish "like a father, the blind, the dumb, the lame, the deformed, the friendless" (Miles, 1999, p. 53). But, there is also reference to an order that there be "no dwarfs, no hump-backed persons, no one of an emaciated constitution, no one who is lame or blind, no one who is an idiot, no woman, and no eunuch, at the spot where the king holds his consultations" (Miles, p. 53).

Some later sources lead us to believe that PWD were oftentimes held in high esteem. For example, a number of tribal groups in East Africa and the southern Pacific were known to treat children with obvious impairments with great kindness and full acceptance (Groce, 1999). Conversely, it is known that PWD have been discriminated against, ranging from minor embarassment to neglect. Although exceptionally rare, a small number of groups have practiced infanticide, usually by abandoning an infant after birth. Outright killing of older children or adults because of disability is almost unheard of. In general, through the pre-industrialized era, even when they were perceived as misfits, PWD were generally maintained in a life-supporting environment (including institutions) and marginally integrated into society (Braddock & Parish, 2001; Scheer & Groce, 1988).

During the industrial era, Euro-American societies began to think of PWD as sick, helpless, and needing to be taken care of. Although Social Darwinism and the eugenics movement gained momentum during the 1800's, this period is best characterized as fostering an institutional service model that continued to call for the segregation and marginalization of PWD. Patients were presumed to be unable to function in their own best interest and were expected to take on the "sick role" (i.e., they are freed from normal social roles and responsibilities). Medical advances and the development of interventions led to the bio-medical model, without attention to the socio-cultural context of the person.

In addition to the features of the bio-medical model that were addressed earlier in this chapter, in this model, providers were presumed to be the expert and likely to view the patient as a compilation of body parts and systems with little attention paid to the whole. This focus on body parts and systems is seen in the rotator cuff tendonitis example provided earlier to illustrate the Nagi model of disability. Although limiting and incomplete in many ways, the bio-medical model is based on the underlying principle of beneficence, and the intention was benevolence.

The view that PWD are sick and a burden is also seen in other, non–Euro-American cultures, although the resulting actions are more extreme. For example, there are reports of killing deformed babies (the Masai tribe), poisoning children who have polio (Ivory Coast), and country-specific holocausts (Nazi Germany) where people without disabilities were killed as well (Braddock & Parish, 2001; Groce, 1999; Ravaud & Stiker, 2001).

J. R. Hanks and L. M. Hanks (1948) hypothesized that the degree to which a society is willing or able to bear the costs incurred in caring for PWD depends upon several interrelating materialistic and cultural factors. Some of these determinants are the relative socioeconomic status of the society (which includes such factors as the number and type of productive units, the need for labor, the amount of economic surplus, and its mode of distribution), the social structure of the society (including whether the society is egalitarian or hierarchical, how it defines achievement, and how it values age and gender/sex), the cultural definition of the meaning of the disability (does the symptom of the disability require magical, religious, medical, legal, or other measures?), and the position of the society in relation to the rest of the world. Although there are significant differences in health status and health care systems, including rehabilitation, among contemporary societies, the differences are most extreme between the "developed" or "industrialized" societies and the so-called developing of Third World societies. These differences, although influenced by socio-cultural practices, primarily reflect the wide economic gap between the two groups (see Chapter 11).

Leavitt (1999) has added to this discussion by noting that general health care and rehabilitation for PWD have historically been a very low priority throughout the world for several reasons. First, the cost-benefit ratio of providing rehabilitation to PWD has always been considered poor compared to other health programs. Second, there has traditionally been an under-estimation of the potential achievements that a disabled person can accomplish. Third, there is a history of negative attitudes toward persons who are disabled. In many societies, PWD have historically been seen to be deviant from the norm and have been considered to have a social stigma or "attitude that is deeply discrediting…a failing, a shortcoming, a handicap" (Goffman, 1963, p. 3). The bio-medical model of disability reinforces this attitude. Fourth, when discrimination limits participation by PWD in various social roles, their plight becomes even more invisible. Fifth, there is an apparent absence of urgency. Rehabilitation is associated with disease and illness that is, for the most part, neither acute, communicable, nor "exciting." The general public will not be at risk, nor will its opposition be mobilized, if rehabilitation services are not given to populations in need. Sixth, on an individual level, mainstream biomedical practitioners tend to reflect a value orientation that stresses mastery of disease and taking personal credit for recovery. In cases in which an individual has a disability, often very little dramatic curing can occur; in some instances, further loss of function is anticipated. Although a wide array of simple and complex technologies are available, the provision of these services does not ensure dramatic results. Thus, many caregivers find rehabilitation frustrating and often not rewarding or worthwhile. Lastly, individuals with disabilities are a disadvantaged minority that is just beginning to assert their rights. In the meantime, their disadvantaged status equates to little political influence when lobbying for the opportunity to affect public policy.

One way to assess societal attitudes cross-culturally and over time is through the language that is used to describe something. Some language used in the past ("moron," "cripple") is not considered "politically correct" in today's environment due to the negative connotation and images associated with these words. But, even in the Euro-American countries, there is disagreement over the most appropriate terminology. Some argue that "person with a disability" should be the preferred term because it places emphasis on the person first and the disability second. However, within the disability subculture, there are those that argue that the phrase "person with a disability" is illogical. To those who follow WHO definitions of *impairment*, *disability*, and *handicap*, then it would be appropriate to say "person with a sensory, cognitive, or motor impairment" and that disability only occurs when one encounters an inhospitable environment. Thus, it is not the person who is disabled (Neufeldt, 1999).

Unfortunately, much of the language that is used to describe, explain, or depict disability and those with disabilities remains predominantly negative, and in many cases, demeaning. As with the WHO definitions, much of this language is grounded in the biases of the bio-medical model (Linton, 1998). Linton (1998) and Zola (1993) offer thoughtful and comprehensive reviews on this topic, including the often stereotype-reinforcing influence of "politically correct" language.

An example from the developing world can be seen by looking at the traditional terms for disability used in China. They are *canfei*, meaning handicap and useless, *canji* meaning handicap and illness, or *canji ren* meaning handicapped and sick people. The term *gong neng zhang ai zhe*, meaning "individuals with disabilities," is rarely used (Liu, 2001). In Bantu (an African language), terms related to physical disability relate to sorcery or reincarnation (Devlieger, 1998). Indeed, the use of language that fosters less-than-ideal images still exists in many places.

Another way to assess societal attitudes is to focus on beliefs about the meaning of disability in a particular culture. This is one component of a society's general belief system about health and sickness, and they have meaning when considering what form of rehabilitation will be developed in a society. The cultural interpretation of disability depends upon how a society attaches value and meaning to a particular type of disability. In summary, there continues to be a range of variation in the language used to describe disability and PWD, and a range of variation in how they are treated. In the last few decades, Western societies have seen an increase in concern and sensitivity toward issues surrounding the presence of disability and increasing public visibility and empowerment of individuals with a disability, along with a concomitant increase in legislation mandating the rights of the disabled (see Chapter 4).

CULTURAL BELIEFS ABOUT DISABILITY AT THE INDIVIDUAL AND FAMILY LEVEL

MEASURING ATTITUDES TOWARD PWD

Currently, psychological research on attitudes toward illness and disability are often measured for a particular disorder (such as AIDS, Parkinson's disease, cardiovascular diseases, etc.). Regarding PWD, the Attitudes Toward Disabled Persons Scale by H.E. Yukor and J.R. Block is commonly used for research (Antonek & Livneh, 1988).

It is important to appreciate that the PWD, their family, and involved rehabilitation professionals may each have a different perspective on the disability. Attitudes toward PWD are first observed in the home (e.g., with the disappointment or even rejection of a child born with a congenital anomaly) and then in society (e.g., as the child enters school). Attitudes toward PWD are generally positively correlated with age and experience, and more positive among women than men. Personality characteristics such as self-esteem and role identity are relevant as well (Aiken, 2002; Tervo, Azuma, Palmer, & Redinius, 2002).

Although there is evidence that attitudes toward PWD are becoming more positive, there is limited theoretical research linking cultural variables with attitudes toward PWD. One such study, "Attitudes Toward Disabilities in a Multicultural Society" (Westbrook, Legge, & Pennay, 1993), investigates the differences in the attitudes of six cultural groups in Australia with regard to 20 diagnoses. Overall, PWD were accepted most by the German community, followed by the Anglo, Italian, Chinese, Greek, and Arabic groups. Interestingly, the results did not show significant differences with regard to the concept of stigma hierarchy—in all communities, people with asthma, diabetes, heart disease, and arthritis were the most accepted, and people with AIDS, mental retardation, psychiatric illness, and cerebral palsy were the least accepted.

There are studies examining attitudes toward PWD for specific cultural groups. Greeks and Greek Americans were compared with regard to attitudes toward PWD, and the analysis indicated that ethnicity accounted for 28% of the variance, with more positive attitudes among Greek Americans (Zaromatidis, Papakai, & Gilde, 1999). Saetermoe, Scattone, and Dim (2001) found that Asian American respondents were more likely to stigmatize PWD than were their African American, Latin American, or Euro-American counterparts. Furthermore, Asian-born participants demonstrated more negative attitudes than the U.S.-born participants, supporting the idea that, for some immigrating groups, acculturation into U.S. culture decreases stigmatization. Iwakuma and Nussbaus (2000) reported that Japanese subjects have a strong sense of shame for having a disability, with the "pollution" of the disability spreading to family members. Japanese folklore associated with disability is illustrated by concepts having to do with death and decay.

Looking at less industrialized societies, Somali immigrant subjects in the U.S. reported that PWD are treated as part of the family and community like any other member (Greeson, Veach, & LeRoy, 2001). Of interest, Nepalese children's attitudes toward PWD were noted to be more positive toward people who are obese than persons with more typically defined disabilities. Obesity in this culture is associated with wealth, power, and food availability; this preference departs from all Western findings (Harper, 1997). This clearly demonstrates the learned, social construction aspect of disability stereotypes.

Do health professionals demonstrate more positive attitudes than the general public? As reported in Aiken (2002), health professionals are similar to the respondents cited above, as they too reported being more accepting of people with asthma, diabetes, heart disease, and arthritis, and less accepting of people with AIDS, mental retardation, psychiatric illness, or cerebral palsy. Basnett (2001) notes that medical professionals are similar to the general population with regard to PWD, and that the dearth of research in this area is likely related to the low priority accorded to disability. A physician with a cervical spinal cord injury, Basnett argues that in Western societies "…health professionals are not just mirrors of society, taking an individualistic interpretation and accentuating it, but are also active promoters of a paradigm that strengthens their own role. That will make understanding disability in terms of social control and oppression much more difficult for individuals trained in that environment" (p. 452). Susan Roush (1993), a physical therapist, suggests that we are similar to other health professionals in our attitudes toward PWD, although she believes that we have a unique background and perspective, as well as a special responsibility to change our own attitudes and those of others.

Methodologic limitations on research regarding attitudes toward disability exist. In the less developed world, especially, the collection of any data regarding PWD, is still in its earliest stages. As recently as 1987, the largest nation in the world, the People's Republic of China (PRC) did its first nationwide count of *canji* adults and children with disabilities in the National Sample Survey of Disabled Persons (Kohrman, 2003). According to Kohrman, it appears that, especially in developing nations, it is the interplay of the global orientation (e.g., the global "disability movement"), and nation-state development, when a collection of bio-statistical data are encouraged. Oftentimes, it is statistics that can foster/mold attention to the issue of disability.

The qualitative research concept of triangulation of data sources is important, especially when doing cross-cultural research and the researcher is less familiar with the gestalt of the community. This may be impractical in some instances. For example, Brown (2001) cited a study by the Ethiopian National Children's Commission, where community leaders felt that the community was sympathetic and ready to assist children with disabilities, but the families had negative attitudes such as feeling ashamed of the child. One does not know the opinion of the families. Similarly yet conversely, Leavitt (1992) based her research on children with disabilities in Jamaica by conducting interviews with family members, but she did not interview key informant community leaders or government officials. In this case, the families were, for the most part, loving and accepting, but believed it was the community and government leaders who were not facilitating integration for children with disabilities into the Jamaican society.

Clearly, one of the greatest methodological concerns is the lack of evidence supporting a direct link between what people say about their attitudes and beliefs, and what they actually do. Assessing attitudes through participant observation is often how judgments are made. In the developing world, there are ample reports of pervasive negative attitudes and behaviors toward PWD. In India, for example, Pinto and Sahur (2001) report that PWD remain highly marginalized. In some villages they are shunned or abused, especially when the disability is thought to be the result of parental sin or God's displeasure. In the cities, there may be increased exposure to people with leprosy, amputations, or visual impairments since it is not uncommon for PWD in India to be beggars. Typically, there have been limited social opportunities and civil rights.

In contrast, Ingstad (2001) has argued that the overwhelming, cross-cultural sense of negativity and rejection of PWD are "myths." They are in conflict with the fact that most families try their best to care for their loved ones with a disability. Furthermore, she argues that these myths undermine the efforts of those people trying to foster a disability rights movement and also serve as an excuse for governments not to address the issues of prejudice and discrimination in education and employment.

BELIEFS ABOUT THE MEANING OF DISABILITY

Although there is most definitely intercultural and intra-cultural variation, three major categories of social beliefs seem to exist cross-culturally and tend to predict how well a PWD will fare in a particular community: valued and disvalued attributes, causality, and anticipated role (Groce, 1999).

VALUED AND DISVALUED ATTRIBUTES

If the society values physical strength and beauty (as defined by that particular culture), then individuals who do not display these attributes will be considered less likable, less worthy, and more disabled. If one's status depends on how well one can lift heavy loads or farm, then one's social status will be diminished with disabilities that interfere with those tasks. If the society favors intellectual capability, such as that needed to be a lawyer or teacher, then being physically limited by a wheelchair might be seen as less significant.

Associated with disvalued attributes is the concept of "otherness" or stigma. Although there is not complete consensus, most often PWD are considered to have the disvalued attribute of an observable deviation from the norm, which typically results in the PWD being branded with stigmata, that is, "marks" or "blemishes." The stigmata are used to assign a negative value to the deviant person (Goffman, 1963). The construction of individual and societal models of stigmatization of PWD seems intimately connected to beliefs concerning causation of disabilities, typically those that are supernatural in origin (see below). As Goffman states, "A disability is often considered evidence of God's displeasure of one's own or one's family's past behavior…a stigmatized individual is presumed to be not quite human, and often a sign of danger" (p. 5). Stigma associated with disability may increase the family's fear of exposure to criticism and disgrace for themselves and their ancestors (Liu, 2001).

In contrast, Leavitt (1992) interviewed family members who had children with a disability in a poor, rural area of Jamaica. A majority of the interviewees did not believe their child was stigmatized. In fact, most noted that their family and neighbors seemed to be quite fond of the child in question. When a subject reported hearing negative comments, it was generally believed to be an isolated incident. Given the likelihood of response bias with this subject matter (e.g., reluctance to admit to negative feelings about a son or daughter to a researcher with whom they did not have an extensive history), however, it is likely that stigma may have been a factor in some of the households.

In most communities, being disabled does make one stand out from the group, and the disability is often an attribute that is disvalued. In Native American communities, being different and calling attention to oneself is particularly stressful (Joe & Malach, 1998). In Korea, deviance tends to lead to isolation, possibly due to uneasiness associated with not knowing what to do. If people help a PWD, there is a tendency for that help to overcompensate and be overprotective, thus infantilizing PWD (Kim-Rupnow, 2001).

Likewise, being labeled as deviant is associated with the notion of contagion. There is fear that a disability might be "caught" or one could become "contaminated." Some Native American parents discourage their children from having any contact with PWD or even touching assistive technology. In Kenya, a hut for a PWD might be built far away from the others, and the person's belongings cannot be touched (Groce, 1999).

Related to attributes is the value associated with gender. In Nepal, there are many more boys reported to have polio than girls. The assumption is that girls do not survive because they are either placed at greater risk by being less well-nourished or not adequately immunized, or they are not given allotted resources to facilitate survival or recovery (Groce, 1999).

CAUSALITY

Causality refers to the cultural explanations for why a disability occurs. Few societies have only one explanation, and there may be different explanations for different disabilities. Causality may be associated with "natural" or "supernatural" factors. The range of variation in the beliefs concerning cause is considerable. Furthermore, people often "hedge their bets," incorporating the notion of multicausality for one diagnosis. Typically, an informant might preface remarks with "I don't know, but maybe…" or "I believe such and such, but my mother (or husband, neighbor, etc.) thinks such and such…" Groce (1999) contends that the need to ascribe causality is related to one's ability to justify demands made on social support networks and community resources.

People from the Euro-American cultures typically ascribe disability to natural causes such as disease (viruses, bacteria), environmental agents (accidents, toxins), or genetic disorders. Nevertheless, people might immediately ask a mother of a child born with a disability if she drank, smoked, or used drugs during pregnancy. A man with paraplegia is oftentimes given more sympathy if the disability is a result of fighting for his country as opposed to a driving accident while he was drunk.

Natural causation is also an explanation used in other cultures, but some explanations are more "scientifically sound" than others. For example, in Jamaica, a scientifically sound natural explanation could be, "fits damage the brain," or "the doctor say long time it take to born… The afterbirth is coming before…I had lots of clots…" (Leavitt, 1992, p. 115).

Still, some naturalistic belief systems are not supported by scientific reality. An example of a disability scientifically understood to be caused by a genetic anomaly but viewed by the mother as having an alternative cause comes from Jamaica. The mother of a daughter with Down Syndrome describes the cause of this disability as follows: "Like how I have the children fast and the food me eat… Me had a problem with me big daughter…sent her to buy shoes and she run away with a guy and she never come back until long after the baby born. I was very worried" (Leavitt, p. 115). In this case, the diagnosis was Down syndrome.

In many Asian cultures, naturalistic explanations often focus on the suspected failure of the mother to follow prescribed healthy practices during pregnancy and the postnatal period. For example, Chan (1998) reports a mother being blamed for her son's epilepsy because she ate lamb, a forbidden food, during pregnancy. In Chinese, epilepsy, *Yang Dian Feng*, translates as "shaking of the lamb." Excessive "cold wind" and shellfish have also been held responsible for disability.

Alternatively, an imbalance of elements, or humors, may be naturalistic causes believed to be responsible for a disability. In much of the world, there is a belief that there needs to be a balance of mutually complementary forces for one to be in harmony with nature. A balance of "hot" and "cold" or *yin* and *yang* are examples (Joe & Malach, 1998; Zuniga, 1998). People of Asian origin may also believe in the need to have harmony by balancing hot and cold and other metaphysical forces of nature. Kim-Rupnow (2001) reports that, in Korea, the mother may be held responsible for a child with a disability if she did something wrong during pregnancy to create an imbalance of metaphysical forces (*myang*). Additionally, there is fairly widespread belief that an illness or condition can be "caught" by touch or sight. Brides and pregnant women in particular are encouraged to avoid being near someone with a disability (Groce, 1999).

In contrast to these naturalistic beliefs are those in which people believe in a supernatural cause for the disability. Not infrequently, supernatural belief systems are associated with witchcraft, spirits, or ancestors who are punishing the PWD or (if a child) the parents because of their "inappropriate" behavior (Groce, 1999; Kim-Rupnow, 2001; Leavitt, 1992; Pinto & Sahur, 2001). These data, however, must be viewed with caution. It is quite possible that informants underreport their belief in supernatural causes or, alternatively, one can believe in the supernatural but not associate it with their personal situation.

In many cultures, religious beliefs are closely associated with a supernatural belief system. Divine intervention is presumed in the Old Testament, when PWD were not allowed to approach the alter, and in the New Testament, when Christ, upon restoring sight to a blind man, is reported to have said "go and sin no more." The Buddhist and Hindu religions also suggest the theory of retribution where a sin in a past life is responsible for a present situation (Miles, 1999). Therefore, the belief in reincarnation (the idea that one's current physical and social state is a reflection of one's conduct in a previous life) places those born with a disability in a troubling situation.

In rural Jamaica, supernatural explanations often include mention of the *duppy* (Leavitt, 1992). The *duppy*, meaning ghost or spirit, is frequently blamed for things that go wrong or are evil. *Duppies* can be visible or invisible, and they can work through people, animals, birds, and plants. *Duppies* live and play around the silk cotton tree and are especially fond of the night. They are thought to be unpredictable, sometimes helpful, and sometimes harmful. "The *duppy*…well, because babies are small, people who pass off like to play with them. That's what cause the life of my last baby… When you leave baby alone, the duppies play with him. The *duppies* want to give assistance" (Leavitt, p. 116).

In India, the belief in karma, or payment for past deeds, underlies the religious belief system (Pinto & Sahur, 2001). Alternatively, as reported in Mexico, God can selectively choose parents who will be particularly kind and protective for "special" children (Madiros, 1989). In Botswana, the birth of a child with a disability can be seen as either God's trust in the parents' ability, or a punishment for a past transgression (Ingstad, 1999).

In Jamaica, the Kumina Queen (a religious leader), who is the "adoptive mother" of a mentally retarded boy, says, "It's a kind of spiritual order...the mother leave him at night and when she coming back for it nobody there to look about the baby. Spirit come and fingle it [plays with it or caring for it]...me give the child sugar and water and the spirit no like that...the father says spirit feed him—him sick and vomit up some green things [the child vomits up the bad spirit food]" (Leavitt, 1992, p. 117).

Additional examples from Jamaica having to do with God's role in a child's disability are: "I just believe God make him and he make everyone of us to his own likeness" and "Sickness is not our fault. God gave it to us. We have faith in God." In contrast, a few people in the Jamaica study specifically stated they did not believe God had any connection to their child's problems. "I don't believe that God make him sick like that. Me say is me the problem come from since me was young" and "God don't make anyone sick. Sickness is from the devil" (Leavitt, 1992, p. 117).

For people of Hispanic origin, one may also become sick (i.e., be punished) if they have sinned or violated a taboo, thereby causing the wrath of God or other source of wickedness. The belief in the evil eye is not uncommon. Generally, this concept implies that an evil spell has been put on another, which causes the victim to fall ill. The motive is usually envy. Other folk beliefs associated with supernatural forces include the notion that a pregnant woman must be careful using a sharp object or the child may be born with a cleft palate, and if she is knitting clothes for the child, she cannot wind the yarn into balls or the child will be born with the cord wrapped around the neck (Zuniga, 1998).

In the highly acclaimed, and very readable book, *The Spirit Catches You and You Fall Down*, Anne Fadiman (1998) describes the cultural conflict between a Hmong family whose daughter, Lia, has a seizure disorder, and her American doctors. The conflict is partly a result of differing views of causality. The Hmong people are an extremely traditional group from Laos, many of whom have unwillingly immigrated to the U.S. as a result of the Vietnam War. The Hmong see illness as a spiritual matter linked to everything in the universe, while the medical community in the U.S. denotes a division between the body and spirit. The Hmong call Lia's illness *quag dab peg*—the spirit catches you and you fall down (i.e., the soul is taken and you cannot get well until the soul is returned).

For the American Indian, supernatural causes of disability may relate to spirit loss, spirit intrusion, spells, or witchcraft (Joe & Malach, 1998).

No matter who or what the "giver" of the disability was, a further question might be for what purpose has the disability been "given." Is it a challenge for the strengthening of a person's soul, a specific lesson to be learned so that progress can be made, an opportunity for a higher being to demonstrate love or power, or an opportunity for an individual to be spurred toward a charitable action (Miles, 1999)?

PERCEIVED ADULT ROLE

The role people can play as an adult and how much they can contribute to the household is the third category of social beliefs to consider when thinking about how a PWD will fare in a particular community. The material conditions of a community are bound to affect belief systems and decisions regarding disability and adult roles, especially in poor communities. If there is a fear of economic cost to the family and no economic gain, this is more likely to result in a negative attitude. In extreme and rare instances, no resources are allocated to the PWD and they are allowed to die.

In the developing world, some PWD may find work outside of the home, but more typically a PWD may contribute by watching children or doing housework or farm work. Some may be assigned tasks that others do not want. For example, Groce (1999) cites a study done in Ecuador where rural families who were introduced to iodized salt for the purpose of eliminating iodine deficiency syndrome (characterized by mild mental retardation and hearing loss), were concerned that there would be no one to collect fire-wood, draw water, or herd animals.

In some societies, PWD were and still are expected to contribute to the family income by their role as beggars. In some cases, begging is clearly associated with disgrace. Conversely, in a rural Mexican community, Gwaltney (1970) describes elderly persons who became blind as a result of onchocerciasis and beg for a living as being treated with respect. These blind villagers derive a sense of approval and purposeful participation in the life of their pueblo, and there has been cultural accommodation on the part of the community.

Ingstad & Whyte (1995) note that in a range of societies, from peoples in Botswana, Uganda, Nicaragua, Sarawak, and others, the acceptance of PWD is not based on their physical or mental condition, but more on the likelihood of their conforming to the defining characteristics of full personhood in the particular society. These characteristics are linked to sociability, kinship identity, the ability to marry and have children, and the ability to contribute to the household economy. If one cannot partake in these obligations, it is up to the family to make it possible. Thus, personhood, in some developing countries, depends more on social identity and the fulfillment of family obligations than on individual ability (Ingstad, 2001). In the U.S., PWD are increasingly demanding that their adult role be the same as it would have been if they did not have a disability, as seen through the previously described social justice view of disability.

CULTURAL RESPONSE TO THE PRESENCE OF DISABILITY AT THE INDIVIDUAL AND FAMILY LEVEL

The preceding section addressed individual and family cultural beliefs associated with disability. Next we turn to the responses (i.e., behaviors or actions) that develop in part from these beliefs and in part secondary to material realities.

An individual with a disability, or their family, is likely to seek some form of intervention in an attempt to "cure" or minimize the effect of having a disability. Beliefs might impact the patient's decision regarding what medicines to use, what foods to eat, or what exercises to do. Behaviors in this regard vary substantially between and among cultures and can be quite different from those held by the Euro-American. Depending upon the individual's socio-cultural background, services may be provided by a Western-style health professional, traditional/indigenous healer, or lay person/family member. Examples of traditional healers include, but are not limited to, curanderos (Mexican American), espiritistas (Puerto Rican), santerios (Cuban), vodoo priests (Haitian), diviners (Southeast Asian American), singers (Native American) and the more generalized herbalists, astrologers, and more. Each has their own repertoire of skills and rituals. In reality, the practical issues of availability, cost, and severity of episode typically account for the choice of practitioner (Leavitt, 2003).

Leavitt (1992) described health behaviors associated with children with disabilities in rural Jamaica. As one might expect, there is a greater tendency for the Jamaican respondents to also use traditional healing practices if they believe in the possibility of a supernatural cause of the disabling condition.

The African heritage is reflected in much of the current Jamaican culture and folk medical belief systems. In particular, the Jamaicans' belief in African forms of witchcraft and animism, or praying to sacrificed animals, is relevant to their behavioral response to the presence of disability. *Obeah*, or the practice of witchcraft, is "essentially a magical means whereby an individual may obtain his personal desires, eradicate ill health, procure good fortune in life and business...evince retribution or revenge upon his enemies, and generally manipulate the spiritual forces...to obtain his will" (Morrish, 1982, p. 41). The *obeah* man or woman keeps his "things" in his *obi* place. These "things" are composed of such materials as blood, feathers, parrots' beak, grave dirt, rum, and eggshells, and his "bush" is a concoction of medicinal herbs. The *obeah* may sometimes cause a problem by "putting" the spirit sickness on a person, or the *obeah* may "work it off." Reportedly, some people visit an *obeah*, even though law forbids it. Strongly linked with the practice of *obeah* is the belief in *duppies* previously described.

Jamaican folk medicine practices can be as simple as the use of a bush tea for a cold, avocado to lower high blood pressure, and pawpaw to get rid of a boil, or as complex as the treatment by an *obeah* man employing many of the previously mentioned materials. Most "bushmen" are not *obeah* men but rather spiritualists who believe that herbs can strengthen the physical body and therefore help to ward off ailments. Often, the spiritualist believes in the necessity of supporting the healing herbs with religious ceremony, charms, fresh air and sunlight, or other foods such as cock soup or roasted animal testes.

Examples of statements concerning the use of indigenous healing practices for the treatment of a child with a disability in rural Jamaica are as follows (Leavitt, 1992):

- "I use baths a whole lot of times, in the night, put wash pan of water over here, and put two sticks and cross them—let it stay overnight, and bathe him in the morning.

- "I put milk in the bath, and no talk with anyone until after the bath.

- "Dig a hole to the level of the waist. Bury him in it for one hour, remove him and stand him.

- "Me use grapefruit juice and brandy to wet his mole [brain]. It helps to keep his brain steady.

- "Yes, I wouldn't hide you that [going to a mother lady], cause I had to try all that because I see and get the vision and maybe it can be a different inferior spirit come along and hurt her.

- "The mother lady sent me to the bush doctor shop. Get some kind oil to use on her and bush to boil" (pp. 124-125).

People of Asian descent and Native Americans are especially likely to consider the interplay between beliefs about cause and traditional healing practices. There is an attempt to regain balance between mind, body, and environment as evidenced by the philosophy underlying energy theory, yin and yang, and the law of five elements (Ling, 2003). The relationship between these beliefs and practice is clearly seen in the Hmong culture.

For the Hmong, traditional healing practices including animal sacrifice and special ceremonies involving such tools as a saber, gong, rattle, finger bells, and a "flying horse" are paramount, as is the role of the *txiv neeb* (indigenous healing practitioner). These are not only very different practices than those used in the U.S., but the Hmong also believe that American doctors remove organs from their patients to eat or sell as food, that they anesthetize patients to allow the patient's soul to escape, and they cut the "spirit-strings" from patients' wrists, thus disturbing their "life-souls" (Fadiman, 1998).

Religion appears to be as important a factor in influencing the caretaker's behavior with regard to treatment practices as it was in influencing the caretaker's belief system. Again, from Leavitt (1992):

- "When the child does not have a *duppy* sickness, the mother takes her to a doctor. But when it is a *duppy* sickness, 'You get a different power to deal with that. Me lay my hand on him and pray...I know when they [the *duppies*] come and run them...I rebuke the spirit and he have to go... Only I is safe to do it, because me only one who feel the holy ghost. I is a Christian...I speak unto God...speak in tongues... It happens at the moment and I interpret the word. The Lord will keep away the *duppies*.'

- "I think God have a different plan for him. I'm praying to see that plan when it come through. I love him [the child] very much—what hope for him I'd like to be around when that hope come through. God will make him better in a way he can help himself.

- "I know the Lord can heal him…I don't know if my faith is strong enough. You need great faith… Darvey [the child] no have faith.

- "I'm a Christian you know, and he weren't like this you know [the child had been functioning at a lower level]. I took him to the Throne of Grace, and I laid on him right here and I prayed on him day and night and I ask God to touch him because he used to run all over the place as though him mad…but I entreated him to God and I laid on down on him and I pray and I say God touch him. I kept on asking the Lord to touch him, and I can see for *sure* him better.

- "The Kumina Queen says, 'You have to call to God before you do anything…me deal with God direct…me no deal with the *duppy* one [obeah man]…me speak seven different languages and speak in tongues…I can't make him [the child] talk, God have to give that'" (pp. 125-126).

Many Hispanic people rely heavily on the Roman Catholic religion to support them during times of stress. Religious beliefs are again closely tied to folk remedies. Rehabilitation professionals are generally familiar with beliefs such as the power of holy water to ward off evil or bringing a sick elder to pray before the image of a saint. At the period of death and dying, the praying of the Rosary and last rites are representative behaviors. Additionally, the "hot/cold" paradigm is relevant to people of Hispanic origin. For example, blood is "hot" and is associated with strength, virility, and machismo. If one is anemic, one might eat more "hot" foods such as those organ meats that are considered blood products.

The prevention of disability rather than treatment of an already existing disability is also associated with folk tales and the behaviors that come from them. The following are examples regarding babies, shared by a group of women in Jamaica who worked with a pregnant Peace Corps volunteer (Thams, 1986):

- Place an opened pair of scissors or a horseshoe over the bedroom door where the baby sleeps to keep away evil spirits.

- *Duppies* are afraid of red. Newborn babies should have a red ribbon tied around their left wrist and wear red clothes to ward off evil spirits.

- Do not let menstruating women hold a baby or it will get stomach cramps.

- If a pregnant woman has sex with a man other than the baby's father, the baby will be handicapped.

- When the baby's navel stump falls off, the mother must bury it outside under a young plant to ensure that the baby will grow strong and healthy.

- Do not cut a baby's hair before he can talk or he will have problems talking.

In summary, the concept of intra-cultural diversity is supported by the range of variation of beliefs and behaviors with regard to disability and rehabilitation. It is easy to imagine how both a traditional people and the Western medical practitioner view the other as strange, ignorant, and stubborn. Conflict can easily arise.

CULTURAL RESPONSE TO THE PRESENCE OF DISABILITY AT THE SOCIETAL LEVEL: A CHANGING PARADIGM

The societal response to the presence of disability continues to evolve, albeit too slowly for many. For example, in the U.S., the Rehabilitation Act of 1973 (United States Access Board, n.d.) calling for civil rights for PWD, the Education for All Handicapped Children Act of 1975 and its subsequent reauthorization as Individuals with Disabilities Education

Act (IDEA) in 1997 (Office of Special Education and Rehabilitative Services, n.d.), and the Americans With Disabilities Act of 1990 and its 2008 amendments (U.S. Department of Justice, n.d.) are revolutionary in that they are based on the philosophy that, in a just society, all individuals must be accorded equal access and opportunity to pursue their individual goals. On one hand, it is argued that PWD have continually experienced more stigma, pervasive prejudice, and discrimination than any other group, including forced sterilization and institutionalization. At least in the industrialized nations, however, the more restrictive bio-medical model of care is generally being replaced with minority group and social justice models. Nevertheless, in today's world, there are barriers to full participation in society. For example, in the U.S., only 55.8% of persons with disabilities aged 16 to 64 are employed (U.S. Department of Labor, n.d.). Additionally, in 2000, 30% of persons with disabilities reported having problems with transportation, with 16% reporting inadequate transportation as a major problem (National Organization on Disability, 2000). Disturbingly, this same data set reveals that the transportation gap between people with disabilities and people without disabilities has actually widened by seven percentage points since 1998. The National Organization on Disability (n.d.) further reports that Americans with disabilities are four times more likely to have special needs that are not covered by their health insurance and more than twice as likely to postpone needed health care because they cannot afford it. For individuals who are also from ethnic minorities, the barriers are even stronger than those for White, middle-class PWD, supporting the idea that some people are faced with a "double burden."

People with disability from ethnic minorities face linguistic and cultural barriers and additional disability-related barriers at all points within the life span. For example, Hampton (2003), who focuses particularly on the plight of PWD who are Asian American, noted that medical expenditures for PWD varied according to ethnicity. In a study published in 1996 (with data from 1987), he notes that White families spent $1,898 per child, but African Americans spent $977 and Asian Americans spent $864. The presumption is that Asian Americans, in fact, have a great need for services, but they are not accessing them secondary to lack of knowledge about health care services or lack of resources. Low utilization of available services has also been reported specifically for Korean and Vietnamese populations (Hampton, 2003; Ling, 2003). Later in life, elder Asian people with disabilities are less likely to have Medicare, pensions, disability insurance, or other benefits; participate in community-based health programs; or live in nursing homes, compared to their White counterparts (Hampton; Leavitt, 2003; Ling).

With regard to special education, in 1990, Asian American students, constituting approximately 3% of the total school population, were thought to be underrepresented in special education (.9%), suggesting that these students were either not being identified or not receiving the services to which they are entitled. Also, these students were identified as not having the language support/modifications and services needed for successful completion of their individualized education plan (IEP) identified goals. Barriers identified by parents of Asian American students with disabilities are language barriers, inappropriate referral and assessment practices, a lack of awareness about educational systems and processes (including their rights), and lack of cultural awareness by professionals (Hampton, 2003).

In contrast to the above data on Asian American experiences in school, African American children are overrepresented in special education. African American students account for about 20% of the special education population across all disabilities. They are 2.4 times more likely than White students to be identified with a diagnosis of mental retardation, and 1.7 times as likely to be labeled as having an emotional or behavioral disorder (Blanchett, 2006). Because many of these referrals are subjective, some believe they are more subject to bias. Furthermore, the in-school and post-school outcomes for African American children in special education are worse when compared to other groups (Blanchett) (see Chapter 8).

Concerning employment opportunities, barriers to meaningful employment for PWD remain substantial. Work can provide both economic security and social and psychological identity. Some PWD may not be able to achieve the employment status that they wish, or return to their previous work after a newly acquired disability. At times, retraining is possible, but the PWD may not find this to be satisfactory. Workplace accommodation remains a challenge in many environments. There are conflicting data about the changes in employment status of PWD since the ADA, but it is generally noted that the changes have been less than anticipated (Smart, 2001). A contributing reason for the disappointing impact of the ADA is that the U.S. Supreme Court has generally endorsed a narrow interpretation of the law that has necessarily limited its applicability (Colker, 2005). Amendments to the ADA were enacted in September 2008 that many hope will clarify its scope and purpose and broaden its impact.

When looking for a job, a Chinese client was frightened about the idea of being "tested" by a government agency and never returned to the counselor's office. Employers may not understand the fear of such intrusions and/or the notion of limited English proficiency. Thus, the employer may presume someone is not cooperative or too severely involved and not worthy of the job. Furthermore, the process of self-directed decision making, favored by the American health care professionals, is an anathema to many Asians who have a worldview that stresses respect for health professionals' knowledge, a collectivist responsibility for one's health and/or the disability, and a belief that the condition was ordained by spirits or the gods, and therefore it would be deemed useless to try dealing with the government (Hampton, 2003).

In summary, language barriers, lack of citizenship, lack of access to insurance, and lack of advocacy skills, as well as a worldview based on different ideals than the norm, are all potential factors that can influence how an individual with a disability or health problem will fare within contemporary society.

Still, there is room for optimism. A new paradigm based on self-determination, self-representation, and human rights is developing. The social justice model of disability is becoming more accepted. The United Nations Year *of* Disabled Persons (as opposed to *for*) in 1981 marked a turning point internationally with regard to the perception of PWD. Originally, the action plan called for bigger institutions and more training of professionals. But, as PWD became more involved themselves, a new model emphasizing cooperation and partnership evolved. The theme of the year became "full participation and equality." The Decade of Disabled Persons (1983-1992) was built upon the promotion of equalization of opportunities and rights for PWD (McColl & Bickenbach, 1998). "Undoubtedly, the major achievement of the Decade was the increased public awareness of disability issues among policymakers, planners, politicians, service providers, parents and disabled persons themselves" (Boutris-Ghali, 1992, p. 4). Antidiscrimination legislation has since been enacted, to varying degrees, throughout the world. In the U.S., the Americans with Disabilities Act (1990) declares that PWD have a right to pursue "equality of opportunity, full participation, independent living, and economic self-sufficiency" (McColl & Bickenbach, p. 159).

ACHIEVING CULTURAL COMPETENCE: THE ROLE OF THE PHYSICAL THERAPIST

What role do physical therapists have in advancing this newer way of approaching the presence of PWD in society? As the world, and likely one's place of employment, becomes increasingly multi-cultural, the need for cross-cultural research investigating the attitudes, beliefs, and behaviors relevant to disability and rehabilitation will become both pragmatic and morally vital.

One possible line of inquiry is to look more formally at attitudes of physical therapists toward PWD and to apply the results to more structured training programs in order to achieve more positive attitudes and behaviors. A second example of needed research is that which addresses ethnic and cultural differences directly related to patient care. Clinicians must acknowledge and accept, rather than ridicule or ignore, differing belief systems and behaviors associated with disability as long as they are not harmful to a person. (Some folk remedies do include arsenic, lead, or opium, and these can be dangerous.) In fact, it may be the physical therapists' professional responsibility to act as a "culture broker," that is, someone who can effectively link the bio-medical world of the health professional with the socio-cultural reality of the client. Using language from earlier in this chapter, this cultural brokering asks professionals to paradoxically fully endorse their role in the bio-medical model and simultaneously embrace the social justice model that rejects much of the philosophy upon which the former is based.

CONCLUSION

The future is likely to see an increasing number of PWD from a range of cultural groups. It is presumed that there will be PWD in every society, and that there will be specific medical care and socio-cultural systems and explanatory models that account for the beliefs about the disability and the cultural patterns of behaviors having to do with disability diagnosis and treatment. The social construction of disability is undoubtedly related in part to the influence of belonging to multiple cultural sub-groups, societal attitudes toward disability, the material realities of the environment, and the adaptation mechanisms that are available for any individual and their family. In removing barriers, disability rights activists, across nations and other sub-groups, are leaning toward theories of social justice, whereby disability is viewed as a form of human variation. That is, a belief that bio-ethics groups and society should promote "not self-sufficiency but self-determination, not independence but interdependence, not functional separateness but personal connection, not physical autonomy but human community" (Asch, 2001, p. 320).

The newest paradigm, focusing on a client or family-centered model, including community-based rehabilitation (CBR), independent living, and paying attention to the client and their family's socio-cultural environment has yet to be embraced by all. The process of change is slow, as evidenced by the many physical, political, societal, and personal obstacles that many PWD face in their everyday lives. Nevertheless, society and the field of rehabilitation are moving in this direction.

Rehabilitation professionals are just beginning to explore the issues associated with disability when viewed from a broader, social perspective. Understanding the inherent bias in their traditional role, as defined within the medical model, and forging new paradigms, skills, and approaches is the challenge for the future. We have a role to play in advancing a modern approach to disability rights and the notion that cultural competence is as important as clinical competence. It is our professional moral imperative to embrace cultural diversity and develop the most appropriate service models and public policy to enhance the lives of all PWD.

REFLECTION QUESTIONS

✔ *Do you ever reflect upon the meaning of a person's disability with regard to their personal life? The impact on the family?*

✔ *Can you imagine someone with a disability choosing to keep their disability status if given the choice?*

✔ *Have you noticed variation among your patients with regard to their attitudes toward the presence of a disability?*

✔ Do you get frustrated when a person with a disability and/or their family believes that the disability is "God's will" and therefore it is not necessary to do a home exercise program?

✔ What are your first thoughts when you see a person with a physical disability? With a developmental disability?

✔ How are people with a disability portrayed in the media?

✔ Do you support the ADA?

✔ Can a person with a physical disability be a physical therapist? How may the rehabilitation environment make accommodations for this therapist?

REFERENCES

Abberley, P. (1987). The concept of oppression and the development of a social theory of disability. *Disability, Handicap and Society, 2*(1), 5-19.

Aiken, L. R. (2002). *Attitudes and related psychosocial constructs: Theories, assessment, and research.* Thousand Oaks, CA: Sage Publications.

Albrecht, G. L., Selman, K. D., & Bury, M. (Eds.). (2001). *Handbook of disability studies.* Thousand Oaks, CA: Sage Publications.

Altman, B. M. (2001). Disability definitions, models, classification schemes, and applications. In G. L. Albrecht, K. D. Seelman, and M. Bury (Eds.), *Handbook of disability studies* (pp. 97-122). Thousand Oaks, CA: Sage Publications.

Antonek, R. F., & Livneh, H. (1988). *The measurement of attitudes toward people with disabilities: Methods, psychometrics, and scales.* Springfield, IL: Charles C. Thomas Publisher.

Asch, A. (2001). Disability, bioethics, and human rights. In G. L. Albrecht, K. D. Seelman, & M. Bury (Eds.), *Handbook of disability studies* (pp. 297-326). Thousand Oaks, CA: Sage Publications.

Basnett, I. (2001). Health care professionals and their attitudes toward and decisions affecting disabled people. In G. L. Albrecht, K. D. Seelman, & M. Bury (Eds.), *Handbook of disability studies* (pp. 450-468). Thousand Oaks, CA: Sage Publications.

Blanchett, W. J. (2006). Disproportionate representation of African American students in special education: Acknowledging the role of white privilege and racism. *Educational Researcher, 35*(6), 24-28.

Block, P., Ricafrente-Biazon, M., Russo, A., Chu, K. Y., Sud, S., Koerner, L., et al. (2005). Introducing disability studies to occupational therapy students. *American Journal of Occupational Therapy, 59*(5), 554-560.

Boutris-Ghali, B. (1992). *Message of the Secretary General: World programme of action opens way to full participation in society in disabled persons.* Bulletin No.2, Publication 64. Vienna, Austria: United Nations Center for Social Development and Humanitarian Affairs.

Braddock, D., & Parish, S. (2001). An institutional history of disability. In G. L. Albrecht, K. D. Seelman, & M. Bury (Eds.), *Handbook of disability studies* (pp. 11-68). Thousand Oaks, CA: Sage Publications.

Brandt, E. N., Jr., & Pope, A. M. (Eds.). (1997). *Enabling America: Assessing the role of rehabilitation science and engineering.* Washington DC: National Academies Press.

Brown, S. C. (2001). Methodological paradigms that shape disability research. In G. L. Albrecht, K. D. Seelman, & M. Bury (Eds.), *Handbook of disability studies* (pp. 145-170). Thousand Oaks, CA: Sage Publications.

Brundtland, G. H. (2002). The future of the world's health. In C. E. Koop, C. E. Pearson, & M. R. Schwarz (Eds.), *Critical issues in global health* (pp. 3-11). San Francisco, CA: Jossey-Bass.

Chan, S. (1998) Families with Asian roots. In E. W. Lynch & M. J. Hanson (Eds.), *Developing cross-cultural competence: A guide for working with children and their families* (2nd ed., pp. 251-344). Baltimore, MD: Brookes Publishing Company.

Colker, R. (2005). The disability pendulum: The first decade of the Americans with Disabilities Act. New York, NY: NYU Press.

Devlieger, P. J. (1998). Physical 'disability' in Bantu languages: Understanding the relativity of classification and meaning. *International Journal of Rehabilitation Research, 21*(1), 51-62.

Eddey, G. E., & Robey, K. L. (2005). Considering the culture of disability in cultural competence education. *Academic Medicine, 80*(7), 706-712.

Evans, N. J. (2008). Theoretical foundations of Universal Instructional Design. In J. L. Higbee & E. Goff (Eds.), *Pedagogy and student services for institutional transformation: Implementing universal design in higher education* (pp. 11-24). Minneapolis, MN: University of Minnesota.

Fadiman, A. (1998). *The spirit catches you and you fall down.* New York, NY: Farrar, Straus and Giroux.

Goffman, E. (1963). *Stigma: Notes on the management of spoiled identity.* Upper Saddle River, NJ: Prentice Hall.

Greeson, C. J., Veach, P. M., & LeRoy, B. S. (2001). A qualitative investigation of Somali immigrant perceptions of disability: Implications for genetic counseling. *Journal of Genetic Counseling, 10*(5), 359-378.

Groce, N. (1999). Health beliefs and behavior towards individuals with disability cross-culturally. In R. L. Leavitt (Ed.), *Cross-cultural rehabilitation: An international perspective* (pp. 37-48). London, England: Harcourt Brace and Company.

Gwaltney, J. L. (1970). *The thrice shy: Cultural accommodation to blindness and other disasters in a Mexican community*. New York, NY: Columbia University Press.

Hampton, N. Z. (2003). Asian Americans with disabilities: Access to education, health care, and rehabilitation services. In L. Zhan, *Asian Americans: Vulnerable populations, model interventions, and clarifying agendas* (pp. 69-88). Sudbury, MA: Jones and Bartlett Publishers.

Hanks, J. R., & Hanks, L. M. (1948). The physically handicapped in certain non-occidental societies. *Journal of Social Sciences, 4*, 11-20.

Harper, D. C. (1997). Children's attitudes toward physical disability in Nepal: A field study. *Journal of Cross-Cultural Psychology, 28*(6), 710-729.

Hemmingsson, H., & Jonsson, H. (2005). An occupational perspective on the concept of participation in the international classification of functioning, disability and health: Some critical remarks. *American Journal of Occupational Therapy, 59*(5), 569-576.

Hughes, B. (2002). Disability and the body. In C. Barnes, M. Oliver, & L. Barton (Eds.), *Disability studies today.* Cambridge: Polity.

Ingstad, B. (1999). Problems with community mobilization and participation in CBR. In R. L. Leavitt (Ed.), *Cross-cultural rehabilitation: An international perspective* (pp. 207-216). London, England: Harcourt Brace and Company.

Ingstad, B. (2001). Disability in the developing world. In G. L. Albrecht, K. D. Seelman, & M. Bury (Eds.), *Handbook of disability studies* (pp. 772-792). Thousand Oaks, CA: Sage Publications.

Ingstad, B., & Whyte, S. R. (Eds.). (1995). *Disability and culture.* Berkeley, CA: University of California Press.

Iwakuma, M., & Nussbaus, J. F. (2000). Intercultural views of people with disabilities in Asia and Africa. In D. O. Braithwaite & T. L. Thompson (Eds.), *Handbook of communication and people with disabilities: Research and application* (pp. 239-256). Mahwah, NJ: Lawrence Erlbaum.

Joe, J. R., & Malach, R. S. (1998). Families with Native American roots. In E. W. Lynch & M. J. Hanson (Eds.), *Developing cross-cultural competence: A guide for working with children and their families* (2nd ed., pp. 127-164). Baltimore, MD: Brookes Publishing Company.

Kielhofner, G. (2005). Rethinking disability and what to do about it: Disability studies and its implications for occupational therapy. *American Journal of Occupational Therapy, 59*(5), 487-496.

Kim-Rupnow, W. S. (2001). *An introduction to Korean culture for rehabilitation service providers.* Buffalo, NY: Center for International Rehabilitation Research Information and Exchange (CIRRIE). CIRRIE Monograph Series.

Kohrman, M. (2003). Why am I not disabled? Making state subjects, making statistics in post-Mao China. *Medical Anthropology Quarterly, 17*(1), 5-24.

Leavitt, R. L. (1992). *Disability and rehabilitation in rural Jamaica: An ethnographic study.* Madison, NJ: Fairleigh Dickinson University Press.

Leavitt, R. L. (Ed.). (1999). *Cross-cultural rehabilitation: An international perspective.* London, England: Harcourt Brace and Company.

Leavitt, R. L. (2003). Developing cultural competence in a multicultural world: Part II. *PT Magazine, 11*(1), 56-70.

Ling, W. (2003). An overview of East Asian cultures for physical therapists. *American Physical Therapy Association, Section on Geriatrics, Cultural Diversity of Older Americans Series,* 1-27.

Linton, S. (1998). *Claiming disability: Knowledge and identity.* New York, NY: NYU Press.

Liu, G. Z. (2001). *Chinese culture and disability: Information for U.S. service providers.* Buffalo, NY: Center for International Rehabilitation Research Information and Exchange (CIRRIE). CIRRIE Monograph Series.

Loveland, C. (1999). *The concept of culture.* In R. L. Leavitt (Ed.), *Cross-cultural rehabilitation: An international perspective* (pp. 15-24). London, England: Harcourt Brace and Company.

Madiros, M. (1989). Conception of childhood disability among Mexican-American parents. *Medical Anthropology, 12*(1), 55-68.

McColl, M. A., & Bickenbach, J. E. (1998). *Introduction to disability and handicap.* Philadelphia, PA: W. B. Saunders.

Michalko, R. (2002). *The difference that disability makes.* Philadelphia, PA: Temple University Press.

Miles, M. (1999). Some influences of religions on attitudes towards disabilities and people with disabilities. In R. L. Leavitt (Ed.), *Cross-cultural rehabilitation: An international perspective* (pp. 49-58). London, England: Harcourt Brace and Company.

Morrish, I. (1982). *Obeah, Christ and rastaman.* Cambridge, UK: James Clarke Lutterworth.

National Organization on Disability. (2000). Access to transportation. Retrieved October 29, 2008, from http://www.nod.org/index.cfm?fuseaction=Feature.showFeature&FeatureID=609

National Organization on Disability. (n.d.). Access to independence: Health care access. Retrieved October 29, 2008, from http://www.nod.org/index.cfm?fuseaction=Page.viewPage&pageId=19

Nagi, S. Z. (1965). Some conceptual issues in disability and rehabilitation. In M. B. Sussman (Ed.), *Sociology and rehabilitation* (pp. 100-113). Washington, DC: American Sociological Association.

Nagi, S. Z. (1969). *Disability and rehabilitation: Legal, clinical, and self-concepts and measurement*. Columbus, OH: The Ohio State University Press.

Nagi, S. Z. (1991). Disability concepts revisited: Implications for prevention. In A. M. Pope & A. R. Tarlov (Eds.), *Disability in America: Toward a national agenda for prevention* (pp. 309-327). Washington, DC: National Academies Press.

Neufeldt, A. (1999). 'Appearances' of disability, discrimination and the transformation of rehabilitation service practices. In R. L. Leavitt (Ed.), *Cross-cultural rehabilitation: An international perspective* (pp. 25-47). London, England: Harcourt Brace and Company.

Office of Special Education and Rehabilitative Services. (n.d.). IDEA. Retrieved November 8, 2008, from http://www.ed.gov/offices/OSERS/Policy/IDEA/the_law.html

Oliver, M. (1990). *The politics of disablement: A sociological approach*. New York, NY: Palgrave Macmillan.

Oliver, M. (2004). The social model in action: If I had a hammer. In C. Barnes & G. Mercer (Eds.), *Implementing the social model of disability* (pp. 18-31). Leeds, West Yorkshire: The Disability Press.

Pinto, P., & Sahur, N. (2001). *Working with people with disabilities: An Indian perspective*. Buffalo, NY: Center for International Rehabilitation Research Information and Exchange (CIRRIE). CIRRIE Monograph Series.

Pope, A. M., & Tarlov, A. R. (Eds.). (1991). *Disability in America: Toward a national agenda for prevention* Washington DC: National Academies Press.

Rauscher, L., & McClintock, M. (1997). Ableism curriculum design. In M. Adams, L. A. Bell, & P. Griffin (Eds.), *Teaching for diversity and social justice: A sourcebook* (pp. 198-230). New York, NY: Routledge.

Ravaud, J. F., & Stiker, H. J. (2001). Inclusion/exclusion: An analysis of historical and cultural meanings. In G. L. Albrecht, K. D. Seelman, & M. Bury (Eds.), *Handbook of disability studies* (pp. 490-512). Thousand Oaks, CA: Sage Publications.

Roush, S. (1993). Shifting the paradigm of disability. *PT Magazine, 1*(6), 48-52.

Saetermoe, C., Scattone, D., & Dim, K. (2001). Ethnicity and the stigma of disabilities. *Psychology and Health, 16*(6), 699-714.

Scheer, J., & Groce, N. (1988). Impairment as a human constant: Cross-cultural and historical perspectives on variation. *Journal of Social Issues, 44*(1), 22-37.

Smart, J. (2001). *Disability, society and the individual*. New York, NY: Aspen Publishers.

Tervo, R. C., Azuma, S., Palmer, G., & Redinius, P. (2002). Medical students' attitudes toward persons with disability: A comparative study. *Archives of Physical Medicine and Rehabilitation, 83*(11), 1537-1542.

Thams, S. (1986). *Jamaican folk tales*. Kingston: Peace Corp Publication.

Tullock, S. (Ed.). (1993). *The Reader's Digest Oxford wordfinder*. Broadbridge, Gloucestershire: Clarendon Press.

United States Access Board. (n.d.). The Rehabilitation Act Amendments of 1973, as amended. Retrieved November 8, 2008, from http://www.access-board.gov/enforcement/Rehab-Act-text/intro.htm

U.S. Department of Justice. (n.d.). Americans With Disabilities Act of 1990, as Amended. Retrieved November 8, 2008, from http://www.ada.gov/pubs/ada.htm

U.S. Department of Labor. (n.d.). Fact sheet: Statistics on the employment rate of people with disabilities. Retrieved October 29, 2008, from http://www.dol.gov/odep/pubs/fact/stats.htm

Verbrugge, L. M., & Jette, A. M. (1994). The disablement process. *Social Science & Medicine, 38*(1), 1-14.

Westbrook, M. T., Legge, V., & Pennay, M. (1993). Attitudes towards disabilities in a multicultural society. *Social Science & Medicine, 36*(5), 615-623.

World Health Organization. (1980). *International Classification of impairments, disabilities, and handicaps: A manual of classification relating to the consequences of disease*. Albany, NY: Author.

World Health Organization. (2000). *Towards a common language for functioning and disablement: ICIDH-2*. Geneva, Switzerland: Author.

World Health Organization. (2001). *International classification of functioning, disability and health (ICF)*. Geneva, Switzerland: Author.

Zaromatidis, K., Papadaki, A., & Gilde, A. (1999). A cross-cultural comparison of attitudes toward persons with disabilities: Greeks and Greek-Americans. *Psychological Reports, 84*(3 Pt 2), 1189-1196.

Zola, I. K. (1993). Self, identity and the naming question: Reflections on the language of disability. In, M. Nagler (Ed.), *Perspectives on disability* (2nd ed., pp. 15-23). Palo Alto, CA: Health Markets Research.

Zuniga, M. (1998). Families with Latino roots. In E. W. Lynch & M. J. Hanson (Eds.), *Developing cross-cultural competence: A guide for working with children and their families* (2nd ed., pp. 209-250). Baltimore, MD: Brookes Publishing Company.

Racial and Ethnic Disparities in Health Status, Health Care, and Physical Therapy

Kristin Lefebvre, PhD, CCS, PT and
Jill Black Lattanzi, EdD, PT

BACKGROUND

Inequities in health are of great concern to medical practitioners, policymakers, and patients in this country. Impacted by provider, patient, and social behaviors; differences in health care access; interventions; and outcomes have resulted in disparities between various groups of people within the U.S. Although linked to patient health risk-behaviors, socioeconomic status, geographic location, and education level, no single variable can account for the inequities we see across a broad spectrum of diseases and medical procedures. Regardless, increasing awareness about this issue and competence of medical practitioners, including the critical domain of cultural competence, is essential to diminishing their presence.

Racial health disparities have emerged from a long history of prejudice and inequity that have existed not only in health care distribution and access, but social status and educational attainment, and were influenced by acts of discrimination and racism. In recent decades, this issue has increasingly garnered the attention of community members, health care providers, government agencies, and insurance payers because of the overall adverse consequences it has on health outcomes. In the mid 1980s, steps were taken to begin to evaluate the extent and impact of the problem of health disparities by the Department of Health and Human Services (HHS). This accelerating consciousness has provided a wealth of literature that supports the presence of disparities among races and ethnicities in the areas of health status, access to care, and health care quality (Gamble & Stone, 2006). Even with the overall decline in mortality throughout the 20th century, African American mortality rates remain 40% higher than the mortality rates of Non- Hispanic Whites (Smith, 2005). Infant mortality rates continue to be substantially greater among minorities (LaVeist, 2005). And finally, not only is there a difference between health measures with regard to race and ethnicity, but the differences continue to widen (Atrash & Hunter, 2005; Jatoi, Becher, & Leake, 2003; LaVeist).

R. L. Leavitt (Ed.).
*Cultural Competence: A Lifelong Journey
to Cultural Proficiency* (pp. 99-120).
© 2010 SLACK Incorporated

Most Americans ultimately believe in equality for all, thus, the presence of racial or ethnic disparities, especially in the area of health care, are very disturbing (Mechanic, 2005). Health disparities are viewed as unfair, affect everyone, and are avoidable (Woodward & Kawachi, 2000). Health disparities are also cost prohibitive, at the individual level due to the adverse impact on employment and greater out-of-pocket expenses, and at the societal level by increasing costs to business and the government (Suthers, 2008). The elimination of health disparities has become a national priority, with the Institute of Medicine (IOM), Congress, HHS, and the National Institutes of Health (NIH) all taking steps to encourage policies that will abolish or, at the very least, minimize them (HHS, 2000; IOM, 2001; LaVeist, 2005). In addition, community groups, funding agencies, health care practitioners, and policymakers are complementing the efforts of these government agencies by uniting to assist with the elimination of such disparities. Physical therapists must recognize their role as a stakeholder in the resolution of health disparities and can join the efforts in the reduction and eventual elimination of health disparities through education and research.

DEFINITIONS OF HEALTH DISPARITIES

Various health care agencies have uniquely defined the problem of health disparities. The IOM defines health disparities as "racial or ethnic differences in the quality of health care that are not due to access-related factors, clinical needs, preferences and appropriateness of intervention" (Smedley, Stith, & Nelson, 2002, p. 3). Alternatively, a widely accepted citation from the National Institutes of Health provides a definition for health disparities as "a difference in the incidence, prevalence, morbidity, mortality, burden of disease and other adverse health conditions that occur among different population groups" (National Center on Minority Health and Disparities [NCMHD], n.d.). Reference to disparities often refers to the role of a person's racial and/or ethnic status in inequities in health, whether referring to prevalence of disease or disease outcomes, and also addresses the variables that lead to these inequities. This chapter will examine health disparities between people of different racial and ethnic groups and the variables that contribute to them. It is important to note that there are also health disparities among other populations, although they are not the focus of this chapter. Examples include health disparities between the lesbian, gay, bisexual, and transgender population as compared to heterosexuals; people with disabilities compared to those without disabilities; and males compared to females.

HISTORY AND GOVERNMENT PERSPECTIVE OF HEALTH DISPARITIES

Health disparities have evolved from a long history of inequities in U.S. social status (see Chapters 7 and 8). In order to appropriately address health disparities, the physical therapist should have an understanding of this history. In addition, an understanding of the history behind the structure and development of current governmental health care agencies combating health disparities is valuable. Governmental policies must be adapted so that effective action can occur (Gamble & Stone, 2006). Therefore, this section will provide an overview of the background of health disparities from both a sociological and governmental policy perspective.

Individuals of a minority race or ethnicity have been subject to limited access to health care, unequal and sometimes very stressful living conditions, and social injustice throughout the history of this country. The first record of slavery in the U.S. is 1619 (Quarles, 1987). For more than 240 years (8+ generations), African Americans inhabited this country as slaves, with limited and segregated access to health care and, at times, brutal living conditions. Finally in 1863, the Emancipation Proclamation freed slaves who lived in states that had not seceded from the Union. Confederate slaves were not liberated until 1865. Yet, following the enactment of the 13th, 14th, and 15th amendments, Southern segregationists began to introduce what became known as Jim Crow laws that would maintain the separation of Blacks from Whites in public locations. These laws were supported by individual state legislatures and by an 1896 U.S. Supreme Court decision, declaring the constitutionality of "separate but equal" facilities. Examples of Jim Crow laws include separation of drinking fountains, waiting rooms, baseball fields, and railroad cars. Jail time was the penalty for disobedience (Black et al., 2003; Smithsonian Museum, n.d.).

The first significant documentation of racial health disparities was found at the turn of the 19th century in literature by W. B. DuBois entitled *The Health and Physique of the Negro American*. The practices and policies of physicians and hospitals, especially in the South, often had adverse outcomes. Minority patients were treated in segregated wards or hospitals of unequal quality. Their subordinate status of secondhand citizenship sometimes excluded them from hospital admission altogether (LaVeist, 2005; Smith, 2005). For example, in November 1931, the Dean of Women at Fisk University in Nashville, TN, Juliette Dericotte, was injured in a car accident in Georgia. Unable to admit Ms. Dericotte to the segregated hospital in the area of Dalton, GA, the local doctor was forced to transfer her to a hospital in Chattanooga, TN almost 50 miles away. Her death was attributed to her inability to access appropriate and timely care for her injuries (Gamble & Stone, 2006).

Dubois' work and publicity of experiences such as what happened to Ms. Dericotte led to some changes. Between the years of 1915 and 1930, over 32 states participated in National Health Week activities, which were designed to bring attention and focus to the health of people of color. In 1930, this initiative was assumed by the U.S. Public Health Service, and two years later, the Office of Negro Health was established, creating the first time since the Civil War that Black health care issues were specifically addressed by the Federal government. Separate health care facilities and medical schools were established for minorities (LaVeist, 2005), and between 1910-1930, the number of minority physicians increased by 25% (Myrdal, 1944), while the number of non-Hispanic White physicians remained constant.

Also during this time, Black attorneys began to challenge the laws enforcing segregation. The tide began to turn in 1946 when the Federal government offered increased funding for hospital expansion under the Hill-Burton Act. In order to obtain funding for building expansion grants available from the government, hospitals were required to eliminate discrimination in employment or provision of health care services. Discrimination based on race in Federal jobs and segregation in Federally funded hospitals such as the Veterans Administration Hospitals was made illegal by President Truman (Smith, 2005). In the 1960s, if a medical school or hospital facility wanted to apply for certain Federal grants or funding, desegregation within the medical school was required (Smith). The Office of Negro Health was closed as a reflection of the attempts to end segregation in all government agencies.

Even with this progress, African Americans continued to battle limited access to health care and medical training. Residency and post-professional training for minority physicians was extremely limited (Myrdal, 1944). Minority physicians were often denied admitting privileges to major hospitals and medical centers even as the American Medical Association and the American College of Surgeons proceeded to standardize medical care in urban medical centers in the early 20th century (IOM, 2001).

The Brown vs. Topeka Board of Education decision in 1954, declaring that segregated schools are not equal, is the landmark decision leading to the desegregation of academic facilities. This has undoubtedly had a significant impact on public policy regarding medical education. Still, today, partially as a result of this history of discrimination, minority physicians make up a smaller percentage of the medical workforce as compared to their population percentage. (See Chapter 8 for a discussion of the concept of affirmative action.) Of the 125 accredited medical schools and 20 accredited schools of Osteopathic medicine in the U.S., only four historically Black programs remain today: Howard University

College of Medicine, Washington, DC; Meherry Medical College, Nashville, TN; Charles R. Drew University of Medicine and Science, Los Angeles, CA; and Morehouse School of Medicine, Atlanta, GA (American Association of Medical Schools, n.d.).

The Civil Rights Act of 1964, the Voting Rights Act of 1965, and the Fair Housing Act of 1968 made it impossible to legally segregate or discriminate on the basis of race across employment, housing, or in public locations. The advent of Medicare in 1965 and the implementation of Medicare non-discrimination provisions specifically attempted to eliminate discrimination within hospitals that accepted Medicare payments. If hospitals wished to receive Medicare reimbursement, they would have to demonstrate no discrimination in the provision of health care based on race. Hospitals were no longer able to segregate racial and ethnic minorities to separate wards of hospitals or inferior levels of care. As a result, the 70 Black-only hospitals in this country either closed or merged with other major medical centers. Ironically, this sometimes caused access problems to those minorities in communities where a health center was eliminated (IOM, 2001).

The historical and personal experiences of Black people within the health care system, including a history of unequal access and mistreatment, is exemplified by what has become known as the Tuskegee Experiment. From the period of 1937-1972, the U.S. Public Health Service involved African American men in research on syphilis. During the 40 years of this experiment, many illiterate African American men, who were often unaware that they even had syphilis, were denied access to appropriate and effective medical treatment. The goal of this research was to provide information regarding the advanced stages of syphilis, which includes dementia, damage to the heart and other vital organs, blindness, and eventual death. By the end of this experiment, a significant number of men had died, infected their wives, or passed on syphilis to their children congenitally. The experiment was finally brought to public attention in 1972, when a writer from The Associated Press, Jean Heller, broke the story of the Tuskegee Experiment in the *Washington Star* (Brunner, n.d.).

As awareness grew of this blight on the medical system, people of color learned to distrust health practitioners of a different race. This feeling of distrust was influenced both by the treatment received in segregated hospitals and doctors offices, and by the research practices exemplified by Tuskegee. Even today, this history has an impact on how African American patients perceive American society and health care providers, and whether they are willing to participate in health-related research (Brandon, Isaac, & LaVeist, 2005). Mistrust has lent to decreased compliance and, at times, lack of seeking preventative care. Distrust of health care practitioners and persistent, although not legal, de facto segregation of minorities continues today and are felt to play a significant role in health disparities (Doescher, Saver, Franks, & Fiscella, 2000; Hughes & Bashi, 1997; Kinder & Mendelberg, 1995; Petersen, 2002).

It is worthy to remember that, up to the Civil Rights movement of the 1960s and 1970s, socially sanctioned segregation and the remnants of Jim Crow public codes not only occurred within health facilities and the health professions, but also in the society at large. Discrimination in Federal housing policies, local housing practices, mortgage lending, and deed restrictions led to overt and covert exclusion of minorities, relegating them to less desirable living situations. Those individuals who live in segregated environments are more often exposed to poor housing conditions and environmental toxins, limited access to employment, and limited access to high-quality education (Alba & Logan, 1993; Atrash & Hunter, 2005; Williams, 1999). Certainly it is arguable that these conditions continue to exist and have a profound impact on health.

In more recent decades, some improvements have been made in the realm of the health of minority patients as a result of Federal policy and legislation. The Civil Rights movement undoubtedly had an impact on issues surrounding unequal treatment, and overall mortality rates have declined substantially for minority individuals over the last 100 years.

Nevertheless, progress has been viewed as inadequate. In 1984, Margaret Heckler, the Secretary of the HHS, established a task force to evaluate the extent of health disparities among individuals of different races and ethnicities in the U.S. The task force released a ten-volume report in 1985 documenting that, although liberated in 1865 and granted citizenship and the right to vote by the 14th and 15th amendments of the Bill of Rights, health disparities among Black, Native American, non-Hispanic White, and Asian/Pacific Islander people are considerable. The report attributed that an excess of 60,000 deaths per year were a result of disparities in health (Gamble & Stone, 2006).

As a result of this report, the Office of Minority Health (OMH), was established under the HHS and was responsible for the implementation of the task force's recommendations in addition to coordination of activities related to addressing health disparities (Gamble & Stone, 2006). Five years later, the NIH established their own Office of Research on Minority Health to promote and support increased research in the area of health disparities. As a result of increased funding and attention to the elimination of health disparities, the decade of the 1990s brought about a deluge of literature on health disparities and the variables that contribute to it.

Concerned over the level of health disparities and their possible impact on the health system, Congress asked the IOM to assess health care quality, access, and use by racial and ethnic minorities in the U.S. in 1999. In response, the IOM released the seminal report called "Unequal Treatment: Confronting Racial and Ethnic Disparities in Healthcare." In 2000, the Minority Health and Health Disparities Research and Education Act of 2000 (P.L. 106-525) established the National Center on Minority Health and Health Disparities (NCMHD) which promotes minority health and leads and coordinates efforts to reduce and ultimately eliminate health disparities (NCMHD, n.d.).

As a result, the field of health disparities has become an area of focus for many researchers. In December 2003, the Agency for Healthcare Research and Quality (AHRQ) released a report on the status of health of minorities in this country entitled "National Health Disparities Report," which drew specific attention to the need for more research in this field (Agency for Healthcare Research and Quality, 2004). Policymakers and entrepreneurs have also realized the effect these disparities have on the health of communities as a whole, and HHS asserts that community and environment play a significant role in health (HHS, 2000).

Identification of health disparities and an agenda to eliminate them continues to be at the forefront of health policy in this country today. Recent "Healthy People" initiatives, have called for a decrease in health disparities by the end of the decade. This document specifically calls on physicians to increase the amount of prevention in their practice, demands communities to enact health-promoting policies into practice in schools and worksites, and encourages scientists to continue with health-improving research to promote equality in health care and the elimination of health disparities (HHS, 2000; Kosoko-Lasaki, Cook, & O'Brien, 2009). Physical therapists can contribute to these goals by adding a focus on community and prevention in their own practice.

OVERVIEW OF GENERAL HEALTH DISPARITIES

Over the past two decades, multiple research studies have provided evidence that health disparities exist across all ages (disparities in asthma treatment in children and cancer in older adults) (Chu, Miller, & Springfield, 2007; Shields, Comstock, & Weiss, 2004), throughout all types of illnesses (diabetes mellitus, coronary artery disease, cancer) (Allen & Szanton, 2005; American Cancer Society [ACS], 2008; Heisler, Smith, Hayward, Krein, & Kerr, 2003; Karter et al., 2002; Lichtman, Krumholz, Wang, Radford, & Brass, 2002), in lab tests (LDL and cholesterol tests) (Safford et al., 2003), in screening procedures (mammogram and Pap tests) (Masi, Blackman, & Peek, 2007; McDougall, Madeleine, Daling, & Li, 2007) and in the availability of surgical procedures (cardiac catheterization and lower extremity bypass procedures) (Hirsch et al., 2001; Kressin & Peterson, 2001).

Health disparities have been found in diseases that effect both women and men, such as breast cancer and prostate cancer, respectively (Cooperberg et al., 2003; Jatoi et al., 2003; Shavers et al., 2004), and disparities are seen in medical procedures that affect the health of populations as a whole, such as influenza immunization for high-risk populations (Egede & Zheng, 2003). In addition, disparities are pervasive among individuals who have health insurance as well as among the uninsured, individuals of high socioeconomic status and low socioeconomic status (Kaplan & Keil, 1993), and individuals in urban and rural geographic locations (Keil & Saunders, 1991) regardless of their socioeconomic status.

DISPARITIES IN PREVALENCE OF DISEASE

Heart disease, cancer, stroke, and diabetes are the leading killers of all individuals, but they are significantly more prevalent among minorities and are the leading causes of death among African Americans. Many correctly argue that most of these diseases and their related disparities are preventable. For example, mortality rates from heart disease are 40% higher for African Americans than non-Hispanic Whites. The death rate from all cancers is 30% higher for African Americans than non-Hispanic Whites, with prostate cancer death rates among African American men being almost double (ACS, 2008; Gamble & Stone, 2006). For each of these chronic disease processes, the disparity between African Americans and non-Hispanic Whites continues to widen (Ferguson et al., 1998; Heisler et al., 2003; Jatoi et al., 2003; Jones et al., 2000; Keil et al., 1993; Lichtman et al., 2002; Ward et al., 2004; Williams & Jackson, 2005).

DISPARITIES IN MEDICAL INTERVENTIONS

Access to preventative medical interventions improves overall health. Yet significant disparities in access to preventative care in the form of medical interventions are prevalent throughout the literature. Carotid endartarectomies, which can prevent transient ischemic attacks and strokes, were performed nearly four times more frequently in Whites than in Blacks, despite twice the incidence of stroke in the latter (Brothers, Robison, Sutherland, & Elliott, 1997). Studies have found that minority patients are much less likely to receive a multitude of preventative vascular screenings and procedures (Huber et al., 1999; Oddone, Petersen, Weinberger, Freedman, & Kressin, 2002; Selby et al., 1996). In the case of lower extremity peripheral arterial disease, minorities are less likely to receive limb-sparing procedures, such as angioplasty and lower extremity bypass (Brothers et al., 1997; Feinglass, Rucker-Whitaker, Lindquist, McCarthy, & Pearce, 2005; Guadagnoli, Ayanian, Gibbons, McNeil, & LoGerfo, 1995; Rucker-Whitaker, Feinglass, & Pearce, 2003). Minorities are also less likely to receive invasive cardiovascular procedures, such as cardiac catheterization, coronary angioplasty, or coronary artery bypass grafting when compared with non-Hispanic Whites (J. Chen, Rathore, Radford, Wang, & Krumholz, 2001; Conigliaro et al., 2000; Ibrahim et al., 2003; Kressin & Petersen, 2001; Schulman et al., 1999; Whittle, Conigliaro, Good, & Lofgren, 1993). Whether it is an inability to physically access care, be referred appropriately by their physician, or the physician's unwillingness, for whatever reason, to do the procedure, there is a chasm between the White and minority races with regard to interventional procedures and preventative care (see Chapter 8).

DISPARITIES IN INSURANCE STATUS

Being among the working poor or being undocumented often leads to lack of health insurance. About one-third, and the largest subgroup among the approximately 46 million people in the U.S. who do not have insurance, is the Hispanic population (U.S. Census Bureau, 2008a). About 41% of Mexican Americans do not have health insurance, the highest percent of all subcultures. African Americans are almost twice as likely as non-Hispanic Whites to be uninsured (Gamble & Stone, 2006). The lack of insurance, in addition to variables such as educational attainment, socioeconomic status, and trust of the health care system, may contribute to the disparities found in medical interventions between individuals of different races and ethnicities.

DISPARITIES IN OUTCOMES

Disparities in health care outcomes exist between individuals of different groups. According to the Center for Disease Control, infant mortality for African Americans is more than twice the infant mortality of the non-Hispanic White population. Infant mortality for babies born to Hawaiian, Puerto Rican, and American Indian mothers is also substantially higher than that of non-Hispanic Whites (Matthews & MacDorman, 2008). In addition, although overall life expectancy has improved for the minority patient over the last 100 years, the life expectancy of the non-Hispanic White ethnicity is significantly higher than that of the African American population (National Center for Health Statistics, 2007). Research has also linked higher infant mortality rates to poverty, where African Americans and other minority groups significantly outnumber non-Hispanic Whites (M. Sims, T. L. Sims, & Bruce, 2007).

With regard to disparities in outcomes of specific disease processes, peripheral vascular disease and diabetes are chronic conditions that can result in amputation because of damage to the vascular system. Utilization of procedures that promote revascularization and prevention of amputation varies. Although it is well known that vascular disease, including lower extremity peripheral vascular disease and cardiovascular disease, occur at a substantially higher rate in minorities (Ayanian, 1993; Burke et al., 1995; Keil et al., 1993), the incidence of amputation and mortality related to vascular diseases among racial and ethnic groups is significantly greater than for non-Hispanic Whites in the U.S. (Dillingham, Pezzin, & Shore, 2005; Ephraim, Dillingham, Sector, Pezzin, & Mackenzie, 2003; Gornick et al., 1996; Tentolouris, Al-Sabbagh, Walker, Boulton, & Jude, 2004).

REHABILITATION/PHYSICAL THERAPY SERVICES AND HEALTH DISPARITIES

Physical therapists play a major role in the health of individuals and society. Although the literature is replete with articles citing health disparities among minority populations, references specific to physical therapy and minority health disparities are difficult to find at the present time. To gain an understanding of how the physical therapy profession might increase its involvement in health disparities research, an evaluation of health disparities specific to the practice of physical therapy is helpful. Physical therapists can evaluate health disparities from the perspective of access, referral patterns, prevention, interventions, and outcomes. Representative studies are summarized below as they relate to the practice of physical therapy. Each one demonstrates evidence of health disparities in areas closely related to physical therapy practice.

DISPARITIES IN REFERRAL TO PHYSICAL REHABILITATION SERVICES

The literature suggests that inequities exist in referral to physical, occupational, and cardiac rehabilitation. Research has found that Medicare patients who are of the White race were more likely to receive physical and occupational therapist services than non-White Medicare patients, even when controlling for functional status and diagnosis (Mayer-Oaks et al., 1992). In another study, Allen, Scott, Stewart, and Young (2004) looked at referrals to cardiac rehabilitation in 253 women who had undergone percutaneous coronary intervention, coronary artery bypass surgery, or a myocardial infarction without intervention. They found that African American women were significantly less likely to receive a referral or to enroll in cardiac rehabilitation, even though the literature supports greater levels of functional disability and higher rates of morbidity and mortality from cardiac disease among minority individuals. These studies suggest the disparity in use of or access to physical and occupational therapist services between minorities and non-minorities and the need for further evaluation.

DISPARITIES IN EVIDENCE OF PREVENTION PRACTICE

Physical therapists have a role in the prevention of chronic diseases such as diabetes and intervene to promote healthy behaviors and practices that may prevent complications. Jiang, Andrews, Stryer, and Friedman (2005) used a dataset to study the hospital admission patterns of a population of patients with diabetes. They found that individuals of a Black or Hispanic race were more likely to experience hospital readmissions for potentially preventable diabetic complications.

DISPARITIES IN PHYSICAL THERAPY INTERVENTION

Research has evaluated the intensity of physical and occupational therapy intervention in Medicare patients with acute hip fractures. By using the American Hospital Association database and calculating the mean number of physical and occupational therapy sessions, the researchers determined that 65% of African American patients and 43% of non-Hispanic White patients received low intensity physical therapist intervention, a statistically significant difference (Hoenig, Rubenstein, & Kahn, 1996). In other words, African Americans were 1.5 times more likely to receive lower intensity physical and occupational therapy when compared to non-Hispanic White patients. Again, this disparity in intensity of services warrants further investigation.

With regard to length of stay, which can be a reflection of quality of care, Lin and Kaplan (2004) compared the length of stay for individuals of varying demographic characteristics who received inpatient rehabilitation following hip or knee arthroplasty. They found that certain patient variables lead to a longer length of stay in the acute rehabilitation environment. The variables evaluated included Black race, indication for surgery, number of co-morbid illnesses, and unmarried marital status. The findings of this research suggest that individuals who are Black might be given the opportunity for knee replacement later in their disease process, thus negatively influencing their outcomes (Lin & Kaplan, 2004). This may also, however, be a reflection of disparities in rehabilitation services provided to minorities within the rehabilitation facilities.

DISPARITIES IN PHYSICAL THERAPY-RELATED OUTCOMES

Although access, prevention, and intervention are areas that would benefit from further scrutiny, most health disparities research in rehabilitation focuses on patient outcomes following rehabilitation. Even when access is considered to be equal, a substantial amount of literature supports health disparities in outcomes, length of stay, and discharge destination based on an individual's race or ethnicity across a variety of conditions such as stroke, arthroplastic surgery, spinal cord injury, and traumatic brain injury.

Disparities in outcome have been found among patients having suffered a stroke who subsequently attended acute inpatient rehabilitation. Stineman et al. (2001) compared rehabilitation outcomes and lengths of stay in the Veterans Administration (VA) health system for 55,438 patients with a stroke diagnosis and found that minority patients experience longer lengths of stay. In addition, individuals of a Black race were found to have lower average functional independence measure (FIM) scores with greater levels of disability at discharge.

In a separate study of functional outcomes for stroke patients who participated in inpatient rehabilitation, although researchers found no differences in the number of interactions or treatment contact hours between individuals of a different race with regard to their time spent in therapy, individuals of a Black race demonstrated a much slower recovery of function than White patients. This was found to continue over the course of the first year following cerebral vascular accident (Horner, Swanson, Bosworth, & Matchar, 2003).

Health disparities in rehabilitation outcomes with a primary focus on employment status and quality of life measures after spinal cord injury have been evaluated in the literature. Researchers have found a difference between career opportunities and finances following injury and current employment rates in minority populations when compared with non-Hispanic Whites. For example, one cohort of participants reflected employment rates after injury of 58% and 47% for Caucasian females and males, respectively, while both minority female and male rates were lower, 38% and 31%, respectively. The disparities in employment rates were found to be consistent even when contributing variables such as level of injury, employment status prior to injury, and level of education were controlled (Krause, Sternberg, Maides, & Lottes, 1998).

In a similar study, Krause, Devivo, and Jackson (2004) used the Model Spinal Cord Injury System to evaluate the impact of health status, economic risk factors, and community integration on mortality following spinal cord injury. The authors found that demographic factors and community reintegration appear to influence mortality following spinal cord injury. In addition, the authors found a significant health disparity in post-injury mortality: Black people experience higher mortality than any other race immediately following spinal cord injury.

Hart, Whyte, Polansky, Kersey-Matusiak, and Fidler-Sheppard (2005) conducted a study with persons who had moderate to severe brain injury. Using four different objective measures (the Community Integration Questionnaire, Aggression and Depression Subscales of Neurobehavioral Functioning Inventory-Revised, Satisfaction With Life Scale, and other questions on demographic and social status), the researchers evaluated a group of 94 individuals with moderate to severe head injury from initial onset of injury to one year follow-up. This study was designed to determine whether pre-injury differences between non-Hispanic White and Black individuals had an impact on outcomes following rehabilitation and community reintegration. Even though individuals of a Black race had a shorter period of post-traumatic amnesia, a faster ability to follow commands, and higher Glasgow Coma Scale scores on admission, they were found to have more difficulty with social integration and experienced lower income than individuals of a non-Hispanic White race at one year post-injury (Hart et al., 2005). Because of the direct role physical therapists play in community reintegration following moderate to severe head injury and spinal cord injury, these findings are troublesome and should lead therapists to reflect upon the possibility of racial disparities in treatment interventions performed during community reintegration and rehabilitation.

VARIABLES CONTRIBUTING TO DISPARITIES

LaVeist (2005) addresses the determinants of health disparities by three distinct categories: socio-environmental, psychosocial/behavioral, and bio-physiological. These categories illustrate the interweaving of social, institutional, provider, and individual level contributions to this phenomenon. No one variable is directly or solely responsible for the presence of health disparities, and defining a cause of health disparities is very complex. LaVeist asserts that a difference in the level of stress, environmental exposures, segregation, and racism have all played a pivotal contributing role. Each of these variables creates an environmental effect that directly impacts the health of minorities.

The IOM evaluates health disparities by grouping confounding variables into three separate categories (Smedley et al., 2002). These categories include patient level variables, health care system variables, and provider level variables. Examples of patient level variables include poor adherence, mistrust, and lack of understanding of provider instructions. Health care system variables could be geographic location and time constraints of providers. Provider level variables include bias, stereotyping, and clinical uncertainty of the physician or health care provider (IOM, 2001).

This portion of the chapter will present bio-cultural, societal, institutional, provider, and individual level variables that contribute to health disparities. It is clear that these variables interact with each other. None alone is likely to be solely responsible for health care disparities. The relative influence of each of these individually remains a mystery. Cultural factors intersect with each of the variables.

BIO-CULTURAL ECOLOGY AND HEALTH DISPARITIES

Because U.S. history is riddled with long standing inequality with regard to the health and social status of minorities, many researchers have looked for genetic differences that could provide a biological definition for this variation. Historical research on minority health (primarily conducted prior to the 20th century) sometimes illustrated an inherent biological inferiority in those of a minority race or ethnicity. Studies reported that minorities were "inherently diseased" and physicians often asserted that minorities had "lack of fitness for freedom and citizenship" (Braun, 2002). A famous text published in the late 19th century titled *Race Traits and Tendencies of the American Negro* speaks specifically to the perception of inferiority among individuals of the Black race during this time period (Gamble & Stone, 2006). Unfortunately, many of these studies were biased, more to accomplish a political and social agenda than to express the truth about the biological difference in race.

Bio-cultural ecology, which includes the effect of biological variation in skin color, heredity, genetics, and drug metabolism (Purnell & Paulanka, 2003) on health could, in theory, contribute to health disparities. Decoding of the human genome has led to a multitude of research that supports the link between genes and disease. A relevant example of this link would include the BRCA gene and breast cancer (Noruzinia, Coupier, & Pujol, 2005). A number of studies are investigating the prevalence and influence of the BRCA gene in specific populations including Ashkenazi Jews (Levy-Lahad et al., 1997), Russians (Tereschenko, Basham, Ponder, & Pharoah, 2002), Japanese (Ikeda et al., 2000), and Hispanics (Weitzel et al., 2007). These genetic links have led many researchers to be interested in investigating whether health disparities in race or ethnicities are related to a genetic predisposition to a disease or greater severity of disease. For example, recent findings have shown that Black women are more likely to present with a more aggressive cancer and at younger ages (Newman, Bunner, et al., 2002; Newman, Mason, et al., 2002; Newman et al., 2006).

Recent advances in pharmacogenomics and ethnic psychopharmacy demonstrate that race and ethnicity, on some occasions, have been linked to drug performance, and yet accommodations are often not made in prescriptive doses (Campinha-Bacote, 2007; Harty, Johnson, & Power, 2006; Kahn, 2006). For example, African American women have been shown to absorb calcium more efficiently than people with lighter skin (Sadler & Huff, 2007). Likewise, differences in methotrexate (often prescribed for rheumatoid arthritis) toxicity exist between Caucasian and African American patients (Ranganathan et al., 2008). In addition, the recent (although controversial) approval of the heart failure regimen BiDil illustrates the interest of the Food and Drug Administration in evaluating the impact of race on drug performance (Bibbins-Domingo & Fernandz, 2007). BiDil was found to be significantly more effective than standard therapy in the African American Heart Failure Trial (A-HeFT), although not effective for White people (Taylor et al., 2004). The biological explanation for this finding is the increased level of nitric oxide in Black people with heart failure (Bibbins-Domingo & Fernandez, 2007). Currently, variability in response to cardiovascular drugs and cardiovascular pharmacogenomics is being studied (El Desoky, Derendorf, & Klotz, 2006).

At present, no statistically significant research exists to provide a solid link between the genes or genetic composition solely on the basis of race, even though significant disparities in the previously mentioned differences in drug performance and disease presence exist. For example, even if genetic composition is identical, phenotype (how genes express themselves) is not the same as genotype, thus indicating that sociological issues, such as elevated stress or decreased access to health care, could impact how disease expresses itself, even among genetically identical individuals, such as twins.

The IOM echoes this belief by declaring race to be a social construct, not a biological one (IOM, 2001) and the American Anthropological Association (AAA) asserts that social beliefs have distorted the true impact of a person's skin color (AAA, 1999). Although skin color has resulted in segregation and division in society, genetics does not provide an absolute explanation for these differences (Braun, 2002). And although the debate regarding race and ethnicity continues in a social context today, the consensus amongst most geneticists and scientists is that race is a social and not biological construct (Braun, 2002; Foster & Sharp, 2002).

Still, the current evidence of differences in pharmacogenomics and the role of genes in health are compelling. As a result, the National Institutes of Health (NIH) announced the formation of the NIH Intramural Center for Genomics and Health Disparities (NICGHD) in March of 2008. By using a genomics approach, this center's main focus will be to act as a catalyst for population and epidemiological research on the interaction of genes and disease and environment. The hope is to optimize the knowledge of genomics to help eliminate health disparities in areas such as obesity, diabetes, and hypertension (NIH, 2008). Future research stands to provide a wealth of knowledge on the link between genetics and disparities in health, but the differences remain to be seen.

SOCIETAL CAUSES OF HEALTH DISPARITIES

Link and Phelan (2002) approach health disparities from the "fundamental social causes" approach. These researchers assert that sociological ideology and constructs have a direct effect on a person's health status. They argue that the ability to avoid disease is not based on a person's biological status, but rather his or her available resources to avoid that disease (such as money, power, prestige, and beneficial social connections). Accordingly, if we do not address how society and community impact health, we will be unable to increase access, affordability, or health-enhancing behavior.

Social issues such as socioeconomic status influence health and contribute to health disparities on multiple levels (see Chapters 4 and 7). Lower socioeconomic status has been related to health disparities through its influence on physician decision making (Bird & Bogart, 2001; vanRyn & Burke, 2000), access to preventative care (Lurie & Dubowitz, 2007), and influence on health risk behaviors (Lantz et al., 2001). In addition, many of the risk factors for vascular disease, such as high body mass index (BMI), elevated blood pressure, and increased cortisol levels, have been found to be significantly higher among individuals of a lower socioeconomic status (E. Chen & Paterson, 2006). It is conceivable that these same issues, especially high-risk behaviors and decreased access to preventative care, also negatively influence the prevention of chronic cardiovascular diseases. This could lend to higher rates of peripheral vascular disease, cardiovascular disease, hypertension, or diabetes, as well as increased number of higher-level amputations.

In addition, educational attainment, which closely links with socioeconomic status, is associated with health status and overall mortality (Jemal et al., 2008). In a recent study of oral health, those with lower educational attainment had more missing teeth in the older age bracket when compared to individuals of higher educational attainment (Paulander, Axelsson, & Lindhe, 2003). Individuals of lower educational attainment are also at greater risk of participation in adverse health behaviors, such as increased alcohol consumption (Gilman et al., 2008), shorter sleep duration (Stamatakis, Kaplan, & Roberts, 2007), and decreased levels of physical activity (Cassetta, Boden-Albala, Sciacca, & Giardina, 2007). Pincus and Callahan (1994) also highlight the increased prevalence of diseases such as hypertension, arthritis, heart disease, back pain, and diabetes associated with lower levels of educational attainment in their review of over 105 journal articles. Educational attainment of minorities is significantly lower than non-Hispanic Whites (U.S. Census Bureau, 2008b) and must be addressed to diminish health disparities and improve the health status of people of color.

Williams and Rucker (2000) support the idea that racial inequities in health should be evaluated from the perspective of racial inequities in social institutions. Racism, for example, is a societal ideology by which categorization of an individual creates a position of subordination of individuals of a minority race. This racial categorization involves a scale in which the non-Hispanic White race is ranked at the top and the Black race at the bottom (Williams, 1999) (see Chapter 8). Williams discusses the impact of racial categories in the absence of biological difference between people of different skin color. For example, minority race has been linked to low-income, greater unemployment, increased poverty, and decreased educational attainment even though there is no biological basis for these social categories (Kinder & Mendelberg, 1995; Williams, 1998).

The reciprocal effect of community on health and health on community creates a reinforcing cycle. The existence of health disparities has a negative effect on society, yet societal structure and ideology stimulate health disparities. The cycle of poor health leading to limited opportunity creates an environment for health disparities and reduced expectations for a long, healthy, and productive life (Bell & Standish, 2005). This higher rate of disease has an impact on a minority individual's ability to participate in health promoting behaviors and contributes to more absenteeism from work and school. In a segregated society, more people of color remain stuck in a cycle that leads them to higher rates of disease, hospitalization, and death (Bell & Standish).

In recognition of the importance of social determinants on health, the 2008 World Health Assembly (of the World Health Organization [WHO]) has recommended three overarching recommendations for closing the health disparities gap (WHO, 2008):

1. Improve daily living conditions, including the circumstances in which people are born, grow, live, work, and age

2. Tackle the inequitable distribution of power, money and resources—the structural drivers of those conditions—globally, nationally, and locally

3. Measure and understand the problem and assess the impact of action

THE PROVIDER RELATIONSHIP TO HEALTH DISPARITIES

Racism, or the ordering of individuals based on race and ethnicity, could be having an impact on provider decision making (IOM, 2001; Smedley et al., 2002). Many individuals may be unconscious of their biases or discrimination toward individuals of different races or ethnicities, but this can still impact practice decisions and outcomes (Schulman et al., 1999; van Ryn & Burke, 2000; van Ryn & Fu, 2003; Williams & Rucker, 2000). Although an individual may like to think of themselves as "color blind," most individuals have preconceived notions about an individual prior to meeting or speaking with them. For example, research has shown that physicians often overestimate levels of literacy, especially among minority patients (Kelly & Haidet, 2007). This finding could directly influence the patient's ability to comply with the medical regimen prescribed. Furthermore, Lopez-Quintero, Crum, and Neumark (2006) found that patients of a minority race were found to be significantly less likely to report receiving smoking cessation counseling from their physician. An unwillingness or inability to provide health education and communicate in a culturally sensitive manner could also be negatively influencing patient perception of care (Collins, Clark, Petersen, & Kressin, 2002; Gordon, Street, Sharf, Kelly, & Souchek, 2006; Johnson, Saha, Arbelaez, Beach, & Cooper, 2004) (see Chapter 9).

INDIVIDUAL LEVEL VARIABLES THAT IMPACT HEALTH DISPARITIES

Patient level variables influence health disparities. For example, individuals of the Black race participate to a greater extent in adverse health risk behaviors, demonstrate decreased compliance with regard to medical treatment, and have concerns about their ability to trust medical providers (Doescher et al., 2000; Halpern et al., 2004; Lantz et al., 2001). Each of these factors can influence the inequality in health care outcomes noted in the literature and should be considered when determining interventions that will reduce health disparities.

The individual brings a culture, a set of beliefs, a communication style, and patterns of behaviors that will influence the degree to which he or she will seek care through the dominant health care system or will comply with the dominant health care recommendations. Differences in health care beliefs and practices may be a large reason why an individual or cultural group may not seek or comply with typical medical practices, including physical therapy. If the health care system is aligned with the individual's cultural beliefs, the individual is more likely to accept, trust, and adhere to health care practitioner recommendations. On the other hand, an individual's health beliefs and preferred health care practices may clash with the institution or provider of health care (Kleinman, 1981). Cultural misalignments between individuals, providers, institutions, and society can contribute to mistrust, miscommunication, and other mismatches that may exacerbate health disparities. Appropriate consideration of culture has the potential to overcome cultural barriers and bridge gaps that otherwise might lead to disparate health care.

Sometimes a lack of trust or comfort with a physician of a different race emerges as an issue with patient adherence (Copeland, Scholle, & Binko, 2003; LaVeist & Carroll, 2002). Unfortunately, the opportunity to access treatment from a physician or physical therapist of minority race is more limited when compared to physicians who are White. According to data from the American Physical Therapy Association (APTA) survey of the profession, the profession of physical therapy continues to consist of an overwhelming number of non-Hispanic White individuals, rating over 91% for each year since 1999 (see Table 1-2 on p. 16). This provides the realization of how difficult it would be for people of color to find a physical therapy practitioner who is of a similar ethnic background.

Now that the extent of health disparities across multiple disciplines has been established, the current focus of NIH research is on the fundamental causes of health disparities. The effort has resulted in the establishment of eight Centers for Population Health and Health Disparities (CPPHD), which were launched in September of 2003. These CPPHDs focus on research that evaluates a combination of population, social, biological, behavioral, and clinical models (Warnecke et al., 2008). The use of a population approach from a public health perspective has been found to be more successful than solely targeting at-risk individuals (Frohlich & Potvin, 2008).

CONCLUSION

THE INSTITUTIONAL RESPONSIBILITY AND HEALTH DISPARITIES

Health care institutions can move toward the elimination of health care disparities by demonstrating a commitment to the provision of culturally competent care and to building healthy relationships with the communities they serve. An institution can make a positive impact on health disparities by identifying the communities within geographic reach of service and exploring their health care needs and desires, including the existing disparities in health care, learning about the community's cultural beliefs and preferred health care practices, and seeking to identify and overcome potential barriers to care (Romeo, 2007). It can demonstrate a commitment to cultural competency by having training for health care providers and staff (Lattanzi & Purnell, 2006). The institution can also demonstrate its dedication to the elimination of health care disparities by observing the HHS National Standards for Culturally and Linguistically Appropriate Services (CLAS) (2001) with all clientele, not only those at high risk (see Chapter 12).

THE PHYSICAL THERAPIST'S RESPONSIBILITY AND HEALTH DISPARITIES

Evidence in the literature supports the presence of health disparities in medical screening, intervention, access, and outcomes in patients who have actively participated in rehabilitation programs, as well as with patients who have diagnoses that predispose them to interaction with physical therapists. By reflecting on the current literature and understanding the opportunities available for further research, there are many areas where physical therapists can initiate research agendas.

The APTA has charged physical therapists with the responsibility of contribution to the elimination of health disparities in their own practices. Guided by RC 41-03 (2005), the APTA has developed strategies and guidelines for identifying and addressing racial and ethnic disparities in access to, utilization of, and outcomes associated with physical therapy services, including disparities in community reintegration that have been identified. They are beginning the process of primary data collection, such as measuring outcomes that include race and ethnicity, to allow for analysis of health disparities in the realm of physical therapy. The APTA has committed itself to making progress toward the elimination of health disparities in our profession.

The culture of the individual patient, physical therapist, physical therapy institution, and society contribute to the existence of health and health care disparities. When cultures clash consciously or unconsciously, overtly or subtly, disparities in health are likely to exacerbate. When physical therapy providers and institutions are able to identify or anticipate the potential clashes and seek ways to overcome potential cultural barriers, whether in the form of access to a minority practitioner, self-reflection and correction of stereotype and bias, or physical ability to access physical therapy, the profession moves toward more culturally congruent care and the elimination of health disparities.

As a physical therapist moves toward culturally competent care with clients, it should enhance the chance that the physical therapy program will have a positive impact on the health and wellness of the client and possibly minimize health disparities. No individual or institution can achieve perfection, but an understanding of the issues can lead to improved interactions with patients as well as other health care providers.

Cultural competence is a step in the right direction, but the challenge is multi-faceted and embedded in historical and societal contexts. Recognition, understanding, and acceptance of these contexts will not only assist the health care provider in identifying his or her own conscious or subconscious contributions to health disparities, but it will also provide a framework by which therapists can identify institutional and society barriers within their own institutions that may be contributing to adverse or unequal outcomes in their practices. Focusing on diminishing health disparities will assist with attaining the ultimate goal of optimal care for every individual who seeks intervention or treatment from the physical therapist.

RESOURCES SPECIFIC TO ADDRESSING HEALTH DISPARITIES

- America's Health Insurance Plans (AHIP) and Cultural Competency has a number of resources including the "Collection and Use of Race and Ethnicity Data for Quality Improvement—2006 AHIP-RWJF Survey of Health Insurance Plans: Issue Brief" and "AHIP's Data as Building Blocks for Change: A Data Collection Toolkit for Health Insurance Plans/Health Care Organizations." They also offer "Quality Interactions" courses for physicians, nurses, and case managers (cross cultural training courses.): http://www.ahip.org/content/default.aspx?docid=10761

- MEDLINEplus Health Information provides information about population groups: http://www.nlm.nih.gov/medlineplus/populationgroups.html

- National Network of Libraries of Medicine has extensive information related to minority health concerns. It includes racial/ethnic group health-related links, language resources including a link to order National Institutes of Health publications in languages other than English, and information: http://nnlm.gov/mcr/resources/community/minority.html

- The Hopkins Center for Health Disparities Solutions (HCHDS) is committed to the elimination of health disparities and provides resources, training, and research to that end. The Center is the recipient of a 5-year grant from the National Center on Minority Health and Health Disparities of the National Institutes of Health: http://www.jhsph.edu/healthdisparities/index.html

REFLECTION QUESTIONS

✔ *Have you recognized the concept of health disparity in your personal or professional life?*

✔ *Do you feel that you have a personal or professional responsibility to work toward greater "health equity" in the U.S.?*

✔ *What do you think are the most important reasons for health disparities in the U.S.?*

✔ *Identify one action you personally can take to minimize health disparities in this country.*

✔ *Identify one action your practice environment can take to minimize health disparities in your professional life.*

REFERENCES

Agency for Healthcare Research and Quality. (2004). *National healthcare disparities report* (No. 05-0014). Rockville, MD: Author.

Alba, R. D., & Logan, J. R. (1993). Minority proximity to Whites in suburbs: An individual-level analysis of segregation. *American Journal of Sociology, 98*(6), 1388-1427.

Allen, J., Scott, L. B., Stewart, K. J., & Young, D. R. (2004). Disparities in women's referral to and enrollment in outpatient cardiac rehabilitation. *Journal of General Internal Medicine, 19*(7), 747-753.

Allen, J., & Szanton, S. (2005). Gender, ethnicity, and cardiovascular disease. *Journal of Cardiovascular Nursing, 20*(1), 1-6.

American Anthropological Association. (1999). AAA statement on race. *American Anthropologist, 100*(3), 712-713.

American Association of Medical Schools. (n.d.). Medical schools. Retrieved June 14, 2006, from http://www.aamc.org/medicalschools.htm

American Cancer Society. (2008). Cancer facts & figures 2008. Atlanta, GA: Author. Retrieved March 17, 2008, from http://www.cancer.org/downloads/STT/2008CAFFfinalsecured.pdf

American Physical Therapy Association. (2005). RC 41-03 racial and ethnic disparities in health care. Retrieved September 23, 2009, from http://www.apta.org/AM/Template.cfm?Section=Home&Template=/CM/ContentDisplay.cfm&ContentID=37522

American Physical Therapy Association (2007). APTA survey of profession demographic characteristics. Retrieved March 3, 2008, from http://www.apta.org/AM/Template.cfm?Section=Surveys_and_Stats1&Template=/MembersOnly.cfm&ContentID=46077

Atrash, H. K., & Hunter, M. D. (2005). Health disparities in the United States: A continuing challenge. In D. Satcher & R. J. Pamies (Eds.), *Multicultural medicine and health disparities* (pp. 3-31). New York, NY: McGraw-Hill.

Ayanian, J. Z. (1993). Heart disease in Black and White. *New England Journal of Medicine, 329*(9), 656-658.

Bell, J., & Standish, M. (2005). Communities and health policy: A pathway for change. *Health Affairs, 24*(2), 339-342.

Bibbins-Domingo, K., & Fernandez, A. (2007). BiDil for heart failure in Black patients: Implications of the U.S. Food and Drug Administration approval. *Annals of Internal Medicine, 146*(1), 52-56.

Bird, S. T., & Bogart, L. M. (2001). Perceived race-based and socioeconomic status (SES)-based discrimination in interactions with health care providers. *Ethnicity and Disease, 11*(3), 554-563.

Black, A., Hopkins, J., Binker, M. J., Frankel, R. P., Jr., Regenhardt, C. E., Brick, C., et al. (Eds.). (2003). Jim Crow laws. In *Teaching Eleanor Roosevelt*. Hyde Park, NY: Eleanor Roosevelt National Historic Site. Retrieved November 15, 2008, from http://www.nps.gov/archive/elro/glossary/jim-crow-laws.htm

Brandon, D. T., Isaac, L. A., & LaVeist, T. A. (2005). The legacy of Tuskegee and trust in medical care: Is Tuskegee responsible for race differences in mistrust of medical care? *Journal of the National Medical Association, 97*(7), 951-956.

Braun, L. (2002). Race, ethnicity and health: Can genetics explain disparities? *Perspectives in Biology and Medicine, 45*(2), 159-174.

Brothers, T. E., Robison, J. G., Sutherland, S. E., & Elliott, B. M. (1997). Racial differences in operation for peripheral vascular disease: results of a population-based study. *Cardiovascular Surgery, 5*(1), 26-31.

Brunner, B. (n.d.). *The Tuskegee Syphilis experiment.* Retrieved September 4, 2008, from http://www.tuskegee.edu/Global/Story.asp?s=1207586

Burke, G. L., Evans, G. W., Riley, W. A., Sharrett, A. R., Howard, G., Barnes, R. W., et al. (1995). Arterial wall thickness is associated with prevalent cardiovascular disease in middle-aged adults. The Atherosclerosis Risk in Communities (ARIC) Study. *Stroke, 26*(3), 386-391.

Campinha-Bacote, J. (2007). Becoming culturally competent in ethnic psychopharmacology. *Journal of Psychosocial Nursing and Mental Health Services, 45*(9), 27-33.

Cassetta, J. A., Boden-Albala, B., Sciacca, R. R., & Giardina, E. G. (2007). Association of education and race/ethnicity with physical activity in insured urban women. *Journal of Women's Health, 16*(6), 902-908.

Chen, E., & Paterson, L. Q. (2006). Neighborhood, family and subjective socioeconomic status: How do they related to adolescent health? *Health Psychology, 25*(6), 704-714.

Chen, J., Rathore, S. S., Radford, M. J., Wang, Y., & Krumholz, H. M. (2001). Racial differences in the use of cardiac catheterization after acute myocardial infarction. *New England Journal of Medicine, 344*(19), 1443-1449.

Chu, K. C., Miller, B. A., & Springfield, S. A. (2007). Measures of racial/ethnic health disparities in cancer mortality rates and the influence of socioeconomic status. *Journal of the National Medical Association, 99*(10), 1092-1100, 1102-4.

Collins, T. C., Clark, J. A., Petersen, L. A., & Kressin, N. R. (2002). Racial differences in how patients perceive physician communication regarding cardiac testing. *Medical Care, 40*(1 Suppl), I27-I34.

Conigliaro, J., Whittle, J., Good, C. B., Hanusa, B. H., Passman, L. J., Lofgren, R. P., et al. (2000). Understanding racial variation in the use of coronary revascularization procedures: The role of clinical factors. *Archives of Internal Medicine, 160*(9), 1329-1335.

Cooperberg, M. R., Lubeck, D. P., Penson, D. F., Mehta, S. S., Carroll, P. R., & Kane, C. J. (2003). Sociodemographic and clinical risk characteristics of patients with prostate cancer within the Veterans Affairs health care system: Data from CaPSURE. *Journal of Urology, 170*(3), 905-908.

Copeland, V., Scholle, S. H., & Binko, J. A. (2003). Patient satisfactions: African American women's views of the patient-doctor relationship. *Journal of Health and Social Policy, 17*(2), 35-48.

Dillingham, T. R., Pezzin, L. E., & Shore, A. D. (2005). Reamputation, mortality, and health care costs among persons with dysvascular lower-limb amputations. *Archives of Physical Medicine and Rehabilitation, 86*(3), 480-486.

Doescher, M. P., Saver, B. G., Franks, P., & Fiscella, K. (2000). Racial and ethnic disparities in perceptions of physician style and trust. *Archives of Family Medicine, 9*(10), 1156-1163.

Egede, L. E., & Zheng, D. (2003). Racial/ethnic differences in adult vaccination among individuals with diabetes. *American Journal of Public Health, 93*(2), 324-329.

El Desoky, E. S., Derendorf, H., & Klotz, U. (2006). Variability in response to cardiovascular drugs. *Current Clinical Pharmacology, 1*(1), 35-46.

Ephraim, P. L., Dillingham, T. R., Sector, M., Pezzin, L. E., & Mackenzie, E. J. (2003). Epidemiology of limb loss and congenital limb deficiency: a review of the literature. *Archives of Physical Medicine and Rehabilitation, 84*(5), 747-761.

Feinglass, J., Rucker-Whitaker, C., Lindquist, L., McCarthy, W. J., & Pearce, W. H. (2005). Racial differences in primary and repeat lower extremity amputation: Results from a multihospital study. *Journal of Vascular Surgery, 41*(5), 823-829.

Ferguson, J. A., Weinberger, M., Westmoreland, G. R., Mamlin, L. A., Segar, D. S., Greene, J. Y., et al. (1998). Racial disparity in cardiac decision making: Results from patient focus groups. *Archives of Internal Medicine, 158*(13), 1450-1453.

Foster, M. W., & Sharp, R. R. (2002). Race, ethnicity, and genomics: Social classifications as proxies of biological heterogeneity. *Genome Research, 12*(6), 844-850.

Frohlich, K. L., & Potvin, L. (2008). The inequality paradox: The population approach and vulnerable populations. *American Journal of Public Health, 98*(3), 216-221.

Gamble, V. N., & Stone, D. (2006). U.S. policy on health inequities: The interplay of politics and research. *Journal of Health Politics, Policy and Law, 31*(1), 93-126.

Gilman, S. E., Breslau, J., Conron, K. J., Koenen, K. C., Subramanian, S. V., & Zaslavsky, A. M. (2008). Education and race-ethnicity differences in the lifetime risk of alcohol dependence. *Journal of Epidemiology and Community Health, 62*(3), 224-230.

Gordon, H. S., Street, R. L., Jr, Sharf, B. F., Kelly, P. A, & Souchek, J. (2006). Racial differences in trust and lung cancer patients' perceptions of physician communication. *Journal of Clinical Oncology, 24*(6), 904-909.

Gornick, M. E., Eggers, P. W., Reilly, T. W., Mentnech, R. M., Fitterman, L. K., Kucken, L. E., et al. (1996). Effects of race and income on mortality and use of services among Medicare beneficiaries. *New England Journal Medicine, 335*(11), 791-799.

Guadagnoli, E., Ayanian, J. Z., Gibbons, G., McNeil, B. J., & LoGerfo, F. W. (1995). The influence of race on the use of surgical procedures for treatment of peripheral vascular disease of the lower extremities. *Archives of Surgery, 130*(4), 381-386.

Halpern, C. T., Hallfors, D., Bauer, D. J., Iritani, B., Waller, M. W., & Cho, H. (2004). Implications of racial and gender differences in patterns of adolescent risk behavior for HIV and other sexually transmitted diseases. *Perspectives on Sexual and Reproductive Health, 36*(6), 239-247.

Hart, T., Whyte, J., Polansky, M., Kersey-Matusiak, G., & Fidler-Sheppard, R. (2005). Community outcomes following traumatic brain injury: Impact of race and preinjury status. *Journal of Head Trauma Rehabilitation, 20*(2), 158-172.

Harty, L., Johnson, K., & Power, A. (2006). Race and ethnicity in the era of emerging pharmacogenomics. *Journal of Clinical Pharmacology, 46*(4), 405-407.

Heisler, M., Smith, D. M., Hayward, R. A., Krein, S. L., & Kerr, E. A. (2003). Racial disparities in diabetes care processes, outcomes, and treatment intensity. *Medical Care, 41*(11), 1221-1232.

Hirsch, A. T., Criqui, M. H., Treat-Jacobson, D., Regensteiner, J. G., Creager, M. A., Olin, J. W., et al. (2001). Peripheral arterial disease detection, awareness, and treatment in primary care. *Journal of the American Medical Association, 286*(11), 1317-1324.

Hoenig, H., Rubenstein, L., & Kahn, K. (1996). Rehabilitation after hip fracture: Equal opportunity for all? *Archives of Physical Medicine and Rehabilitation, 77*(1), 58-63.

Horner, R. D., Swanson, J. W., Bosworth, H. B., & Matchar, D. B. (2003). Effects of race and poverty on the process and outcome of inpatient rehabilitation services among stroke patients. *Stroke, 34*(4), 1027-1031.

Huber, T. S., Wang, J. G., Wheeler, K. G., Cuddeback, J. K., Dame, D. A., Ozaki, C. K., et al. (1999). Impact of race on the treatment for peripheral arterial occlusive disease. *Journal of Vascular Surgery, 30*(3), 417-425.

Hughes, M. A., & Bashi, V. (1997). Gobalization of the changing U.S. city. *Annals of the American Academy of Political and Social Sciences, 551*, 105-120.

Ibrahim, S. A., Whittle, J., Bean-Mayberry, B., Kelley, M. E., Good, C., & Conigliaro, J. (2003). Racial/ethnic variations in physician recommendations for cardiac revascularization. *American Journal of Public Health, 93*(10), 1689-1693.

Ikeda, N., Miyoshi, Y., Yoneda, K., Shiba, E., Sekihara, Y., Kinoshita, M., et al. (2000). Frequency of BRCA1 and BRCA2 germline mutations in Japanese breast cancer families. *International Journal of Cancer, 91*(1), 83-88.

Institute of Medicine. (2001). *Crossing the quality chasm: A new health system for the 21st century*. Washington, DC: Author.

Jatoi, I., Becher, H., & Leake, C. R. (2003). Widening disparity in survival between White and African-American patients with breast carcinoma treated in the U. S. Department of Defense Healthcare system. *Cancer, 98*(5), 894-899.

Jemal, A., Thun, M. J., Ward, E. E., Henley, S. J., Cokkinides, V. E., & Murray, T. E. (2008). Mortality from leading causes by education and race in the United States, 2001. *American Journal of Preventive Medicine, 34*(1), 1-8.

Jiang, H. J., Andrews, R., Stryer, D., & Friedman, B. (2005). Racial/ethnic disparities in potentially preventable readmissions: The case of diabetes. *American Journal of Public Health, 95*(9), 1561-1567.

Johnson, R. L., Saha, S., Arbelaez, J. J., Beach, M. C., & Cooper, L. A. (2004). Racial and ethnic differences in patient perceptions of bias and cultural competence in health care. *Journal of General Internal Medicine, 19*(2), 101-110.

Jones, M. R., Horner, R. D., Edwards, L. J., Hoff, J., Armstrong, S. B., Smith-Hammond, C. A., et al. (2000). Racial variation in initial stroke severity. *Stroke, 31*(3), 563-567.

Kahn, J. (2006). Race, pharmacogenomics, and marketing: Putting BiDil in context. *American Journal of Bioethics, 6*(5), W1-W5.

Kaplan, G. A., & Keil, J. E. (1993). Socioeconomic factors and cardiovascular disease: A review of the literature. *Circulation, 88*(4 Pt 1), 1973-1998.

Karter, A. J., Ferrara, A., Liu, J. Y., Moffet, H. H., Ackerson, L. M., & Selby, J. V. (2002). Ethnic disparities in diabetic complications in an insured population. *Journal of the American Medical Association, 287*(19), 2519-2527.

Keil, J. E., & Saunders, D. E., Jr. (1991). Urban and rural differences in cardiovascular disease in Blacks. *Cardiovascular Clinics, 21*(3), 17-28.

Keil, J. E., Sutherland, S. E., Knapp, R. G., Lackland, D. T., Gazes, P. C., & Tyroler, H. A. (1993). Mortality rates and risk factors for coronary disease in Black as compared with White men and women. *New England Journal of Medicine, 329*(2), 73-78.

Kelly, P. A., & Haidet, P. (2007). Physician overestimation of patient literacy: A potential source of health care disparities. *Patient Education & Counseling, 66*(1), 119-122.

Kinder, D. R., & Mendelberg, T. (1995). Cracks in American apartheid: The political impact of prejudice among desegregated Whites. *Journal of Politics, 57*(2), 402-424.

Kleinman, A. (1981). *Patients and healers in the context of culture: An exploration of the borderland between anthropology, medicine, and psychiatry.* Berkeley, CA. University of California Press.

Kosoko-Lasaki, S., Cook, C. T., & O'Brien, R. L. (2009). Cultural proficiency in addressing health disparities. Sudbury, MA: Jones and Bartlett Publishers.

Krause, J. S., Devivo, M. J., & Jackson, A. B. (2004). Health status, community integration, and economic risk factors for mortality after spinal cord injury. *Archives of Physical Medicine and Rehabilitation, 85*(11), 1764-1773.

Krause, J. S., Sternberg, M., Maides, J., & Lottes, S. (1998). Employment after spinal cord injury: Differences related to geographic region, gender, and race. *Archives of Physical Medicine and Rehabilitation, 79*(6), 615-624.

Kressin, N. R., & Petersen, L. A. (2001). Racial differences in the use of invasive cardiovascular procedures: Review of the literature and prescription for future research. *Annals of Internal Medicine, 135*(5), 352-366.

Lantz, P. M., Lynch, J. W., House, J. S., Lepkowski, J. M., Mero, R. P., Musick, M. A., et al. (2001). Socioeconomic disparities in health change in a longitudinal study of U.S. adults: the role of health-risk behaviors. *Social Science & Medicine, 53*(1), 29-40.

Lattanzi, J. B., & Purnell, L. D. (2006). *Developing cultural competence in physical therapy practice.* Philadelphia, PA: F.A. Davis.

LaVeist, T. A. (2005). *Minority populations and health: An introduction to health disparities in the United States.* Hoboken, NJ: Jossey-Bass.

LaVeist, T. A., & Carroll, T. (2002). Race of physician and satisfaction with care among African-American patients. *Journal of the National Medical Association, 94*(11), 937-943.

Levy-Lahad, E., Catane, R., Eisenberg, S., Kaufman, B., Hornreich, G., Lishinsky, E., et al. (1997). Founder BRCA1 and BRCA2 mutations in Ashkenazi Jews in Israel: Frequency and differential preference in ovarian cancer and in breast-ovarian cancer families. *American Journal of Human Genetics, 60*(5), 1059-1067.

Lichtman, J. H., Krumholz, H. M., Wang, Y., Radford, M. J., & Brass, L. M. (2002). Risk and predictors of stroke after myocardial infarction among the elderly: Results from the Cooperative Cardiovascular Project. *Circulation, 105*(9), 1082-1087.

Lin, J. J., & Kaplan, R. J. (2004). Multivariate analysis of the factors affecting duration of acute inpatient rehabilitation after hip and knee arthroplasty. *American Journal of Physical Medicine and Rehabilitation, 83*(5), 344-352.

Link, B. G., & Phelan, J. C. (2002). McKeown and the idea that social conditions are fundamental causes of disease. *American Journal of Public Health, 92*(5), 730-732.

Lopez-Quintero, C., Crum, R. M., & Neumark, Y. D. (2006). Racial/ethnic disparities in report of physician-provided smoking cessation advice: Analysis of the 2000 National Health Interview Survey. *American Journal of Public Health, 96*(12), 2235-2239.

Lurie, N., & Dubowitz, T. (2007). Health disparities and access to health. *Journal of the American Medical Association, 297*(10), 1118-1121.

Masi, C. M., Blackman, D. J., & Peek, M. E. (2007). Interventions to enhance breast cancer screening, diagnosis, and treatment among racial and ethnic minority women. *Medical Care Research and Review, 64* (5 Suppl), 195S-242S.

Matthews, T. J., & MacDorman, M. F. (2008). Infant mortality statistics from the 2005 period linked birth/infant death data set. *National Vital Statistics Reports, 57*(2), 1-32.

Mayer-Oakes, S. A., Hoenig, H., Atchison, K. A., Lubben, J. E., De Jong, F., & Schweitzer, S. O. (1992). Patient-related predictors of rehabilitation use for community-dwelling older Americans. *Journal of the American Geriatrics Society, 40*(4), 336-342.

McDougall, J. A., Madeleine, M. M., Daling, J. R., & Li, C. I. (2007). Racial and ethnic disparities in cervical cancer incidence rates in the United States, 1992-2003. *Cancer Causes & Control, 18*(10), 1175-1186.

Mechanic, D. (2005). Policy challenges in addressing racial disparities and improving population health. *Health Affairs, 24*(2), 335-338.

Myrdal, G. (1944). *An American dilemma: The Negro problem and modern democracy.* New York, NY: Harper & Brothers.

National Center for Health Statistics. (2007). *Health, United States, 2007 with chartbook on trends in the health of Americans.* Hyattsville, MD: Author. Retrieved September 24, 2009, from http://www.cdc.gov/nchs/data/hus/hus07.pdf

National Center on Minority Health and Disparities. (n.d.). Web site. Retrieved August 14, 2006, from http://ncmhd.nih.gov

National Institutes of Health. (2008). NIH launches center to study genomics and health disparities: Geneticist Charles Rotimi to lead research on diseases affecting minority groups. Retrieved December 20, 2008, from http://www.nih.gov/news/health/mar2008/nhgri-17.htm

Newman, L. A., Bunner, S., Carolin, K., Bouwman, D., Kosir, M. A., White, J., et al. (2002a). Ethnicity related differences in the survival of young breast carcinoma patients. *Cancer, 95*(1), 21-27.

Newman, L. A., Griffith, K. A., Jatoi, I., Simon, M. S., Crowe, J. P., & Colditz, G. A. (2006). Meta-analysis of survival in African American and White American patients with breast cancer & ethnicity compared with socioeconomic status. *Journal of Clinical Oncology, 24*(9), 1342-1349.

Newman, L. A., Mason, J., Cote, D., Vin, Y., Carolin, K., Bouwman, D., & Colditz, G. A. (2002b). African-American ethnicity, socioeconomic status, and breast cancer survival. *Cancer, 94*(11), 2844-2854.

Noruzinia, M., Coupier, I., & Pujol, P. (2005). Is BRCA1/BRCA2-related breast carcinogenesis estrogen dependent? *Cancer, 104*(8), 1567-1574.

Oddone, E. Z., Petersen, L. A., Weinberger, M., Freedman, J., & Kressin, N. R. (2002). Contribution of the Veterans Health Administration in understanding racial disparities in access and utilization of health care: A spirit of inquiry. *Medical Care, 40*(1 Suppl), I3-I13.

Paulander, J., Axelsson, P., & Lindhe, J. (2003). Association between level of education and oral health status in 35-, 50-, 65- and 75-year-olds. *Journal of Clinical Periodontology, 30*(8), 697-704.

Petersen, L. A. (2002). Racial differences in trust: Reaping what we have sown? *Medical Care, 40*(2), 81-84.

Pincus, T., & Callahan, L. F. (1994). Associations of low formal education level and poor health status: Behavioral, in addition to demographic and medical, explanations? *Journal of Clinical Epidemiology, 47*(4), 355-361.

Purnell, L. D., & Paulanka, B. J. (2003). *Transcultural healthcare: A culturally competent approach* (2nd ed.). Philadelphia, PA: F.A. Davis.

Quarles, B. (1987). *The Negro in the making of America.* New York, NY: Collier.

Ranganathan, P., Culverhouse, R., Marsh, S., Mody, A., Scott-Horton, T. J., Brasington, R., et al. (2008). Methotrexate (MTX) pathway gene polymorphisms and their effects on MTX toxicity in Caucasian and African American patients with rheumatoid arthritis. *Journal of Rheumatology, 35*(4), 572-579.

Romeo, C. (2007). Caring for culturally diverse patients: One agency's journey toward cultural competence. *Home Healthcare Nurse, 25*(3), 206-213.

Rucker-Whitaker, C., Feinglass, J., & Pearce, W. H. (2003). Explaining racial variation in lower extremity amputation: A 5-year retrospective claims data and medical record review at an urban teaching hospital. *Archives of Surgery, 138*(12), 1347-1351.

Sadler, C., & Huff, M. (2007). African-American women: Health beliefs, lifestyle, and osteoporosis. *Orthopedic Nursing, 26*(2), 96-101.

Safford, M., Eaton, L., Hawley, G., Brimacombe, M., Rajan, M., Li, H., et al. (2003). Disparities in use of lipid-lowering medications among people with type 2 diabetes mellitus. *Archives of Internal Medicine, 163*(8), 922-928.

Schulman, K. A., Berlin, J. A., Harless, W., Kerner, J. F., Sistrunk, S., Gersh, B. J., et al. (1999). The effect of race and sex on physicians' recommendations for cardiac catheterization. *New England Journal of Medicine, 340*(8), 618-626.

Selby, J. V., Fireman, B. H., Lundstrom, R. J., Swain, B. E., Truman, A. F., Wong, C. C., et al. (1996). Variation among hospitals in coronary-angiography practices and outcomes after myocardial infarction in a large health maintenance organization. *New England Journal of Medicine, 335*(25), 1888-1896.

Shavers, V. L., Brown, M. L., Potosky, A. L., Klabunde, C. N., Davis, W. W., Moul, J. W., et al. (2004). Race/ethnicity and the receipt of watchful waiting for the initial management of prostate cancer. *Journal of General Internal Medicine, 19*(2), 146-155.

Shields, A. E., Comstock, C., & Weiss, K. B. (2004). Variations in asthma care by race/ethnicity among children enrolled in a state Medicaid program. *Pediatrics, 113*(3 Pt 1), 496-504.

Sims, M., Sims, T. L., & Bruce, M. A. (2007). Urban poverty and infant mortality rate disparities. *Journal of the National Medical Association, 99*(4), 349-56.

Smedley, B. D., Stith, A. Y., & Nelson, A. R. (2002). *Unequal treatment: Confronting racial and ethnic disparities in health care.* Washington, DC: National Academies Press.

Smith, D. B. (2005). Racial and ethnic health disparities and the unfinished civil rights agenda. *Health Affairs, 24*(2), 317-324.

Smithsonian Museum of National History. (n.d.). Separate is not equal: Brown vs. the Board of Education. Retrieved November 15, 2008, from http://americanhistory.si.edu/brown/history/3-organized/legal-campaign.html

Stamatakis, K. A., Kaplan, G. A., & Roberts, R. E. (2007). Short sleep duration across income, education, and race/ethnic groups: Population prevalence and growing disparities during 34 years of follow-up. *Annals of Epidemiology, 17*(12), 948-955.

Stineman, M. G., Ross, R. N., Hamilton, B. B., Maislin, G., Bates, B., Granger, C. V., et al. (2001). Inpatient rehabilitation after stroke: A comparison of lengths of stay and outcomes in the Veterans Affairs and non-Veterans Affairs health care system. *Medical Care, 39*(2), 123-137.

Suthers, K. (2008). Evaluating the economic causes and consequences of racial and ethnic health disparities. *Issue Brief.* Retrieved September 24, 2009, from http://www.apha.org/NR/rdonlyres/26E70FA0-5D98-423F-8CDF-93F67DE319FE/0/CORRECTED_Econ_Disparities_Final2.pdf

Taylor, A. L., Ziesche, S., Yancy, C., Carson, P., D'Agostino, R., Jr., Ferdinand, K., et al. (2004). Combination of isosorbide dinitrate and hydralazine in Blacks with heart failure. *New England Journal of Medicine, 351*(20), 2049-2057.

Tentolouris, N., Al-Sabbagh, S., Walker, M. G., Boulton, A. J. M., & Jude, E. B. (2004). Mortality in diabetic and nondiabetic patients after amputations performed from 1990 to 1995: A 5-year follow-up study. *Diabetes Care, 27*(7), 1598-1604.

Tereschenko, I. V., Basham, V. M., Ponder, B. A., & Pharoah, P. D. (2002). BRCA1 and BRCA2 mutations in Russian familial breast cancer. *Human Mutation, 19*(2), 184.

U.S. Census Bureau. (2008a). Income, poverty and health insurance coverage in the United States: 2007. Retrieved September 22, 2009, from http://www.census.gov/prod/2008pubs/p60-235.pdf

U.S. Census Bureau. (2008b). Educational attainment in the United States: 2007. Retrieved September 4, 2008, from http://www.census.gov/population/www/socdemo/education/cps2007.html

U.S. Department of Health and Human Services. (2000). *Healthy people 2010: Understanding and improving health* (2nd ed.). Washington, DC: Author.

U.S. Department of Health and Human Services, Office of Minority Health. (2001). *National standards for culturally and linguistically appropriate services in health care: Final report.* Washington, DC: Author. Retrieved September 24, 2009, from http://www.omhrc.gov/assets/pdf/checked/finalreport.pdf

van Ryn, M., & Burke, J. (2000). The effect of patient race and socio-economic status on physicians' perceptions of patients. *Social Sciences and Medicine, 50*(6), 813-828.

van Ryn, M., & Fu, S. S. (2003). Paved with good intentions: Do public health and human service providers contribute to racial/ethnic disparities in health? *American Journal of Public Health, 93*(2), 248-255.

Ward, E., Jemal, A., Cokkinides, V., Singh, G. K., Cardinez, C., Ghafoor, A., et al. (2004). Cancer disparities by race/ethnicity and socioeconomic status. *CA: A Cancer Journal for Clinicians, 54*(2), 78-93.

Warneke, R. B., Oh, A., Breen, N., Gehlert, S., Paskett, E., Tucker, K. L., et al. (2008). Approaching health disparities from a population perspective: The National Institutes of Health Centers for Population Health and Health Disparities. *American Journal of Public Health, 98*(9), 1608-1615.

Weitzel, J. N., Lagos, V. I., Herzog, J. S., Judkins, T., Hendrickson, B., Ho, J. S., et al. (2007). Evidence for common ancestral origin of a recurring BRCA1 genomic rearrangement identified in high-risk Hispanic families. *Cancer Epidemiology, Biomarkers and Prevention, 16*(8), 1615-1620.

Whittle, J., Conigliaro, J., Good, C. B., & Lofgren, R. P. (1993). Racial differences in the use of invasive cardiovascular procedures in the Department of Veterans Affairs medical system. *New England Journal of Medicine, 329*(9), 621-627.

Williams, D. R. (1998). African-American health: The role of the social environment. *Journal of Urban Health, 75*(2), 300-321.

Williams, D. R. (1999). Race, socioeconomic status, and health. The added effects of racism and discrimination. *Annals of the New York Academy of Sciences, 896*, 173-188.

Williams, D. R., & Jackson, P. B. (2005). Social sources of racial disparities in health. *Health Affairs, 24*(2), 325-334.

Williams, D. R., & Rucker, T. D. (2000). Understanding and addressing racial disparities in health care. *Health Care Financing Review, 21*(4), 75-90.

Woodward, A., & Kawachi, I. (2000). Why reduce health inequalities? *Journal of Epidemiology and Community Health, 54*(12), 923-929.

World Health Organization. (2008). Closing the gap in a generation: Health equity through action on the social determinants of health. Retrieved February 14, 2009, from http://whqlibdoc.who.int/publications/2008/9789241563703_eng.pdf

Poverty and Health

SOCIAL STATUS DIFFERENCES IN LEADING HEALTH INDICATORS

Rebecca Reviere, PhD and
Valerie R. Stackman, MA

Health is an intimate personal experience that is lived in the body, but even at its most individual, health is also a social phenomenon. Individual health is a result not only of personal biology and behavior, but also of one's placement in the system of social stratification. In this chapter, the focus is on the impact of poverty on health. There are many ways to measure health, and by any standard, the poor are worse off. They have higher mortality and morbidity rates, lower self-reported health, and higher rates of disabilities. These differences in health are a result of many factors, some of which poor individuals control and some that they cannot.

We start with the definition and the distribution of poverty and with a discussion of health. Next, the *Healthy People 2010* initiative is used to examine the interrelationships between social class and the federal governments' chosen indicators. We suggest that individual health incubates in families and neighborhoods, filters through the life course, and resides in the individual. We acknowledge that power and the ability to make healthy choices are not equitably distributed and that this has implications for health.

BACKGROUND

Once a clear system of stratification emerged in early human groups, there was a recognition that those with "less" had poorer health, and early documentation of this has existed since the 1200s (Farmer, 2001). More recent evidence for the link between income and mortality has been accumulating since the 1960s (Marmot et al., 1991) with a set of longitudinal studies of British civil service workers. These findings consistently revealed a steady gradient: employees with higher ranks lived longer than those in lower ranks. In other words, workers with higher occupational positions had lower mortality rates for all causes, and specifically from coronary heart disease. This held true despite steady work and access to the British National Health Service and for diseases not related to smoking cigarettes (Marmot, 2003). These seminal studies are generally considered the beginnings of the accumulation of data documenting these relationships. Later studies in the U.S. report basically the same inverse relationship between mortality and social position without the constant of national health insurance.

R. L. Leavitt (Ed.).
*Cultural Competence: A Lifelong Journey
to Cultural Proficiency* (pp. 121-136).
© 2010 SLACK Incorporated

In this chapter, the focus is only on those who are at the bottom of the social hierarchy: the poor. In the U.S., absolute poverty (where individuals lack basic necessities such as clean water and food) is practically nonexistent. Individuals are poor on a relative basis; they generally do not lack for the vital requirements for life. Those who are lowest on the socioeconomic scale have access to food programs, clean water is readily available, and most have housing. Conditions may not be as dire as in other countries, but the availability of economic resources is still a strong predictor of both mortality and morbidity rates.

DEFINING POVERTY

Socioeconomic stratification is the unequal access to society's rewards and resources (Eaton & Muntaner, 1999). Often called *socioeconomic status* (SES), this stratification reflects differences in education, occupation, and economic resources such as wealth and income. Although education is a very important predictor of health outcomes, here the focus is primarily on the absence of any substantial income that results, for most, in poverty. In the U.S., the federal government establishes the official poverty line each year based on a formula established 50 years ago. The idea then, and now, was that the poverty threshold should reflect the cost of feeding a family from an economic food plan that "reflects the different consumption requirements of families in relation to their size and composition, and the sex and age of the family householder" (U.S. Census Bureau, 2009, p. 5).

According to these calculations, 12.3% of the U.S. population (36.5 million people) lived below the official poverty line in 2006 (U.S. Census Bureau, 2007a, p. 11). In other words, a single poor person had an income below $10,400, and a family of four had an income below $21,200 (U.S. Department of Health and Human Services [HHS], 2009). The poverty line has consequences beyond the designation that someone is poor. It defines eligibility for many state and federal governmental services that are crucial for many poor families, such as Head Start, Job Corps, and the Food Stamp Program, although the exact formula may vary from program to program.

DISTRIBUTION OF POVERTY

Poverty is not randomly distributed through the population of the U.S., but it is clearly concentrated in certain locations and certain groups. Regionally, 10.7% of Northeastern, 9.4% of Midwestern, 13.5% of Southern, and 12.1% of Western populations live below the poverty line. Among those in central cities and among those outside metropolitan areas, the poverty rates are 16.5% and 14.2%, respectively. Although urban poverty is more visible, rural residents are more likely to be poor than urban residents (Fisher, 2007; Institute for Research on Poverty, 2004). Furthermore, because of their isolation, they have less access to needed services and programs. In 2007, people with disabilities also had an increased rate of poverty at 30.4% as compared to 10.5% of persons without disabilities (Centers for Disease Control and Prevention [CDC], 2009a).

In particular, gender, age, and race/ethnicity are important predictors of poverty. More women (14.5%) than men (11.7%) of all ages are poor (US Census Bureau, 2008a), largely because of wage differentials and caregiving responsibilities throughout the life cycle. In persons 65 years of age and over, 9.4% are in poverty, but the gender variation is considerable: 11.5% of women over 65 are poor compared with 6.6% of men (U.S. Census Bureau, 2007b). Women's higher rates of poverty have serious consequences for their families. More than any other group, children are at risk of living in poverty. Among children under age 18, 14.1 million children (19.0%) lived in poverty in 2008 (Institute for Research on Poverty, 2004; U.S. Census Bureau, 2007b). Specifically, 43.8% of children of female-headed households were below the poverty line in the last twelve months, compared to 8.6% of married-couple families, according to the U.S. Census Bureau (2006a).

In persons under 18 years of age, Asian American children have the lowest rate of poverty at 11.3% compared to African American children at 33.6%, Hispanic American children at 28.2%, and White American children at 14.5% in 2007 (U.S. Census Bureau, 2007c).

In adults ages 18 to 64, the total poverty rate is 10.8%. White Americans in particular have the lowest rate of poverty (8.7%) compared to African Americans (19.9%), Asian Americans (9.4%), and Hispanic Americans (17.3%) (U.S. Census Bureau, n.d.). African Americans are three times more likely to live in severe poverty (less than 50% of the poverty threshold) than Whites.

LOW-WAGE WORK

Work has always been considered as an essential and honorable way to provide for a family (Shulman, 2003). However, for the 30 million adults working in low-wage jobs in the U.S., this is an illusion; the reality is that they can barely scrape by. For this segment of the population, wages are inadequate; schedules are rigid; conditions are stressful, unsafe, and/or unhealthy; and benefits are inadequate or lacking. Further, these are the jobs that command little respect and confer little dignity (Shulman). Of those Americans who do not have health insurance, 80% are in working families, and over half, including two-thirds of uninsured children, live in families headed by workers with incomes below 200% of the poverty line (Shulman). These numbers destroy the stereotype that the poor are lazy; many of the working poor commute between second and third jobs and still fail to reach the American dream.

A snapshot of the nation's values and future is seen in this portrait of poverty. The large numbers of poor women and minorities reflect the pervasiveness and persistence of sexism and racism in the U.S. (Williams & Harris-Reid, 1999). The lack of a living wage for millions of Americans suggests preferences for supporting big businesses rather than working people. The large numbers of poor children represent not only a failure of present policies to ameliorate living conditions for the most dependent, but also a health vulnerability for the future. Poor children grow up to be adults who are less healthy and more prone to disabilities than more advantaged children. In addition to the dangers and stressors of low wage work, these workers rarely have ready access to the health care system because they have no health insurance.

DEFINING AND MEASURING HEALTH

Health is a complex, multidimensional phenomenon and can be measured in many ways, both general and specific. In general terms, health can be assessed in terms of self-reported health; specific measurements include such things as infant mortality and specific causes of death (Graham, 2004). The health of the elderly is often measured by the ability to complete activities of daily living independently (i.e., eating, dressing, bathing, toileting, transferring). The World Health Organization (WHO) defines health as "a state of complete physical, mental, and social well-being and not merely the absence of disease or infirmity" (1946). This definition suggests that not only physical health needs to be considered, but also mental health and social role and relationship functioning. By every measure, poorer individuals have poorer health.

When looking broadly at self-reported health, there are marked differences between groups. For example, men report better health than women on average (U.S. Census Bureau, 2006b). Non-Hispanic Whites are more likely to report that their health status as excellent (37.1%), compared to 31.3% of Blacks. Also, more Blacks report poor health (4.6%) than any other racial group (U.S. Census Bureau, 2006b). Expectedly, older individuals are less likely to report excellent health and more likely to report poor health (U.S. Census Bureau, 2006b). This is influenced, in part, by their functional abilities.

The relationship between social class and risk of death is evident regardless of how social class is measured (Weitz, 2006). Kitagawa and Hauser (1973) reported that death rates from most major causes were higher for those in lower social classes. The impact of poverty on mortality is evident from birth. The infant mortality rate (the number of babies per 1,000 that die before the first birthday) is considered particularly sensitive to poverty. Even though the nation's infant mortality rate is down, African Americans and American Indians/Alaska Natives have more than double the rates of Whites. Low birth weight is an important predictor of infant mortality, and twice as many low birth weight babies are born to African American women at 14% than to White women at 7% (CDC, 2009b). However, these differences by social class persist even among babies of normal birth weight and among mothers of different races and similar educations. Clearly, both poverty and race are relevant to infant mortality.

Mortality among children in all socioeconomic groups has seen dramatic reductions. However, children in higher socioeconomic groups have experienced much larger declines than those in lower social classes, especially with regard to injury and natural-cause mortality (Singh & Kogan, 2007).

Chronic diseases account for 70% of all deaths in the U.S. These degenerative diseases, such as heart disease, hypertension, diabetes, and cancers, develop slowly and persist over time, and rates of these conditions vary by placement in the stratification system. For example, mortality rates from heart diseases and cancers are significantly higher for African Americans than for Whites (CDC, 2009b). Black men die from prostate cancer at a rate more than double that for White men, and Black women have a higher death rate from breast cancer than White women, despite similar rates of mammography-screening (CDC, 2009b). Hispanics living in the U.S. are almost twice as likely to die from diabetes than non-Hispanic Whites are (CDC, 2005).

Physical health and life expectancy are strongly and positively related to position within society's economic and social hierarchy (Weitz, 2006). There are multiple and interrelated causes of these persistent differentials, and the exact pathways have yet to be mapped. There are many vectors into the body—we make no attempt to provide a comprehensive explanation for the consistent health disadvantage of economic marginalization. Surely, a multitude of individual, family, and neighborhood factors contribute. We also recognize that social policies underlie many of the conditions that persist for the poor in this country.

As medical sociologists, we take a biosocial view of health, recognizing that health resides in a body that exists in a stratified social world. We recognize the power differential that accompanies the inequitable distribution of income and wealth in this country and argue that individual health results from individual behaviors that may be constrained by lack of choices, from community level variables, and from social policies (e.g., those that make health care or food vouchers available).

In this chapter, the sociological dynamics surrounding individual health are spotlighted. If the focus is only on the individual when examining health, the importance of considering social forces and social contexts that constrain individual behavior is lost. Clearly individuals have responsibility for their behaviors—people do put cigarettes and cookies in their mouths; however, when the power and freedom of the individual is overstated, it implies that the victim is to be blamed for their illnesses and disabilities (Farmer, 2001).

THE INFLUENCE OF POVERTY ON HEALTH DISPARITIES

The U.S. government, through the Office of the Surgeon General, devised a *Healthy People* plan to improve the health of individuals, communities, and the nation in 1979 (HHS, 2005). The current *Healthy People 2010* targets health disparities by gender, race or ethnicity, disability, location, sexual orientation, education, or income as a primary goal.

Further, it sets out a list of leading health indicators that gage our nation's overall health. These descriptors are targeted for change based on their ability to motivate action, the availability of data to measure progress, and their importance as public health measures (CDC, 2007a). We use these as an outline for examining health differentials between the poor and the non-poor. The health indicators are as follows:

- Physical activity
- Overweight and obesity
- Tobacco use
- Substance abuse
- Responsible sexual behavior
- Mental health
- Injury and violence
- Environmental quality
- Immunization
- Access to health care

These are discussed in the order presented in the *Healthy People* document. We do not evaluate these indicators according to governmental timelines or outcomes but supply details from studies that are considered reliable and that highlight the social impacts on health. While we appreciate that not all African Americans, Hispanics, and Native Americans are poor, race/ethnicity is often used as a proxy for poverty since the federal government generally does not provide statistics on the relationship between social class and race/ethnicity (see Chapter 6).

PHYSICAL ACTIVITY

The relationship between exercise and health is well documented. Higher levels of exercise are associated with lower risks of hypertension, diabetes, osteoporosis, colon cancer, coronary heart disease, anxiety, and depression (Boutelle, Jeffery, & French, 2004), yet fewer than 25% of all Americans exercise at an adequate rate for health advantage. One study found that those who maintained an exercise program over time were likely to be employed, more affluent, White, better educated, a nonsmoker, and a less frequent TV watcher, and to have a lower body mass index (Boutelle et al.).

It may be that neighborhood characteristics are better predictors of regular exercise than individual characteristics (Ohio State University, 2008). It is easy to imagine a poor neighborhood where mothers keep their children indoors, and no one willingly goes for a run at night. In these conditions, television is the most common alternative, and there is an inverse relationship between SES and television watching among children (Evans & Kantrowitz, 2003). Recognizing the importance of social cohesion in a neighborhood, researchers suggest that individuals, particularly women, exercise more when they live in neighborhoods where they trust their neighbors and see them as helpful (Ohio State University).

OVERWEIGHT AND OBESITY

A normal or lean body mass is considered crucial to good health, and a diet high in vegetables and fruits and low in fats and sugars is associated with healthy body weight. On the other hand, overweight, and particularly obesity, is also associated with higher risks of heart disease, high blood pressure, diabetes, arthritis-related disabilities, and some cancers (CDC, 2007b) and is reported to increase health care costs even more than smoking cigarettes (Rand Corporation, 2008).

In the U.S., about 34% of adults ages 20 and over are obese, but the rate and the health impacts of obesity are not evenly distributed across the social spectrum. Obesity is concentrated among the poor. For example, prevalence of overweight among adolescents is more than 50% higher in poor families relative to non-poor families (Miech et al., 2006). Over half of Black women and Mexican American women ages 40 to 59 are obese. Geography is also predictive—the five poorest states are in the top ten states for obesity rates (U.S. Department of Housing and Urban Development [HUD], 2006; Yang, Lynch, Schulenberg, Diez-Roux, & Raghunathan, 2008).

When looking at variations by race/ethnicity in some of these weight-related diseases, there are dramatic differences. For example, low income individuals have three times the rate of heart disease compared to more affluent individuals (CDC, 2007b). Rates of high blood pressure for African Americans are 15% higher than for Whites (CDC, 2009c). African Americans, Hispanics, American Indians, and Alaska Natives living in the U.S. all have significantly higher rates of diabetes than Whites (CDC, 2005). They are also more likely to live below the poverty line.

This uneven distribution of obesity and associated health risks is not simply the result of poor choices at meal time. Individuals choose foods for a variety of reasons, such as cost, availability, and culture. Healthy foods are, by and large, more expensive than less healthy choices. Vegetables, for example, are much more costly than calories from oil, butter, and sugar (Yale University Rudd Center for Food Policy and Obesity, 2008), and nutrition assistance programs do not usually provide vouchers for fresh fruits and vegetables. It may be nearly impossible to afford a healthy diet on a food stamp budget, for example.

Poor urban neighborhoods are packed with fast food, take-out restaurants, and convenience stores. Individuals with limited incomes may have little choice but to eat cheaper foods that are calorie-dense and nutrient-poor compared to healthier but more expensive fare like fruits and vegetables, lean meats, and fish. Further, food manufacturers increasingly add high fructose corn syrup and palm oil to food, both of which are related to rapid weight gain, and these food additives are more common in cheaper, processed foods (Weitz, 2006).

Reduced access to healthy foods and the ready availability of cheap, fast foods creates a diet that predisposes individuals to weight problems and poorer health throughout the life course (Yale University Rudd Center for Food Policy and Obesity, 2008). As rates of overweight and obesity increase among children, their health problems also increase. The foods that children eat contribute to their development both physically and educationally, and obesity in children can lead to lifelong health risks. The interplay between individual behavior and structural constraints is demonstrated (Farmer, 2001): poorer individuals may make bad choices, but they have fewer good choices in the first place.

Food insecurity is an issue associated with obesity. The U.S. Department of Agriculture Report for 2007 showed the number of children and adults experiencing a substantial disruption in the amount of food they typically eat more than doubled from the year before and is now 36.2 million. That is, 12.2% of Americans do not have the money or assistance to get enough food to maintain an active, healthy life, and almost one-third of these went hungry at some point (U.S. Department of Agriculture, 2008).

TOBACCO USE

Tobacco causes far more premature deaths in the U.S. than any other legal or illegal drug (Weitz, 2006), accounting for one of every five deaths a year. Current smokers have less education and lower incomes than nonsmokers, and individuals who live below the poverty line smoke more than those living at or above the poverty level (Yang et al., 2008). The nicotine in cigarettes is more addictive than heroin (Weil & Rosen, 1998), and the tobacco lobby is quite powerful. But smoking and acceptance of smoking is declining in the U.S., and morbidity patterns should begin to reflect these changes in coming years.

SUBSTANCE ABUSE

The category of substance abuse implies a law violation and a potential brush with the criminal justice system. While substance abuse does have clear and potent health ramifications, the punishment system in place for drug violations can create more problems than the drugs themselves in the lives of the individuals involved. Considering this, a thorough discussion of the interplay between illegal drug use, opportunity, association, demography, health outcomes, and poverty is beyond the scope of this chapter. Nevertheless, the drug with the most health impact, tobacco, has been discussed.

RESPONSIBLE SEXUAL BEHAVIOR

Responsible sexual behavior per se is not as important as the result of irresponsible sexual behavior, that is, sexually transmitted diseases (STDs). Syphilis and gonorrhea are more concentrated in the South than in the North and among women of color, especially at younger ages (CDC, 2007c). This correlates with the distribution of poverty and the associated lack of quality, available health care services, information, and resources.

The most lethal STD is HIV/AIDS, and poverty is a significant risk factor for infection and for inadequate treatment (Farmer, 2001). In 2006, African Americans accounted for 42.7% of persons reported to be living with AIDS, compared to 34.4% of White Americans, and 18% for Hispanic Americans (U.S. Census Bureau, 2008b). Women were twice as likely to contract AIDS through heterosexual contact than through injection drug use; men were three times more likely to contract AIDS through male-to-male sexual contact than through injection drug use (U.S. Census Bureau, 2008b). Poorer women have less power to insist on condom use, especially when they feel physically or economically threatened. HIV risk then depends, to a degree, less on knowledge of how the virus is transmitted— most of these infected women knew a great deal about the disease. It depends on freedom to make choices, and poverty is the great limiting factor of freedom (Farmer, 2001). Finally, socioeconomic problems associated with poverty not only increase risk but also decrease access to high-quality health care and effective treatments.

MENTAL HEALTH

Despite its importance to well-being, mental health is largely ignored as a health outcome. This may be, in part, because mental health and mental disorders are not as easily operationalized as physical health problems. A mental disorder exists when the failure of a person's psychological system to perform its expected functions impinges harmfully on the person's well-being in their social context (Horowitz, 2002; Wakefield, 1999). Mental disorders, then, involve both internal dysfunctions and socially defined notions of inappropriateness and are often a response to stressful life events and on-going stressors (Horowitz).

In general, the poor, the poorly educated, and women have higher rates of depression, the most common mental disorder. The poor also have higher rates of the most serious mental illness, schizophrenia (Cockerham, 2006) than the non-poor. Mood disorders and anxiety, on the other hand, are more common in the middle and upper classes. In general, however, researchers have found that social class is inversely related to mental distress (Eaton & Muntaner, 1999).

There are two dominant explanations for this social class differential in serious mental illness: social selection and social causation. The social selection hypothesis suggests that persons with mental disorders drift into lower social classes because of their inability to work and complete regular daily activities. A variation of selection, social "residue," is the opposite, where the mentally healthy individuals in the lower class are upwardly mobile, leaving the mentally disordered behind in the lower class. The social causation hypothesis, on the other hand, suggests that the poor have fewer economic or social resources to contend with the on-going stressors of a life of deprivation (Cockerham, 2006).

Clearly if mental health problems are linked with stressful life environments, those on the fringes of society are more vulnerable. Not only are their living conditions likely to be more dangerous, precarious, and tiring, but they also have fewer resources to cope with these situations. Further, there are fewer available, accessible, and acceptable treatment options for those who may normalize distress and depression as a regular part of daily life. High stress levels alone are considered a significant risk factor for ill-health, but when combined with unhealthy behaviors (smoking, low levels of physical activity) and low socioeconomic status, this disadvantaged segment of the population has an even greater increased risk of death (Krueger & Chang, 2008).

INJURY AND VIOLENCE

The poor have higher unintentional injury rates (federal statistics sometimes use the term *accidents*). This is most obvious when looking at injury rates among children. Unintentional injuries disproportionately affect poor children and are more likely to be fatal. Children from low-income families are twice as likely to die in a motor vehicle crash and four times more likely to drown (National SAFE Kids Campaign, 2004). They are five times more likely die in fires (National SAFE Kids Campaign), often traced to faulty electrical heating and electrical equipment (Sandel, Sharfstein, & Shaw, 1999). Hazardous living conditions such as overcrowded and rundown housing, dangerous and unsafe neighborhoods, busy and littered streets, and inadequate supervision contribute to these deaths. Low-income families are also less likely to be able to afford protective gear and safety devices or to have quick transportation to medical facilities after an injury (National SAFE Kids Campaign).

Workers in low-wage jobs are also at higher risk for injuries (Evans & Kantrowitz, 2003; Shulman, 2003). For example, poultry processing is one of the most dangerous (and poorly paid) jobs in the country. Poultry workers perform repetitive, dangerous physical motions in cold rooms at increasingly faster line speeds. These conditions have resulted in an injury rate that is twice the rate of other manufacturing jobs (Shulman). Other low-wage workers such as nursing aides, home health care workers, and orderlies suffer an increased likelihood of back injuries due to constant lifting.

The urban poor often live in violent neighborhoods where they are more likely to be victims and agents of violence. Neighborhoods with high densities of poverty offer fewer opportunities to engage in and fewer adults to model positive alternative behaviors. While these crimes are not limited to the poor by any means, Black males ages 18 to 24 have the highest homicide victimization and offending rates (Bureau of Justice Statistics [BJS], 2008). Homicide is now the leading cause of death for Black males between the ages of 15 and 24 and the second for Black women in that age group (BJS).

In addition, child abuse and neglect and violence against women are more likely to be reported among those with fewer resources. Women who are dependent either financially or psychologically are more vulnerable to abuse and less able to escape. Violence against women can take many forms, but the ultimate is death. Women are much more likely to be killed by an intimate partner or a family member than men (30% versus 5%, respectively).

Despite mandatory reporting laws, little is known about the true prevalence of child maltreatment and neglect. In 2006, 3.3 million referrals involved alleged abuse of 6 million children. Neglect was most commonly reported, and parents were the most likely perpetrators (HHS, 2006). There is no single causal pathway to the mistreatment of children; variables related to the child, to the parent, and to the community are all involved.

Neighborhoods with high crime rates, a lack of available social services, and high unemployment rates are linked to higher risk for children. However, the most frequently and persistently noted risk factor is poverty (Bethea, 1999). Both the stress of trying to raise a child in desperate situations and the scrutiny from social service agencies are responsible. Economic security is not the only solution for parents who abuse or neglect their children, but increased resources would reduce some of the burden these parents face.

ENVIRONMENTAL QUALITY

Researchers now link conditions of the proximate environment to individual level health outcomes. Individuals and families who are poor are more likely to live in areas with sub-optimal environmental conditions, and both specific conditions and an accumulation of exposures reduce health quality (Augustin, Glass, James, & Schwartz, 2008; Evans & Kantrowitz, 2003). The focus here is on issues of housing and environmental degradation, especially air quality.

Housing

Poor families live in more dilapidated and dangerous housing in more unsafe neighborhoods than families with greater resources. The impact of rundown homes is most visible in growing children who are more vulnerable to environmental dangers, spend more time indoors, and engage in risk-taking behaviors. For example, children in poor neighborhoods are more likely to be hospitalized for asthma attacks (Claudio, Tulton, Doucette, & Landrigan, 1999). Asthma rates increase for individuals living in homes that are damp, have inadequate heat, and have rodent infestations, and living in neighborhoods they perceive are unsafe (Rosenbaum, 2008). Children in substandard housing also have increased risk of viral or bacterial infections and a greater chance of suffering mental health and behavioral problems (Harker, 2006).

Lead poisoning rates among Hispanic and Black children are roughly double than those among White children (HUD, 2006). Lead poisoning is more serious for children because their nervous systems are more sensitive. Levels build up over time, resulting in reduced IQ, slow growth, hearing problems, behavioral and cognitive problems, and kidney damage. The problem is more common in cities, near highways, and in older homes.

HUD (2006) found that unintentional injuries were associated with housing quality, and children and older adults are at higher risk as mentioned earlier. Falls are the major cause of nonfatal injury in children: high porches, windows, broken stairs, fire escapes, balconies, and even furniture can be dangerous if safety measures are not in place. Poor ventilation of appliances can lead to poisoning and wiring problems can lead to fires. Simple safety measures such as baby gates and window latches may be too expensive for a poor family, and families who rent may have few options in improving their homes if the landlord will not cooperate.

It is estimated that living in substandard housing leads to an average of 25% greater risk of disability or severe ill health across a person's lifespan. Those who suffer housing deprivation as children are more likely to suffer ill health in adulthood, even if they live in non-deprived conditions later in life (Marsh, Gordon, Heslop, & Pantazis, 2000). This may be a direct effect of physical damage to the body from years of substandard housing, and there may also be an indirect effect on education. Poorer households have fewer books and home computers, for example (Evans & Kantrowitz, 2003), and may be in areas where noise interferes with concentration and learning.

Housing quality and costs continue to be a problem for the poor. Households with a single minimum wage earner are not able to afford even a modest two-bedroom rental apartment at today's rents anywhere in the country (Joint Center for Housing Studies, 2007). This housing squeeze results in long commutes between more affordable housing, work places, and schools, or doubling up with friends and family members. Household crowding is associated with more pest infestations, noise, stress, and clutter; these can be associated with both chronic and communicable diseases. Further, the adverse impacts of crowding manifest differently for women and men—women living in crowded environments report more depression than men, while men report more withdrawal (Regoeczi, 2008).

The homeless represent an extreme picture of the relationship between poverty and health—they have higher rates of chronic diseases, acute illness, and mortality (Hwang, 2000). Their lives are littered with difficulties in everyday activities that eventually influence health (i.e., eating, washing, sleeping, dressing). Skin conditions such as frostbite, lice, scabies, and eczema are common. Homeless women face additional risks from violence and rape; birth control and sanitary supplies are not readily available. Homeless children are also more likely to have asthma, diarrhea, fever, and ear infections (to name a few) and to have more delays in immunizations and routine screenings than homed children (Weinreb, Goldberg, Bassuk, & Perloff, 1998). Substance abuse, mental illness, and dual diagnosis (having both) are common and usually untreated. Because access to health care is so difficult, all homeless are more likely to use the emergency room as their primary care facility and are less likely to comply with prescribed medication regimes and to return for follow-up visits (Hwang).

Environmental Degradation

Disproportionately high pollution levels plague poor communities, and race again predicts which populations are hardest hit. African Americans and Hispanics, for instance, are much more likely than Whites to live in areas where air pollution levels pose health risks. The differences in community health is so striking that the term *environmental racism* was coined to highlight the disproportionate burden of environmental pollution experienced by racial and ethnic minorities (Weitz, 2006, p. 427) who are more likely to live near toxic waste sites, garbage dumps, liquor stores, lead paint, and otherwise contaminated land.

Poor air quality contributes to respiratory illnesses, heart diseases, and cancers. Asthma, an increasingly prevalent disorder, can be triggered or worsened with exposure to air pollutants. In the U.S., air pollution is estimated to be associated with 50,000 premature deaths and an estimated $40 billion to $50 billion in health-related costs annually (CDC, 2009b). Millions of tons of toxic pollutants are released into the air each year from automobiles, industry, and other sources, and families with more resources move to areas where the air is breathable. Poorer families do not have these choices, and a disproportionate number of the poor live in areas with unacceptably bad air quality.

IMMUNIZATION

Vaccinations protect children in the U.S. from more than a dozen serious diseases, but compared with children living at or above the poverty level, children below the poverty level have significantly lower coverage for all vaccines (including DTP3, polio, Hib, MCV, and hepatitis B). Differences in series coverage among Black and White children disappeared with controls for income (CDC, 1998, 2007d).

ACCESS TO HEALTH CARE

Ironically, *Healthy People* lists this as an important indicator of our nation's well-being since U.S. citizens do not have universal access to health care, leaving many uninsured or underinsured. Health care in the U.S. is some of the most expensive in the world, and many find it difficult or impossible to negotiate and pay for the intricacies of the health care industry. This is seen even in the most basic preventive care—childhood vaccinations.

Next we examine four aspects of using (or not using) the health care system: affordability, accessibility, quality, and willingness.

Affordability

The U.S. is the only industrialized country that does not guarantee health care to its citizens (Weitz, 2006). This leaves individuals and their employers to find a way to provide insurance to cover health care costs. About 60% of the U.S. population has employment-based insurance, about 9% purchase their own insurance, and roughly 27% are covered by government insurance programs (Medicare, Medicaid, or military health benefits). That leaves approximately 47 million Americans, almost 16% of the U.S. population, without health insurance coverage.

Insurance coverage varies by income, race/ethnicity, nationality, gender, and age. Those with household incomes of less than $25,000 have the highest rates of no health care coverage (24.9%); those with household incomes of $25,000 to $49,999, the second highest rates (21.1%), and those who make $75,000 or more have the lowest rates (8.5%) (U.S. Census Bureau, 2007a). Only about 15% of Whites do not have coverage, while about 33% of Hispanics and 19% of African Americans are without insurance (U.S. Census Bureau, 2007a). Those who are foreign-born are less likely to have health insurance coverage (33.8%) as compared to those who are native to the U.S. (13.2%) (U.S. Census Bureau, 2007a). Because they are concentrated in unskilled agricultural jobs, migrant workers have very low rates of insurance coverage (Bollini & Siem, 1995). Women have higher rates of any kind of health insurance coverage than men (U.S. Census Bureau, 2007a), largely because many social programs are more generous to pregnant women and children than to men. Older individuals are generally covered by Medicare.

Even families with basic insurance may face difficulties paying for health care needs. The cost of co-payments, required premiums, and deductibles may make the health care they have unaffordable (Cockerham, 2006). Further, insurance may not pay for all needed supplies and medicines. One study (Himmelstein, Warren, Thorne, & Woolhandler, 2005) reported that roughly 50% of their sample filing for bankruptcy (most of whom were middle or working class) had medical problems that were prime contributors to their financial problems. The study cited gaps in insurance coverage, out-of-pocket expenses, loss of coverage and income due to job loss resulting from the health condition, and medical bills as significant factors in the decision to file. While those who file for bankruptcy are not poor, this study does indicate the precarious situation that individuals face with health care costs, despite being insured.

Accessibility

Who gets health care in the U.S.? Each year roughly 27% never see a doctor, although this rate decreases as people get older (U.S. Census Bureau, 2006b). Women are more likely to visit a physician than men (32.5% to 21.4%, respectively) (U.S. Census Bureau, 2006b). Hispanics may not visit physicians because of immigration issues and language barriers. Those who live in the southern (19.0%) or western (17.9%) regions of the country are less likely to get health care than those who live in the northeast (12.3%) or the midwest (11.4%), possibly because of distance to the provider (U.S. Census Bureau, 2007a).

Lack of transportation makes accessing health care facilities difficult. Without a car, individuals must rely on other people, public transportation, medical transport, or taxis, and most of these cost money. Travel may be particularly difficult for those in rural areas if the nearest health care facility is a great distance away. Migrant workers are often isolated from access to prevention and treatment services, making them vulnerable to health problems such as poor birth outcomes (Gwyther & Jenkins, 1998). Delaying treatment only exacerbates the condition, leaving the individual in need of more extensive care in the long run.

If individuals are not able to visit a health care facility when problems arise, they seek treatment when the condition is advanced. The emergency room may be their best and only option at that point. Marginalized patients also may substitute the emergency room for regular health care visits because waits are relatively short, and it is always open and accessible (Abraham, 1994). Of course, overloading the emergency room with nonurgent cases may seem to make little sense, but for an individual who cannot afford more routine care, it may be the quickest option to see a health care provider.

Quality of Care

The poor use different sources of health care than the non-poor. Quality of care is difficult to measure, but by any definition, the "Medicaid mills"—practices that cater to the poor—give inferior care. They have been associated with shorter visits, inadequate preventive care and physician-patient communication, and less reliable access to hospital facilities (Abraham, 1994). In addition, longer waits for appointments and in the waiting room make seeking health care more onerous. Longer waits for physician visits, for whatever reasons, may contribute to worsening illnesses and injuries and, again, treatment may be more intensive, prolonged, and expensive. Migrant workers and foreign-born residents are particularly vulnerable to care that does not meet their needs. Many of these individuals may not speak English, and translators may be unavailable. In addition, cultural differences can present a challenge. If the family has a set of expectations that providers do not understand or respect, this discrepancy may produce another barrier to appropriate health care and its associated health outcomes.

Willingness

Poor individuals may feel little motivation to use health care services. Having little success in other endeavors, they often feel hopeless in the face of negotiating an unfamiliar medical bureaucracy, and for good reason. The facilities available to the poor are often crowded public clinics where service is fragmented, providers discourteous and impersonal, and waits interminable. When attention is forthcoming, the interaction is often controlled by staff who directly and indirectly indicate status and knowledge differences. These encounters can leave the individual feeling out of place and unserved. The inhospitality of these settings, coupled with travel and financial problems, can discourage the poor from visiting medical offices early or often. As a result, treatment is often delayed until the problem is much more serious.

CONCLUSION

In this chapter, we looked at the effect of poverty on health indicators in the U.S. Regardless of the index, those who are economically marginalized fare worse. Women have higher morbidity rates than men, and people of color have higher morbidity and mortality rates than Whites. Children suffer disproportionately.

Poverty impacts health, but it also influences everyday interactions. Waiting in long lines that may or may not lead to the needed services, listening to young grocery clerks check off food voucher items, and taking three buses to work are not activities for those with choices. The ongoing indignities and insults to the poor may be as debilitating in the long run as dangerous neighborhoods. And it is particularly ironic that the poor and uneducated must try to navigate confusing forms, requirements, and guidelines to try to access the services and programs that are available. One expert on women and poverty stated, "show me the poor woman who finds a way to get everything she's entitled to in the system, and I'll show you a woman who could run General Motors" (Abraham, 1994). It is not surprising that feelings of confusion and humiliation sometimes lead to anger, disengagement, and fatalism—if there is nothing I can do to improve my situation, why not eat fried foods?

The importance of social factors in individual health is stressed and alludes to the inequitable distribution of power that limits individual choice. If families live in poor and violent neighborhoods with little or no access to groceries with fresh vegetables or the gym, their higher rates of obesity are not entirely their fault.

Although we may imply that poverty is all or nothing in this chapter, in fact, the population of the poor is more fluid. People move in and out of poverty. It seems clear, however, that poverty often stays with individuals. The life course perspective implies that early events influence later events, and this is true for children who grow up in poor families and carry the health burden even in later life.

Along with reducing health disparities, the other goals of *Healthy People 2010* are to increase life expectancy and improve the quality of life for all citizens. This goal is realistic only if policymakers consider the impact of stratification on individual lives. Programs that promote exercise are bound to fail in unsafe neighborhoods, HIV education programs are irrelevant to women who cannot afford to leave abusive boyfriends, and admonishments from physicians for medication compliance are useless for patients who cannot afford the full supply of pills.

The health burden of poverty may fall disproportionately on the poor, but the effects of this inequity reach everyone. The U.S. has higher infant and overall mortality rates and lower life expectancy than most other industrialized nations, although our health care costs are far more (Syme, 2008). Although stratification and the associated health gradient will never be eliminated, programs and policies can reduce the health burden and improve quality of life. Work that pays a living wage, national health insurance, quality education, and safe neighborhoods are not impossible goals. When we refuse to see the problems of the poor, we cannot reduce health disparities or improve quality of life, and the growing gap between the haves and the have-nots in the U.S. makes seeing and solving those problems more pressing than ever.

REFLECTION QUESTIONS

✔ *Have you considered the impact of poverty or limited economic resources for your clients?*

✔ *What stereotypes do you hold about people from an impoverished background?*

✔ *Are you aware of the* Healthy People 2010 *document? Have you thought about how to incorporate this document into your professional practice?*

✔ *Are you involved with any health promotion/wellness programs as a physical therapist?*

REFERENCES

Abraham, L. K. (1994). *Mama might be better off dead: The failure of health care in urban America*. Chicago, IL: University of Chicago Press.

Augustin, T., Glass, T. A., James, B. D., & Schwartz, B. S. (2008). Neighborhood psychosocial hazards and cardiovascular disease: The Baltimore memory study. *American Journal of Public Health, 98*(9), 1664-1670.

Bethea, L. (1999). Primary prevention of child abuse. *American Family Physician, 59*(6), 1577-1585.

Bollini, P., & Siem, H. (1995). No real progress towards equity: Health of migrants and ethnic minorities on the eve of the year 2000. *Social Science & Medicine, 41*(6), 819-828.

Boutelle, K. N., Jeffery, R. W., & French, S. A. (2004). Predictors of vigorous exercise adoption and maintenance over four years in a community sample. *International Journal of Behavioral Nutrition and Physical Activity, 1*(1), 13.

Bureau of Justice Statistics. (2008). Homicide trends in the United States. Retrieved January 17, 2008, from http://www.ojp.usdoj.gov/bjs/pub/pdf/htius.pdf

Centers for Disease Control and Prevention. (1998). Vaccination coverage by race/ethnicity and poverty level among children aged 19-35 months—United States, 1997. *Morbidity and Mortality Weekly Report, 47*(44), 956-959.

Centers for Disease Control and Prevention. (2005). National diabetes fact sheet: General information and national estimates on diabetes in the United States, 2005. Atlanta, GA: Author. Retrieved March 13, 2008, from http://apps.nccd.cdc.gov/DDTSTRS/template/ndfs_2005.pdf

Centers for Disease Control and Prevention. (2007a). About Healthy People 2010. Retrieved May 14, 2008, from http://www.cdc.gov/nchs/healthy_people/hp2010.htm

Centers for Disease Control and Prevention. (2007b). Chronic disease prevention and health promotion. Retrieved January 17, 2008, from http://www.cdc.gov/nccdphp

Centers for Disease Control and Prevention. (2007c). Cigarette smoking among adults—United States, 2006. *Morbidity and Mortality Weekly Report, 56*(44), 1157-1161. Retrieved November 8, 2007, from http://www.cdc.gov/mmwr/preview/mmwrhtml/mm5644a2.htm

Centers for Disease Control and Prevention. (2007d). Vaccination coverage among children in kindergarten—United States, 2006-07 school year. *Morbidity and Mortality Weekly Report, 56*(32), 819-821.

Centers for Disease Control and Prevention. (2009a). Disability and functioning (adults). Retrieved January 17, 2008, from http://www.cdc.gov/nchs/fastats/disable.htm

Centers for Disease Control and Prevention. (2009b). National Vital Statistics Reports: Births: Final data for 2006. Volume 57. Number 7. Retrieved November 16, 2009, from http://www.cdc.gov/nchs/data/nvsr/nvsr57/nvsr57_07.pdf

Centers for Disease Control and Prevention. (2009c). High blood pressure facts. Retrieved May 16, 2008, from http://www.cdc.gov/bloodpressure/facts.htm

Claudio, L., Tulton, L., Doucette, J., & Landrigan, P. J. (1999). Socioeconomic factors and asthma hospitalization rates in New York City. *Journal of Asthma, 36*(4), 343-350.

Cockerham, W. C. (2006). *Sociology of mental disorder* (7th ed.). Upper Saddle River, NJ: Prentice Hall.

Eaton, W. W., & Muntaner, C. (1999). Socioeconomic stratification and mental disorder. In A. V. Horowitz & T. L. Scheid (Eds.), *A handbook for the study of mental health: Social contexts, theories, and systems* (pp. 259-283). New York, NY: Cambridge University Press.

Evans, G. W., & Kantrowitz, E. (2003). Socioeconomic status and health: The potential role of environmental risk exposure. In P. R. Lee & C. L. Estes. *The nation's health* (7th ed., pp. 93-119). Sudbury, MA: Jones and Bartlett Publishers.

Farmer, P. (2001). *Infections and inequalities: The modern plagues.* Berkeley, CA: University of California Press.

Fisher, M. (2007). Rural residents: Cause or effect from poverty. *Perspectives on Poverty, Policy, and Place, 4*(2), 2-5.

Graham, H. (2004). Social determinants and their unequal distribution: Clarifying policy understandings. *Milbank Quarterly, 82*(1), 101-124.

Gwyther, M. E., & Jenkins, M. (1998). Migrant farmworker children: Health status, barriers to care, and nursing innovations in health care delivery. *Journal of Pediatric Health Care, 12*(2), 60-66.

Harker, L. (2006). *Chance of a lifetime: The impacts of bad housing on children's lives.* Retrieved September 9, 2008, from http://image.guardian.co.uk/sys-files/Society/documents/2006/09/12/Lifechancereport.pdf

Himmelstein, D. U., Warren, E., Thorne, D., & Woolhandler, S. (2005). Illness and injury as contributors to bankruptcy. *Health Affairs,* Suppl Web Exclusives, W5-63–W5-73.

Horowitz, A. V. (2002). *Creating mental illness.* Chicago, IL: University of Chicago Press.

Hwang, S. W. (2001). Homelessness and health. *Canadian Medical Association Journal, 164*(2), 229-233.

Institute for Research on Poverty. (2004). Who is poor? Retrieved March 12, 2008, from http://irp.wisc.edu/faqs/faq3.htm

Joint Center for Housing Studies. (2007). *The state of the Nation's housing, 2007.* Cambridge, MA: Harvard University Press.

Kitagawa, E. M., & Hauser, P. M. (1973). *Differential mortality in the United States: A study in socioeconomic epidemiology.* Cambridge, MA: Harvard University Press.

Krueger, P. M., & Chang, V. W. (2008). Being poor and coping with stress: Health behaviors and the risk of death. *American Journal of Public Health, 98*(5), 889-896.

Marmot, M. G. (2003). The influence of income on health: Views of an epidemiologist. In P. R. Lee & C. L. Estes. *The Nation's health* (7th ed., pp. 79-92). Sudbury, MA: Jones and Bartlett Publishers.

Marmot, M. G., Smith, G. D., Stansfeld, S., Patel, C., North, F., Head, J., et al. (1991). Health inequalities among British civil servants: The Whitehall II study. *Lancet, 337*(8754), 1387-1393.

Marsh, A., Gordon, D., Heslop, P., & Pantazis, C. (2000). Housing deprivation and health: A longitudinal analysis. *Housing Studies, 15*(3), 411-428.

Miech, R. A., Kumanyika, S. K., Stettler, N., Link, B. G., Phelan, J. C., & Chang, V. W. (2006). Trends in the association of poverty with overweight among U.S. adolescents 1971-2004. *Journal of the American Medical Association, 295*(20), 2385-2393.

National SAFE KIDS Campaign. (2004). Children at risk fact sheet. Washington, DC. Retrieved November 16, 2009, from http://www.preventinjury.org/PDFs/CHILDREN_AT_RISK.pdf

Ohio State University. (2008). Neighborhoods play key role in how much people exercise, study says. *Science Daily.* Retrieved August 1, 2008, from http://www.sciencedaily.com/releases/2008/03/080317123252.htm

Rand Corporation. (2008). Health and health care. Retrieved March 17, 2008, from http://rand.org/research_areas/health

Regoeczi, W. C. (2008). Crowding in context: An examination of the differential responses of men and women to high-density living environments. *Journal of Health and Social Behavior, 49*(3), 254-268.

Rosenbaum, E. (2008). Racial/ethnic differences in asthma prevalence: The role of housing in neighborhood environments. *Journal of Health and Social Behavior, 49*(2), 131-145.

Sandel, M., Sharfstein, J., & Shaw, R. (1999). *There is no place like home: How America's housing crisis threatens our children.* San Francisco, CA: Housing America.

Shulman, B. (2003). *The betrayal of work: How low-wage jobs fail 30 million Americans.* New York, NY: The New Press.

Singh, G. K., & Kogan, M. D. (2007). Widening socioeconomic disparities in U.S. childhood mortality, 1969-2000. *American Journal of Public Health, 97*(9), 1658-1665.

Syme, S. L. (2008). Reducing racial and social-class inequalities in health: The need for a new approach. *Health Affairs, 27*(2), 456-459.

U.S. Census Bureau. (2006a). United States children characteristics: 2006 American community survey. Retrieved April 30, 2008 from http://factfinder.census.gov/servlet/STTable?_bm=y&-geo_id=01000US&-qr_name=ACS_2006_EST_G00_S0901&-ds_name=ACS_2006_EST_G00_&-redoLog=false

U.S. Census Bureau. (2006b). Health status, health insurance, and health services utilization: 2001. *Current Population Reports.* Retrieved March 23, 2008, from http://www.census.gov/prod/2006pubs/p70-106.pdf

U.S. Census Bureau. (2007a). Income, poverty, and health insurance coverage in the United States: 2006. *Current Population Reports.* Retrieved March 23, 2008, from http://www.census.gov/prod/2007pubs/p60-233.pdf

U.S. Census Bureau. (2007b). Annual social and economic (ASEC) supplement: POV01. Retrieved May 13, 2008, from http://pubdb3.census.gov/macro/032007/pov/new01_100_01.htm

U.S. Census Bureau. (2007c). Annual Social and Economic (ASEC) Supplement: POV03: People in families with related children under 18 by family structure, age, and sex, iterated by income-to-poverty ratio and race: 2007. Retrieved November 16, 2009, from http://www.census.gov/hhes/www/macro/032008/pov/new03_100.htm

U.S. Census Bureau. (2008a). United States: S1701: Poverty status in the past 12 months. Retrieved November 16, 2009, from http://factfinder.census.gov/servlet/STTable?_bm=y&-geo_id=01000US&-qr_name=ACS_2008_3YR_G00_S1701&-ds_name=ACS_2008_3YR_G00_&-redoLog=false

U.S. Census Bureau. (2008b). Annual Statistical Abstract: Table 178: Estimated numbers of persons living with Acquired Immunodeficiency Syndrome (AIDS) by year, age, and selected characteristics: 2000 to 2006. Retrieved November 16, 2009, from http://www.census.gov/compendia/statab/tables/09s0178.pdf

U.S. Census Bureau. (2009). How the Census Bureau measures poverty. Retrieved January 17, 2008, from http://www.census.gov/hhes/www/poverty/povdef.html#1

U.S. Census Bureau. (n.d.). Historical poverty tables: Table 3. Retrieved January 17, 2008, from http://www.census.gov/hhes/www/poverty/histpov/hstpov3.html

U.S. Department of Agriculture. (2008). More American kids went hungry last year. Retrieved December 14, 2008, from http://www.msnbc.msn.com/id/27771447

U.S. Department of Health and Human Services. (2005). Healthy People 2010. Retrieved March 12, 2008, from http://www.healthypeople.gov/default.htm

U.S. Department of Health and Human Services. (2009). Prior HHS poverty guidelines and *Federal Register* references. Retrieved May 13, 2008, from http://aspe.hhs.gov/poverty/figures-fed-reg.shtml

U.S. Department of Health and Human Services, Administration for Children and Families. (2006). Summary: Child maltreatment 2006. Retrieved September 1, 2008, from http://www.acf.hhs.gov/programs/cb/pubs/cm06/summary.htm

U.S. Department of Housing and Urban Development. (2006). *Healthy home issues: Injury hazards.* Washington, DC: Office of Healthy Home and Lead Hazard Control.

Wakefield, J. C. (1999). The measurement of mental disorder. In A. V. Horowitz & T. L. Scheid (Eds.), *A handbook for the study of mental health: Social contexts, theories, and systems* (pp. 29-57). New York, NY: Cambridge University Press.

Weil, A. T., & Rosen, W. (1998). *From chocolate to morphine: Everything you need to know about mind-altering drugs* (3rd ed.). New York, NY: Mariner Books.

Weinreb, L., Goldberg, R., Bassuk, E., & Perloff, J. (1998). Determinants of health and service use patterns in homeless and low-income housed children. *Pediatrics, 102*(3 Pt 1), 554-562.

Weitz, R. (2006). *The sociology of health, illness, and health care: A critical approach* (4th ed.). Belmont, CA: Wadsworth Publishing.

Williams, D. R., & Harris-Reid, M. (1999). Race and mental health: Emerging patterns and promising approaches. In A. V. Horwitz & T. L. Scheid (Eds.), *A handbook for the study of mental health: Social contexts, theories, and systems* (pp. 295-314). New York, NY: Cambridge University Press.

World Health Organization. (1946). Preamble to the Constitution of the World Health Organization as adopted by the International Health Conference, New York, 19-22 June, 1946; signed on 22 July 1946 by the representatives of 61 States (Official Records of the World Health Organization, no. 2, p. 100) and entered into force on 7 April 1948.

Yale University Rudd Center for Food Policy and Obesity. (2008). Food prices. Retrieved November 10, 2009, from http://yaleruddcenter.org/what_we_do.aspx?id=85

Yang, S., Lynch, J., Schulenberg, J., Diez-Roux, A., & Raghunathan, T. (2008). Emergence of socioeconomic inequalities in smoking and overweight and obesity in early adulthood: The national longitudinal study of adolescent health. *American Journal of Public Health, 98*(3), 468-477.

8

Understanding Racism

Joseph W. Smey, EdD, PT

INTRODUCTION

I began studying racial attitudes and behavior among college students in the late 1970s. In some aspects, it is clearly a different world now than it was then. Shifts in U.S. demographics are quite visible: Hispanic and Asian populations are increasing dramatically, and there are a rising number of mixed-race children being born. Surprising to many, the country has recently made history by electing a person of color as President of the U.S. The substantial progress that has been made in recent years has provided the opportunity for some to ignore this country's long history of racial prejudice, discrimination, and subordination and to argue that it is now time to finally put issues of race behind us and move ahead as a colorblind society. The notion of a colorblind society is one in which everyone is treated equally and group membership based on color is de-emphasized. A colorblind society focuses on attributes other than the color of one's skin. However, this approach fails to recognize that color/ethnicity is a characteristic of one's cultural heritage and identity. Furthermore, it is impossible to ignore past injustices, and this approach would legitimize and perpetuate a racist society (Brown et al., 2003; Lopez, 2006). On the contrary, it is critical that we continue to address the issues of race and racism because of their powerful role as deterrents of equity and social justice. America remains a nation divided, as well as a highly segregated and racially stratified country.

PURPOSE

The purpose of this chapter is to address key issues pertaining to race, human behavior, and health. Selected demographic, socioeconomic, and health-related statistics and the concepts of individual, cultural, and institutional racism will be presented to illustrate present-day inequities. The chapter will describe some of the forces that exist that serve to maintain a White-dominated society and will consider how racism differentially affects the identity development of White people and people of color. The process of individual and organizational change to promote equity and remove barriers to greater opportunity for under-served and disenfranchised groups will also be discussed. It is critical to recognize that although this chapter deals exclusively with racism, much of the discussion also applies to other -*isms* that exist in our society (e.g., sexism, heterosexism, anti-Semitism, classism, ableism, ageism, and others).

R. L. Leavitt (Ed.).
*Cultural Competence: A Lifelong Journey
to Cultural Proficiency* (pp. 137-158).
© 2010 SLACK Incorporated

DEMOGRAPHICS

More than half of the U.S. population traces its ancestry to White men, women, and children from Europe who came through Ellis Island between 1892 and 1954. However, more than 80% of the immigrants in the 1980s and 1990s trace their ancestry to Asia, Mexico, the Caribbean, or Central and South America (Migration Policy Institute, 2008). Today, about one out of every three people in the U.S. is a person of color. The U.S. Census Bureau reported that as of July 2008, the Hispanic population increased to 15.1% (estimated total population of 45.5 million) and is the largest minority group in the U.S. Blacks (single race or multiracial) were reported to be second at 13.5% (40.7 million), followed by Asians at 5% (15.2 million). The population of Whites (single race and not of Hispanic origin) totaled 199.1 million, or 66% of the population, down from 211 million (or 75%) reported in the 2000 U.S. Census. It is estimated that 45% of children under age five are from a racial or ethnic minority (U.S. Census Bureau, 2008). Hispanics are the fastest-growing minority group, up 3.3% in 2007 from the previous year. Asians are the second fastest growing, up 2.9% from the previous year. During the same one-year period, the White population grew by only 0.3% (U.S. Census Bureau, 2008). With current birth rates and immigration patterns, early estimations that Whites will be in the minority by the year 2050 appear to have missed the mark (Henry, 1990; Hodgkinson, 1985; Kinney, 1990). The U.S. Census Bureau now estimates that Whites will no longer be the majority by 2042, eight years ahead of the previous schedule (Varnon, 2008).

This trend is the same around the globe. In the year 1900, White people represented approximately 30% of the total population worldwide. This number has been steadily shrinking and is projected to be 9% by the year 2010. These significant changes are occurring at a time when national boundaries are more fluid and the notion of the world as a global village is becoming a reality.

DIVERSITY AMONG HEALTH PROFESSIONALS

While dramatic demographic changes are occurring, diversity among health professionals has changed little, and people of color are not represented in proportion to their population. In 2007, Hispanics comprised 5.6% of all health professionals: only 5.2% of physicians, 2.5% of pharmacists, 4.6% of the registered nurses, and 5.3% of physical therapists. Blacks comprised 10.2% of all health professionals: 15.6% of physicians, 5.9% of pharmacists, 9.9% of registered nurses, and 3.5% of physical therapists (U.S. Department of Labor, 2008). Thus, a largely White population of professionals has responsibility for the health and well being of a multicultural society. It is suggested that part of the solution to improving health care for the under-served is to increase diversity within health care professions (Schroeder, 1996).

RACIAL INEQUITY

People of color (Blacks, Hispanics, American Indians, and Alaska Natives) experience a multitude of inequities in health, education, and employment. Asians are the exception as data across these variables are generally usually quite favorable for this group in comparison to the total U.S. population (U.S. Census Bureau, 2007).

According to the U.S. Census Bureau (2007), the average family median income in 2005 for Blacks was $30,858 and $35,967 for Hispanics, as compared to $50,784 for Whites. In 2006, there were 22.5% of Hispanics, 25% of Native Americans, and 20% of Blacks living at the poverty level as compared to 8% of Whites. In 2003, 17.3% of Blacks and 30% of American Indians and Alaska Natives had no health insurance in comparison to 12% of Whites. Hispanics, the most uninsured group overall, varied within subgroups, ranging from 22.8% (Cubans) to 37.6% (Mexicans) (U.S. Census Bureau).

In the past, the "all-American" child came from an "intact middle-class" family. Today's reality is dramatically different, especially for people of color. In 2002, 38% of Black and 65% of Hispanic children lived with two married parents as compared to 77% of White children under the age of 18 (U.S. Department of Health and Human Services [HHS], Office of the Assistant Secretary for Planning and Evaluation [ASPE], 2008). Teen pregnancy rates for Black and Hispanic teens were more than two and one-half times the rate for White teens. Although the pregnancy rate for teenagers 15 to 19 years old has generally been going down, the U.S. rate remains the highest among industrialized nations (Boonstra, 2002; HHS, ASPE, 2008; Ventura, Abma, Mosher, & Henshaw, 2006).

Differences among groups based on color are also seen in education. Although 81% of Whites graduated from high school in 2004, only 55% of Hispanics, 74% of African Americans, and 76% of American Indians and Alaska Natives received high school diplomas. While 24.6% of all White adults 25 years and over completed four or more years of college, 10% of Hispanics, 14% of American Indians and Alaska Natives, and 14.5% of Blacks completed bachelor's degrees (HHS, Office of Minority Health [OMH], 2008a, 2009).

Related to socioeconomic status and education, persons of color are more likely to be victims of violent crime, robbery, car theft, and aggravated assault. Homicide victimization rates for Blacks in 2005 were six times higher than the rates for Whites with most intra-racial murders. Homicide is the leading cause of death among African American males between the ages of 15 and 34, with Blacks 5.4 times more likely than Whites to die of homicide (U.S. Department of Justice, 2007, 2009a). Rates for men in prison also vary greatly. In 2007, there were 4,618 Black male prisoners per 100,000 Black males, 1,747 Hispanic men in prison per 100,000 Hispanic males, and 773 White males in prison per 100,000 White males (U.S. Department of Justice, 2009b).

HEALTH AND HEALTH CARE

Differences in health status between White and non-White persons is stark, as illustrated by infant mortality rate (IMR), life expectancy, mortality, and death rate (see Chapter 6). The IMR for Blacks is more than twice that of Whites. For Hispanics, it is 1.4 times the IMR of Whites, with Puerto Ricans having the highest IMR among Hispanic subcultures (HHS, OMH, 2008a, 2009). The average life expectancy for Blacks is 71.8 years, compared to 77.4 years for Whites (HHS, Centers for Disease Control and Prevention [CDC], National Center for Health Statistics, 2007). Life expectancy is correlated with the presence of chronic diseases, including diabetes, heart disease, cancer, and stroke. The incidence of diabetes in Hispanic and African Americans is approximately 50% and 70% higher, respectively. The death rate for Blacks due to diabetes is more than twice that for Whites and 1.5 times more likely for Hispanics than Whites (HHS, OMH, 2001). Mortality rates due to heart disease for Blacks are 30% higher than for Whites. Blacks are 30% more likely to die of cancer than Whites and 80% more likely to die of stroke (National Institute of Neurological Disorders and Stroke, 2003).

Data related to HIV/AIDS shows a similar pattern. In 2006, 47% of all reported new cases of HIV/AIDS were among African Americans, largely associated with injection drug use or sex with an injecting drug user. Hispanic men were 2.6 times as likely to die of HIV/AIDS as White men, and Hispanic women were four times as likely to die of HIV/AIDS as White women (HHS, OMH, 2001, 2008a, 2008b, 2009).

While some may attribute these differences in statistics to biological or genetic factors, *Unequal Treatment: Confronting Racial and Ethnic Disparities in Health Care* (Smedley, Stith, & Nelson, 2002) makes it clear that people of color have less access to costly health care, even when their insurance and income are the same as for Whites. They often receive fewer tests and less sophisticated treatment for their ailments, including heart disease, cancer, diabetes, and HIV/AIDS—those same ailments for which disparities in prevalence have been reported. The report concludes that, while things such as socioeconomic status, genetics, clinical appropriateness, patient preference, risk behavior, and differences in the health care system contribute to difference in health status across racial and ethnic groups, *racial biases and prejudice on the part of caregivers plays an important role* [emphasis added] (Smedley et al., 2002).

The American Medical Association (AMA) did a search of the literature on racial and ethnic disparity in health care from 1984 to 1994, restricting the study to the *New England Journal of Medicine* (*NEJM*) and *Journal of the American Medical Association* (*JAMA*) (AMA, 1995). The review found that Blacks consistently received care that differed from that of Whites. Blacks were less likely to receive hip and knee joint replacements, have cardiac surgery for heart disease, or obtain organ transplants and sophisticated testing procedures, but they were more likely to undergo hysterectomies and amputations. Gornick et al. (1996) studied 26 million Medicare beneficiaries in 1993 and determined that *both race and income have effects on access and quality of care, but race was the overriding determinant of disparities in the level of health care received* [emphasis added]. Numerous others have linked race with disparities in the provision of appropriate screening, diagnostic testing, and/or management for heart disease, stroke, diabetes, HIV/AIDS, and asthma (AMA, 2002). Disparities in the provision of coronary revascularization procedures have been linked with higher mortality rates among Blacks (Conigliaro et al., 2000; Ibrahim et al., 2003; Peterson et al., 1997). Disparities in cancer care have been associated with higher deaths among people of color (Bach, Cramer, Warren, & Begg, 1999; Shavers & Brown, 2002) and disparities in the care to HIV clients have been linked to survival rates among people of color (Bennet et al., 1995, Cunningham et al., 2000). Race has also been shown to negatively influence surgical procedures for treatment of peripheral vascular disease even though the rate of amputations is over two times higher for Blacks (Brothers, Robison, Sutherland, & Elliott, 1997; Guadagnoli, Ayanian, Gibbons, McNeil, & LoGerfo, 1995; Lefebvre & Lattanzi, 2007; Rucker-Whitaker, Feinglass, & Pearce, 2003).

Furthermore, studies have found that racial and ethnic minorities have lower levels of trust and satisfaction with their physicians than do Whites (Blendon et al., 2007; Hunt, Gaba, & Lavizzo-Mourey, 2005) and that Blacks in particular actually receive lower quality health care than Whites.

In summary, racial and ethnic disparities in health status and quality of care have been widely demonstrated. These disparities are seen across a wide range of diseases and clinical services and across a range of clinical settings. They exist even when access and clinical factors such as age and severity of disease are taken into account (AMA, 2002; HHS, OMH, 2008a, 2008b; Smedley et al., 2002). The reasons for these disparities are complex and not fully understood. Socioeconomic inequality, individual behavior, and cultural ways of life each contribute (Smedley et al., 2002; Stepanikova, Mollborn, Cook, Thom, & Kramer, 2006). Of particularly concern and relevance is the fact that even with equivalent levels of access to care, people of color receive lower quality and quantity of health care services compared to Whites (AMA, 2002). As Escarce, Epstein, Colby, & Schwartz (1993) note, race might possibly unconsciously influence physicians' clinical decisions that are not justified by medical need.

The data above illustrate that, for millions, the land of opportunity has been elusive. Although an increasing number of upwardly mobile people of color have been able to move into the middle class, the U.S. remains a largely segregated society, and equality does not exist for a good number of Americans. For people of color, social reality contrasts sharply with America's social ideology. A key question to be considered is, to what extent are racial prejudice, discrimination, and racism impacting these health relevant data?

UNDERSTANDING RACIAL PREJUDICE AND STEREOTYPING

The word *prejudice* stems from the Latin *praejudicium*, which means pre-judge or to form an opinion without sufficient knowledge or experience. While prejudices are sometimes positive, racial prejudice as defined by Allport (1954) is a negative attitude toward people solely on the basis of skin color. Whites with racial prejudice have unfavorable attitudes and negative beliefs toward people of color that are not founded upon actual experience but rather upon notions that are shared and transmitted within a particular society. These negative feelings and thoughts are generalized by one's racial identity, as determined principally by skin color, the shape of one's nose, and the features of one's hair (Allport, 1979; Allport & Kramer, 1946; McDonald, 1970). Without question, this is something we learn from family and through cultural influences. By the age of four, children (Black or White) establish a sense of White superiority as they select, accentuate, and interpret sensory data from their experiences with parents, schools, and religious and social organizations (Allport 1954; Tatum 1997). This prejudice serves to reinforce the sense of White privilege (see below) and sends negative messages to people of color that can have a profound negative effect on their identity development and feelings of self worth.

The practice of making sweeping generalizations about members of outside groups without regard to individual differences is known as stereotyping. Stereotyping is symptomatic of the closed and rigid thinking associated with racial prejudice. According to Katz & Allport (1931), with stereotyping, we respond to individuals as a personification of the symbols we have attached to them as a result of fixed values, attitudes, and beliefs. These stereotypes are sustained by selective perception and selective forgetting (Allport, 1954). Common stereotypes in the U.S. ascribed to Asians are that they are smart and work hard; to African Americans that they are very good at sports and dancing; and to Hispanics that they are good lovers. Stereotypes, omissions, and distortions all contribute to the development of prejudice.

Kramer (1949), Katz and Stotland (1959), Rokeach (1968), and Secord and Backman (1964) defined different levels of racial prejudice. These authors, using what Kramer called an "age-old trichotomy," described prejudice in terms of three distinct levels: cognitive, emotional, and conative.

The *cognitive* dimension of prejudice is linked to unfounded judgments. This dimension deals with thought processes that incorporate unsubstantiated information to develop perceptions, beliefs, and exceptions with regard to particular individuals and groups. The style of thinking associated with this dimension of racial prejudice is closed-mindedness and inflexibility. For example, Whites may believe that Blacks are not as bright, less motivated to achieve, and would much rather take a "hand-out" than earn their own way. Once learned, such opinions are unlikely to change in the face of evidence to the contrary.

The strong feelings often associated with racial prejudice are the *emotional* dimension. These feelings stem from a variety of early life experiences involving family and friends and the way people of color are portrayed through such communication vehicles as the news media, television, movies, and advertising. The emotional dimension is salient when Whites believe that Blacks and Hispanics are dangerous and are to be avoided because they are more apt to commit crimes and steal from Whites. A White person approaching a group of Black or Hispanic youths loitering on the street and feeling nervous, suspicious, or fearful is another example.

The *conative* dimension of prejudice is an individual's desire or impulse directed at the targeted group, regardless of whether the impulse is carried out. This component is not an action or behavior but instead an attitude suggesting how one might act in certain situations involving a group or "typical" individuals belonging to that targeted group (Harding, Proshansky, Kutner, & Chein, 1968). For example, Whites might report an opinion (positive or negative) about their willingness to move into a home next to a person of color, have their child date a person of color, or enjoy having people of color as close personal friends. However, what is said in public when confronted with a hypothetical situation is often inconsistent with actions when presented with the real possibility. Therefore, the measures of the conative dimension of racial prejudice are no substitute for observable action.

THE COMPLEX NATURE OF RACIAL PREJUDICE

A commonly noted characteristic of racial prejudice is its extreme complexity (Adorno, Frenkel-Grunswick, Levinson, & Sanford, 1950; Kramer, 1949). Historians feel that racial prejudice results from the failure of the U.S. society to understand the beginnings of slavery, resistance of Whites to racial integration, and class differences that form along racial lines. Sociologists consider social structure itself and cultural patterns to be the cause, while psychologists look to personality characteristics and the inability of people to recognize individuals for what they are. Historically, research into racial prejudice has been troubled by the failure to thoroughly consider the interrelations of the dimensions of racial prejudice and the relationships of this attitude to racial discrimination and other associated behaviors (Brighman, Woodmansee, & Cook, 1976; Ehrlich, 1973; Rokeach, 1968).

Adorno et al. (1950), over a half century ago, portrayed the structure of an individual's ideology as a series of levels: "What the individual consistently says in public, what he says when he feels safe from criticism, what he thinks but will not admit to himself, what he is disposed to think or to do when he feels safe from criticism, what he is deposed to think or to do when various kinds of appeals are made to him" (p. 4). Contradictions and inconsistencies among these levels in part result from the interactions of this powerful attitude known as prejudice, with other critical instincts and extrinsic factors associated with an individual, such as culture, language, social class, education, and the economic and political environment. Although more than 50 years have passed since Adorno et al., a full and complete understanding of the very complex attitude of prejudice still eludes historians, sociologists, and psychologists.

PERSONAL DIMENSIONS INVENTORY MODEL

The Personal Dimensions Inventory (PDI), developed by Arredondo et al. (1996), has considerable utility for those in physical therapy and the health professions seeking to understand racial prejudice. The PDI sheds light on how a single attitude (i.e., racial prejudice) can appear so complex. It does so by placing race in the context of other critical variables that contribute to individual differences and shared identity. Arredondo et al. (1996) have used the PDI to define competencies required to assist people in developing capabilities with regard to people of different cultural, ethnic, and racial backgrounds. Adaptations of these competencies were endorsed by the American Psychological Association (APA) Council of Representatives in 2002 (APA, 2003; Arredondo & Perez, 2003). By explaining the interaction of multi-cultural group identity and other dimensions of human diversity, the PDI provides direction for those seeking to improve their interpersonal effectiveness in today's multi-cultural society. The PDI model suggests that race, along with the other important variables that contribute to personal identity, can be categorized in three dimensions:

1. Dimension A includes race along with such things as age, culture, ethnicity, gender, language, physical disability, sexual orientation, and social class. Like race, each of these factors is largely a characteristic that one is born with or grows into. These characteristics are fixed and largely visible differences that engender stereotyping and labeling.

2. Dimension C, on the other hand, encompasses historical movements or eras that profoundly influence society. These are events over which one has little control (economic depression or armed conflict). Dimension C places individuals in context, grounded in historical, political, sociocultural, and economic events. According to Arredondo et al. (1996), Dimension C suggests that there are many factors that surround us over which we have no control, but that nevertheless affect us. The economic recession in the U.S. beginning in 2007, the wars in Iraq and Afghanistan, and global terrorism are contemporary examples that shape our attitudes toward individuals who have identities different from our own.

3. Finally, Dimension B is included last as it theoretically represents the "consequences" of the interaction of Dimensions A and C. These consequences include a number of qualities over which one may have some control (e.g., educational background, geographic location, income, marital status, religion, work experience, citizenship status, military experience, and recreational interests). Historically, political, socio-cultural, and economic events in Dimension C together with race, age, culture, ethnicity, gender, language, and physical disability from Dimension A, intersect and enhance or limit what happens to the individual along Dimension B. Considering the interaction of Dimensions A and C allows for a better appreciation of how people become who they are.

The three dimensions of the PDI model illustrate the complexities of humanity. The model helps place race in a broader and more complete framework and makes it easier to appreciate why the stereotypical labels of identity are limiting and counterproductive. For the physical therapist, the PDI model provides direction for those wishing a fuller understanding of themselves, their co-workers and patients, and those who desire to become more culturally competent health care providers.

UNDERSTANDING DISCRIMINATION AND RACISM

Action that is prejudicial and directed categorically or individually is defined as discrimination (Merriam-Webster, 1983). Discrimination stemming from racial prejudice is called *racial discrimination*, and one particularly oppressive type of racial discrimination is racism. Racism involves the use of power or influence (i.e., economic, political, emotional, etc.) differentially to the advantage of one racial group and to the disadvantage of another. Racism is defined in the Merriam-Webster Online Dictionary (2009) as "a belief that race is the primary determinant of human traits and capacities and that racial differences produce an inherent superiority of a particular race." James Jones (1972, 1981, 1986, 1988) defines racism as "the exercise of power against a racial group defined as inferior...with the intentional or unintentional support of the entire culture" (Jones, 1981, p. 28).

In summary, the term *racism* is used to describe behavior that can result from the interaction of racial prejudice with key personal variables such as authority, status, and control. It may be intentional or unintentional and can have a profound sociological and psychological effect on individuals. In reality, there is more than one kind of racism, including individual racism, cultural racism, and institutional racism.

INDIVIDUAL RACISM

Individual racism is no doubt the easiest form of racism to identify and comprehend. Wijeyesinghe, Griffin, and Love (1997) define individual racism as "the beliefs, attitudes, and actions of individuals that support or perpetuate racism" (p. 89). A demeaning racial joke told at the expense of a person of color, racial epithets written on the blacktop of a local playground, or the provision of poor service at a hotel or restaurant just because the customer is a person of color are clear and all too familiar examples of individual racism that occur on a regular basis. Perpetrators of individual racism send messages that "non-Whites" are less-than-equal people to be mocked, demeaned, and segregated. With individual racism, the rationalization for the bias is the acceptance of unfounded beliefs and/or the misapplication of well-founded scientific theories (Halstead, 1988). A physical therapist who consciously or unconsciously considers a particular person of color as less intelligent, less educated, and less refined at first glance simply because of the stereotypes the provider holds for all individuals of that particular race can very well result in the provision of a lower level of care. This is individual racism, an action by an individual physical therapist.

CULTURAL RACISM

Cultural racism is subtle, pervasive, and insidious. It involves individual and institutional expression of the idea that cultural practices of the normative group are superior to those that are associated with other groups. That is, there is a sense that White cultural norms (social customs, manners and behavior, moral beliefs, language and leisure activities) are correct. There is a lack of acceptance of those things that are not part of the historic White American culture. This has become known as the concept of "White is Right" (Halstead, 1988; Tatum, 1997). With cultural racism, the dominant culture dictates cultural norms, beliefs, and values associated with right and wrong, good or bad, desirable or not (Charlton, 2000; Schmidt, 2005). Bell (1997) emphasized that cultural racism, like the other types of racism, is often the result of unconscious attitudes and behaviors.

Cultural racism is reinforced through advertising, the media, and entertainment. The subliminal message seen in much advertising is that light-skinned Blacks are more attractive than those with darker skin. Advertisements for sporting goods send the message that Blacks belong on the basketball court or football field, but not in the boardroom. With cultural racism, a physical therapist might view differences in the cultural background or health practices of a patient in some way as flawed or inferior to that of the White majority. This belief may lead the therapist, consciously or unconsciously, to offer shorter clinical visits and fewer appointments. It might also lead the therapist to conclude that the patient would be better served to abandon his or her own culture and practices in exchange for those of the White majority. As generation after generation acculturates to accept the norms and beliefs of the dominant culture as "normal and right," "good and attractive," "loyal and patriotic," cultural racism is perpetuated.

INSTITUTIONAL RACISM

Institutional racism is a third type of racism. It too is insidious and omnipresent in the institutions that make up American society. A few of the American "institutions" are the government and educational, health care, judiciary, and religious systems. Institutional racism is when the White majority, consciously or unconsciously, establish policies and practices in the institutions that are oriented toward and serve to reinforce the advantages of the White majority. By creating institutional rules and regulations that serve the White majority, minority groups are discriminated against by institutions rather than individuals. Institutional racism, although sometimes not consciously perpetuated, is systematic and is sustained over a long period of time. People in an institution who recognize the discriminatory nature of particular policies and practices and either seek to perpetuate them or fail to act to correct them are guilty of institutional racism. It is the most dangerous form of racism when considering present-day racial inequities because of the pervasive role American institutions have on everyone's lives.

Physical therapy admissions policies and practices that lack evidence for predicting success, yet simultaneously advantage graduates from affluent White communities over those from under-funded urban school systems populated largely by Black and Hispanic students, are an example of institutional racism. Such would also be the case with health care administrators who continue, in the face of a largely White work force, to depend upon the "good-old-boy's network" rather than affirmative action for their hiring.

Two contemporary examples of institutional racism from the American judicial system further illustrate the concept. First is the unfair mandatory prison sentencing guidelines for using powder cocaine versus crack cocaine. A defendant with 50 grams of crack received the same penalty as one with 5,000 grams of powder, even though crack is just adulterated powder. A large majority of crack users are Black, often from low socioeconomic environments, and most powder cocaine convictions involve White and more well-to-do individuals. In a move to eliminate this institutional racism (i.e., a 20+-year-old policy of using mandated Federal judicial guidelines), the U.S. Supreme Court ruled in December 2007 to change the guidelines in order to reduce the disparities that have been consistent along racial lines (Cose, 2007). In the future, individual judges have leeway to determine sentences.

The second contemporary example of institutional racism in the U.S. legal system was seen in the disparate charges in the 2007 case of the "Jena Six" (Jena, LA). In this case, six African American teenage boys were charged with attempted murder (as adults) after jumping a White boy, who was not seriously hurt. In contrast, the White teenage boys who hung a rope from a tree to symbolize the past history of lynching in the South and to intimidate their Black classmates were not arrested. The Jena Six case led to the largest civil rights protests in years. Many editorialists and activists viewed the arrests of the African American boys and subsequent charges as excessive and racially discriminatory. The case remained in the news for many months, and Congressional hearings were held concerning the incidents. In December 2007, one Black student pleaded guilty to a juvenile charge of second-degree battery and was to serve an 18-month sentence (Wikipedia, 2009).

WHITE PRIVILEGE

Intimately associated with racism in the U.S. is the concept of "white privilege." Indeed racism is, in part, a result of "White privilege." Peggy McIntosh (1989), author of a classic article promoting diversity and social justice, describes "White privilege" as an invisible package of unearned assets available to Whites each day, but about which they are conditioned to be ignorant of and oblivious to. What McIntosh and others who have worked to promote diversity and social justice have come to recognize is that White people are often blind to the fact that in the U.S., there is a heavily White-dominated system that clearly favors Whites over others. Being White in a White-dominated society, it is extremely difficult to recognize the influence of White privilege. For example, if White, I can be pretty sure of shopping without being followed or harassed by a salesperson, seeing people who look like me in history books and news magazines, and not being asked to speak for all people of my racial group. The experience of non-Whites in the U.S. is of frequently being looked upon with suspicion while shopping, rarely seeing people who look like themselves in history books or news magazines, and being asked to speak for all members of their minority group.

Being "successful" in life is due to more than just intelligence, ingenuity, and hard work. Rather, it has as much, if not more, to do with a social system that provides concrete benefits, and psychological freedoms for people who represent the norm. White people are often oblivious to their unearned assets and benefits while others are being oppressed (McIntosh, 2004).

How can one begin to recognize the advantages Whites experience in society that others do not? How do these privileges work to reinforce racially stratified communities?

An educational simulation game designed by R. Garry Shirts (1969) called StarPower, has been used by me and by my colleagues to do just that. We have used StarPower to help allied health students, physical therapists, and other health professionals engaged in racism awareness studies to gain insight into how White privilege works.

All participants are told from the start that the game involves trading chits (poker chips) of different values, that the distribution of chits is random, and that success in the game depends upon hard work and savvy trading. Participants are given visible symbols that they wear as large buttons, depending upon their respective group placement. Certain participants are rewarded and others penalized or handicapped unknowingly. Selected participants are placed in positions where they are unknowingly given the higher valued chits, rewarded unfairly throughout the game, and eventually grouped together in a high "achievement" group labeled "Squares." These Squares are continuously praised for their hard work and success. Conversely, those remaining participants who are unknowingly given the lower valued chips and unknowingly penalized or handicapped throughout the simulation are grouped into middle and low groups labeled "Circles" and "Triangles," respectively. The Circles, representing the middle class or silent majority, are nearly ignored by the workshop leaders throughout the game, while the lower Triangle group is constantly criticized for being lazy and not caring.

The StarPower simulation game resembles real-life social situations for the participants. The interactions occurring throughout the game parallel those in society related to racial inequality, racial prejudice, and racism. As the simulation draws to the end, the "high achieving" Squares are given the opportunity to change the rules any way they like. The Squares typically change the rules at the close of the game to benefit their group, attributing their success to good luck and the way they played the game. Squares are always the last group to discover that the game was rigged to their advantage. Members of the Circle group usually continue to compete to the end of the game, strive to move up to the Square group, and, if they do advance through a good fortune in their trading, usually act exactly like their new Square neighbors. Members of the Circle group usually discover that the game is rigged earlier than the Squares yet much later than participants in the Triangle group. Triangles, purposefully dealt a bad hand throughout the game, often become angry and typically quickly look for ways to break the rules of the game or to mount a "revolution" against the dominate Squares. Alternatively, some Triangles become apathetic, indifferent, and withdrawn. They express frustration toward both Squares and Circles as they see Squares as having been dealt an unfair advantage in a rigged game. Circles that advance to Square status are typically viewed by Triangles as selling out to their former colleagues.

In our experience, the StarPower simulation and debriefing fosters self-reflection and insight; powerfully, it gets White participants to more willingly identify White privilege in their own lives. That is, there is increasing recognition of the benefits accorded to Whites in a White-dominated society. White participants report growing up in the comfort and safety of the White suburbs. They talk about the well-funded school systems they attended, the extracurricular activities available to them, and their comfort with their predominately White classmates. Participants recognize that their teachers expressed high expectations for their success and were able to focus on helping, rather than diverting their attention to coping with behavior issues, high absenteeism, and a large percentage of students who fail to progress. Students are able to take credit for their past successes without being afraid of others attributing their success to affirmative action and racial quotas. There is recognition that they receive praise for their achievements without having to bear the humility of being told that they are a "credit to their race." Given their new discoveries of how White privilege works for them, they begin to understand that they have been given advantages in a game that does not provide an even playing field for all.

I grew up with "White Privilege." I grew up in a community where I was respected and admired for whom I was—a White middle-class male who kept out of trouble. There were always White people in positions to help push me ahead in life and others out in front helping to pull me along. There was an expectation that things would work out well for me. My high school language teacher reassured my dad that I would do well in life, in spite of my near failing grades in freshman Latin. I grew up where family and friends helped me obtain part-time and summer jobs, and where I did not have to worry about housing, a solid school system, transport to and from extracurricular activities, or spending money for recreational purposes. I had White coaches making phone calls on my behalf to White college admission officers to assist with my admission, and White faculty and academic advisors in college making key contacts to help solidify my commission as an officer in the U.S. Public Health Service and admission to graduate school. That is White privilege. A brief interview with two White male hospital administrators resulted in my appointment as Chief of Physical Therapy in a 450-bed hospital. Soon after that, I was offered a tenure-track faculty appointment without a formal interview. That is White privilege. While I have always believed that my hard work and some good fortune paid off for me in life, certainly the invisible "push" from those in my family and my community and invisible "pull" from others in higher places (i.e., my White privilege) was a tremendous help along the way. I was made to feel comfortable, confident, and supported by others throughout life. I often wonder what my life would have been like had I been Black and grown up poor in an urban, high crime neighborhood a short drive from my home and attended a poorly funded school system that provided few avenues for extracurricular activities? What would life be like if I grew up as a middle-class Black male yet had the disadvantages of being a person of color in a White-dominated society where unearned privileges were only given to White people?

AFFIRMATIVE ACTION

Recognition of White privilege and an uneven "playing field" makes it easier to understand why affirmative action has become part of today's culture. This nation's history of racial prejudice and the existence of a racially-stratified society led to passage of the Civil Rights Act of 1964 (1964). This statute outlawed racial segregation; prohibited discrimination on the basis of race, color, religion, sex, or national origin in public facilities, government, and employment; and invalidated the Jim Crow laws still prevalent in the South. Jim Crow laws, defined by each state, allowed for separation of Blacks from Whites in public locations. Title VII of the Act had the first reference to "affirmative action" as a remedy that could be used to combat institutional discrimination. An Executive Order by President Lyndon Johnson and subsequent orders from the Secretary of Labor in the early 1970s made affirmative action a tool to redress disparities in gender and race within America's public and private institutions (Fullinwider, 2009).

While nondiscrimination policies called for by the Civil Rights Act are designed to prohibit discrimination, it is affirmative action that requires purposeful activities to accomplish a specific end. Nondiscrimination policies alone ignore America's long history of racial prejudice and subordination and thus cannot achieve equal treatment for all. Affirmative action, by contrast, specifies that positive initiatives be taken to increase the representation of women and people of color in employment, education, and business, from which they have historically been excluded (Harvey, 2004).

Over the past 30 years, thanks in part to affirmative action, larger numbers of Blacks and Hispanics (males and females) have moved into the middle class, earned college degrees, and advanced to higher status and higher paying jobs once held almost exclusively by White males. With this progress, the rationale today for affirmative action programs has begun to address the strategic mission and goals of American institutions rather than just redressing past inequities. Affirmative action now includes the goal of creating a more diverse work force in business and industry to strengthen an organization's competitiveness and improve its financial success. In education, enrolling a more diverse student body is expected to enhance learning and better equip all students to deal with the challenges in a global society. Regardless of whether to compensate for past discrimination or for the future good of institutions and society, affirmative action is not without great controversy (Harvey, 2004). Whites who are blind to their "White privilege" have historically been reluctant to accept the concept of affirmative action and frequently refer to it as "reverse discrimination."

Those who oppose affirmative action argue that racial preferences are wrong. One assertion is that people of color who are not disadvantaged no longer need nor deserve special attention to get ahead. Additionally, it has been argued that those who are disadvantaged have to learn to help themselves, as they claim Whites in this country have done for centuries, and handing unearned advantages to people of color teaches Blacks and Hispanics how to be dependent rather than self-reliant. Still, another argument is that affirmative action hurts all people of color as it stigmatizes all members of that group and devalues what many high-achieving people of color accomplish on their own. What most opponents (particularly White people) fail to recognize is that unearned advantages by Whites in the form of White privilege have been an acceptable way of life for White Americans for centuries and is also essentially a form of affirmative action.

Three important U.S. Supreme Court cases involving race and educational institutions have helped shape the landscape as to what does and does not constitute an acceptable affirmative action program. In the 1968 case of Green vs. New Kent County, VA, the court found that Virginia's "freedom of choice" plans that allowed pupils to choose their school were ineffective at decreasing school segregation. With "freedom of choice" in place, only a small number of Black students (15%) chose to attend the formerly all-White New Kent High School, while 85% of Black pupils elected to remain at their all-Black George W. Watkins School. The Supreme Court concluded that the "freedom of choice" plan was not an effective strategy and that the officials were obligated to take positive steps to integrate the schools (Virginia Historical Society, 2004). In the 1978 Regents of the University of California v. Bakke case, the high court ruled that affirmative action in higher education could not consider race-conscious admissions to fill quotas. However, the courts did state that admission policies can take race into account as a vehicle to attain the educational benefits of diversity. The more recent 2003 Grutter v. Bollinger case banned the use of rigid formulas and the awarding of points to students of color in making admissions decisions at the University of Michigan. The court did, however, permit colleges to consider race in their "holistic review" of all applicants (Buck, 2007; Glater, 2006).

Interpretation of these landmark decisions has helped inform decision makers in higher education, employment, business, and government as to what affirmative action can be. The Green case signifies that "free choice" programs that follow a colorblind strategy are not affirmative action as they only reinforce the status quo rather than stimulate diversity. One needs to take action to eliminate segregation. The Bakke decision makes it clear that affirmative action is not a quota system. Race-based admissions and employment decisions must be part of a larger and more thoughtful program designed to enrich the learning and work environment for all. Lastly, the Grutter decision continues to support race-conscious policies when used as a mechanism to help guarantee a college education to all competitive individuals. It supports the notion that race can be a consideration to ensure the admission of talented and qualified individuals of every race and ethnicity (Schmidt, 2008).

Affirmative action can take many forms. These may include the following:

- Strategic recruitment of applicants for employment from under-represented groups

- Considering race among other factors in hiring

- Initiatives to develop a culturally-sensitive work environment
- Providing employee training and employee development opportunities for all members of the work force
- Providing support to under-represented groups for upward and lateral mobility within the organization

In education, affirmative action can be measures to attract academically competitive students of color to an applicant pool, considering race as one factor in admissions decisions, creating retention programs that include development of culturally competent schools, and providing support for students of color in gaining further education and/or job placement.

THE DEVELOPMENT OF RACIAL IDENTITY

A part of exploring the nature of prejudice and racism is understanding how each person develops a "racial identity." Personal identity, as noted above in the discussion of the PDI model, is shaped by the complex interplay of individual characteristics, family dynamics, historical factors, and environmental contexts including the social and political times. Children move through the preschool years, to adolescence, and onto adulthood with an evolving personal identity. One's identity is fluid, and certain components can be more or less significant at any given time and/or place. Ponterotto, Utsey, and Pederson (2006) describe many theoretical models of racial identity development. The model of Helms (2006) provides a good representation of these models. The salient features of this model are summarized in Table 8-1.

In retrospect, it was the response to two questions posed to a class of physical therapy students at the University of Connecticut in the mid-1970s that sparked my interest in the study of racial identity and prejudice. This experience also is a powerful illustrator of White racial identity development. As part of a campus-wide Metanoia Day (day of reflection), all faculty were encouraged to discuss ways to help alleviate racial tension on campus and to promote greater appreciation for cultural diversity. My class of 30 White

---

TABLE 8-1

STAGES OF IDENTITY DEVELOPMENT

DOMINANT GROUP MEMBERS

A. Encapsulation: Comfortable with status quo

B. Disintegration: Clash with previous perspective; feel guilt and anger

C. Reintegration: Resolve discomfort and guilt; return to first stage

D. Pseudo-independence: Actively seek information about other group and identify more with that group

E. Autonomy: Positive identity with own group; unwilling to accept subordinate status of the other group; social activists

OPPRESSED GROUP MEMBERS

A. Conformity; Accept negative images of own group

B. Dissonance: Clash with previous perspective; feel confusion; need to know more

C. Resistance and immersion: Actively reject dominant society; anger at being oppressed

D. Internalization: Positive identity with own group; willing to reconnect with dominant group but with equal status

E. Commitment: Positive identity with own group and members of the dominant group in state of autonomy; social activists

Adapted from Helms, J. E. (2006). An update of Helms' White and people of color racial identity models. In J. G. Ponterotto, S. O. Utsey, & P. B. Pederson. *Preventing prejudice: A guide for counselors, educators, and parents* (2nd ed., pp. 81-198). Thousand Oaks, CA: Sage Publications.

physical therapy students was taken aback by the fact that the issue of race was raised. They were very quick to acknowledge, when asked, that they had no racial prejudices. The students went on to look around the room during several minutes of awkward silence after being asked a second question. Was the lack of diversity in their classes an issue? They had apparently never noticed the Whiteness of their class before as this is just the way things were for them. Through nonverbal behavior and the choice of language used in the responses that followed, the message was clear. Each of these students existed in the White egocentric world so typical of the students who had sat in these seats for years before. They were the "cream of the crop," admitted to what was widely known to be a very competitive academic program. The unspoken assumption was that this group of 30 White students (mostly women) was very special and that people of color could not compete.

Over the years, similar questions have been posed each semester to groups of predominantly White allied health students participating in racism awareness studies at the University of Connecticut. What was it like to grow up White in America? The responses from the students have varied little over the years. To grow up White in America is "to be normal," "to be average," and to "fit in." When encouraged to go further, students acknowledge that to grow up White in America is to be "popular," "fortunate," and "successful." Answers to a subsequent question of "when did you first recognize you were White?" always take more thought by the students. Respondents often recall a very early encounter with someone "who was different," "who was an outsider," or "who did not fit in." The discussion around this second question seems to always flow naturally into a discussion of a third question: "What it is like to grow up Black in America?" To White students in the class, growing up Black means being "an outsider," "different," "not normal," "less fortunate," and "less successful."

From this discussion, students are helped to understand that from a very early age, whether it is recognized or not, White children are continuously bombarded with often unconscious yet very powerful messages that shape White social identity. Whites are repeatedly reminded that to be White in America is to be "right," "desirable," and "superior." Simply because of the color of one's skin, White people are granted freedoms and privileges (i.e., "White privilege") and are given myriad opportunities. This "rightness of whiteness" has a profound influence on who one is and who one will become. These benefits are taken for granted without much thought and are usually attributed to one's own efforts, hard work, and good fortune. Those engaged in racism awareness studies can generally recognize the "rightness of whiteness" advantages with time and a bit of open-mindedness and self-examination.

Just as the Triangles in the StarPower game were first to see the Squares for whom they really were, people of color seem to be much more aware of the benefits of being White than are White people themselves. Whites have much more difficulty seeing their ties to racism and find it easy to avoid any consideration of what costs might exist by living in a racist society. Once students in the racism awareness training begin to consider that people of color are disadvantaged and hurt by racism, their level of personal discomfort seems to rise. When White students reflect upon how people of color are still made to feel uncomfortable traveling outside of their own neighborhoods; are at times stopped by the police for no apparent reason; are frequently looked upon with suspicion in shops and malls; and are still denied housing, jobs, and other opportunities based upon the color of their skin, a new level of awareness occurs. This new insight can result in depression, guilt, and feelings of anger. An individual's first recognition that White people, intentionally or unintentionally, benefit from racism while people of color are disadvantaged by it can be a very painful revelation. One large hurdle for White individuals in their racism awareness studies is to get past the realization that Whites are not bad people just because of their many White advantages.

As previously mentioned, Black racial identity development is different than White racial identity development. Beverly Tatum (1997) describes how young children naturally focus on obvious physical differences and, in particular, the color of one's skin and the style of one's hair and dress. A White child at the age of three might naively ask in a very loud voice for all to hear why a Black passerby's skin is so dark or why their hair is so tightly curled. White children, as they mature, are taught to keep their curiosity about people of color quiet as this might be perceived as insulting. However, the curiosity remains. Black children similarly might ask why their friend's skin is several shades darker or lighter than their own or why people use the color label Black when most in this group are actually brown or tan.

Children begin to understand the concept of race around the age of six or seven. The White child begins to learn to accept power and superiority as a fact of life. Children of color, in contrast, begin to feel less desirable and, in many ways, inferior as they are immersed in a White-dominated culture where White supremacy is the natural order of things. Lighter skin tones and straighter hair are seen as an advantage as they are closer to being White. As children move toward adolescence, patterns of racial and cultural identity and stereotyping continue. Black youths begin to think of themselves in terms of their race as they recognize that this is the way others view them. What becomes apparent at this later stage of development is that people of color get bombarded with powerful and often less-than-subtle messages that influence their identity and begin to reinforce their sense of being subordinate (Feagin, 2000). Black and White children begin to learn the advantages of being White as they are exposed to more stereotypes. More consistent segregation begins later in elementary school, according to Tatum (1997), with social gatherings and friendships beginning to form along racial rather than solely gender lines.

Students of color continue to recognize that they are viewed as outsiders as they learn of prejudicial statements about them and become recipients of acts of racism by the White community. Anger and resentment builds as young Blacks become more aware of their systematic exclusion from many of the opportunities their White peers enjoy. Tatum (1997) and Fordham and Ogbu (1986) have observed that Black youth begin to react to the stresses of racism by distancing themselves from the White-dominant group and begin to congregate with their peers for support. They undergo a socialization process that leads them to assign greater value on being "authentically Black" rather than "acting White." It becomes increasingly important for Black youth to sound Black, dress Black, and to congregate with Blacks to preserve their self-identity and protect themselves psychologically. Tatum titles her book (1997) *Why Do All the Black Kids Sit Together in the Lunchroom?* as a way to let the reader know that segregation is a reality. But, the rhetorical question she then poses is why do all the White kids sit together in the lunchroom?

A race-conscious society cannot address racism without considering White and Black racial identity as the two are inextricably connected. White people have difficulty seeing their "Whiteness" because they want to believe that what they have achieved is based on merit and not privilege. Black people and others who are "different" typically are very keenly aware of these "differences."

This idea is easily illustrated: ask a White college student to describe their identity and they will talk about their gender, age, and perhaps their height and body build, and they describe their likes, dislikes, hobbies, and interests. They rarely identify themselves as White as they take their race for granted in this predominantly White society. Whites often reach adulthood without thinking much if anything at all about their racial group as their race is the norm and in their mind is not important. Ask a Black, Hispanic, Asian, or Native American student to describe their identity and they will most likely identify their race, color, or ethnicity as one of the very first and most important identifiers. For them, these traits are of major importance as they have been made to feel different and not the norm.

Understanding the idea of different identity development based on color is relevant to this chapter because it impacts the health-related behaviors of individuals. Successful strategies to combat racism must, in some way, lead individuals to explore their racial identity, open up their thinking, remove their blinders, and see the world from a broader perspective.

CHANGING FOR THE BETTER

Considerable debate exists regarding initiatives to eliminate barriers to upward mobility for people of color and to establish a more culturally integrated society. For change to occur, people must recognize that racism today has become camouflaged in everyday practices, policies, notions, and ideas (Bonilla-Silva, 2003; Goodman, 2000; Schmidt, 2005). It is very difficult to change what you choose not to see or recognize. White Americans use several distancing strategies, often unconsciously, to avoid taking responsibility for the presence of individual, cultural, and institutional racism. For example, the concept of "blaming the victim" is common. "Blaming of the victim" in this context occurs when White individuals fail to take responsibility for their own actions but rather attribute a discriminatory action or resulting disparity to a person of color. For example, if a patient of color does not "follow" the physical therapist's instructions, the therapist may presume it is due to some contributory behavior that results from being less intelligent, not interested in getting better, or to a flawed cultural background. It is far easier to "blame the victim" rather than seek out and be open to an understanding of the true underlying causes for an action. In fact, the physical therapist may lack any sense of cultural competence, (i.e., the ability to communicate effectively or address alternative health seeking behaviors that the patient may find more appealing).

While conservatives and liberals are polarized with regard to their stand on promoting diversity, leaders in educational institutions, employers, government agencies, and professional and accrediting bodies are now recognizing the critical value of understanding and managing diversity and are beginning to take action (Orlando, 2000; Parker, 2004). The result is that more programs are in place to increase self-understanding and promote positive relations among people with different cultural ways of life. Racism awareness and cultural competency training are occurring so that institutions can operate and compete in an ever-more diverse society.

To increase the likelihood for success, it is important to understand how to stimulate and control positive change. This is particularly true when dealing with emotionally-laden issues such as racial prejudice, discrimination, and racism. Hardiman (1982) and Helms (2006) have set forth models of White racial identity development that include steps to assist a White person in changing from being part of the problem to someone who opposes institutional racism and is part of the solution. These models have similarities and some differences, yet all include the recognition that this is a difficult journey requiring a paradigm shift (Ponterotto et al., 2006).

A particularly useful theoretical behavioral model, described by Lewin (1951) over a half century ago, identifies three stages for change that can assist in combating racism:

1. An "unfreezing" state where the need for change is realized and motivation for change begins

2. The "change" state where new responses are evidence based on new information

3. A "refreezing" state when the changes and the new patterns of behavior are stabilized and integrated

UNFREEZING: FEELING THE PRESSURE FOR CHANGE

To stimulate change on the individual level, one first needs to reach the "unfreezing" state; that is, to experience a critical level of disequilibrium and a desire to change. One needs to compare one's own true attitudes, beliefs, and behaviors relating to color and race against what they believe to be nonracist attitudes, beliefs, and behaviors and, with a new level of insight, come to the realization that change is necessary. This self-examination and the cognitive dissonance it creates provide the desire for change. This stage is marked by a growing consciousness of racism and White privilege and often results from personal friendships with people of color or contact with key individuals who are willing to be mentors through the change process.

Additionally, the "unfreezing" stage can be facilitated through teaching media and discussion relating to the civil rights movement. Powerful images and discussion about the Jim Crow era in the South, the Civil Rights movement of the 1960s, the nonviolent fight against White oppression led by Martin Luther King Jr., as well as a review of present-day health-related disparities are usually enough to create the disequilibrium and pressure within people necessary for change. While this step brings out a range of emotions from denial and depression to guilt and anger, this tension is necessary for individuals to be open to a different look at the world.

REORIENTATION AND CHANGE

The next step in the process is actual change that requires one to reorient their thinking and accept a new paradigm. As White individuals begin to recognize how powerful a force racism is in their lives and the lives of their friends and family, they are able to identify many of the racist elements in their environment that serve to reinforce White supremacy. They become more aware of the stereotypes, omissions, and distortions in the media, advertising, and entertainment industry. The discomfort of being confronted with this new reality about racism begins to be transformed into action.

The process of reorientation continues through additional discussion about the elements and dynamics of racism (e.g., through statistical information regarding the disparity that currently exists for people of color in socioeconomic status and health). Discussion further highlights the long-term nature of racial disparity in our society and helps bring the issues of racial prejudice and racism to a conscious level of awareness. The StarPower simulation described earlier (Shirts, 1969) helps students gain further insight into White privilege and how institutional racism works. This simulation arouses great emotion, as the frustrations experienced closely parallel those associated with racial conflict in the community. A greater level of insight becomes apparent, facilitating a transformation of thinking about the way the American society works.

Individuals at this phase are often very eager to share their new-found awareness and view of the world with others. They are often overzealous in their efforts and are frequently met with opposition by family, friends, and colleagues. They experience being kidded by friends and confronted by die-hard racists who remain steadfast in the assertion that the blame for inequity rests entirely on the shoulders of people of color. "Transformed" individuals discover that many White people view racism as a thing of the past and are unwilling to attribute any of the causes of today's racial inequity to themselves or recent generations of Whites. "Blaming the victim" may be a typical and frequent reaction from others, often accompanied by stereotyping and unfounded assertions about the root causes of the systematic inequities that exist for people of color today. These discussions often become heated and can repel the new racism awareness convert into solitude and silence—there is often considerable social pressure to revert back to their former selves.

Because these early attempts to spread the word about racism can be very frustrating and feel like swimming upstream against a very strong and steady current, it is important to identify and seek out allies for support. For example, in Connecticut, several members of the Connecticut Physical Therapy Association formed the Cultural Diversity Committee. A group such as this can provide a vehicle for those who have worked on the issue of racism to continue to learn, deal with frustrations, and provide mutual support and encouragement to one another.

RE-FREEZING AND A NEW IDENTITY

Lewin's final stage of change in one's White identity is when one feels comfortable about a new awareness of racism and recognizes that changes in identity will remain a work in progress. This stage brings with it the understanding that the fight against racism needs to be integrated into one's daily life. At this point of new White identity, the individual has a much clearer picture of who they are and are not. They shed their fear of acknowledging who they were and where they have come from in the identity development process. With this stage, one becomes more adept at picking battles to fight racism and more comfortable and confident in interacting in a multiracial setting. Speaking out against individual racist acts such as stopping people from telling racist jokes no longer is uncomfortable. White people in this stage can confront stereotyping and acts of discrimination as they encounter them and hold perpetuators accountable for their acts. With this final stage of White identity development, individuals feel energized and recognize the real power they possess to fight racism.

Yet, people understand that combating racism one person at a time is demanding and can be extremely frustrating. One begins to realize that greater results can be achieved by focusing on institutional racism as one identifies it within their communities, at work, or in professional and civic organizations. Such things as altering hiring policies and practices, increasing the diversity represented in public relations and advertising materials, and modifying employee reward systems have the possibility of having a profound, positive, and lasting effect long after any one person is gone. For organizations to be culturally competent, these and more action steps are required (see Chapter 12).

CONCLUSION

Racism is often subtle, most often unconscious and unintentional, and is ingrained in the fabric of American culture and American institutions. For this reason, most White people find it comfortable riding the wave of White privilege and give little consideration to breaking the self-perpetuating pattern that has worked for White Americans for centuries. To foster improved patient care and remain competitive in the health care marketplace, heath care providers have increasingly begun to recognize the critical value of positive race relations, cross-cultural training, and cultural competence. There is, as well, a growing consensus that efforts to create culturally competent health care providers should be done in concert with efforts to create culturally competent health care organizations and systems (Arrendondo & Perez, 2003; Bruhn, 1996; Cross, Bazron, Dennis, & Isaacs, 1989).

Physical therapists should be encouraged to undergo introspective examination of personal values and behaviors and understand their potential cultural biases that could affect behavior. This, in conjunction with a thorough exploration of objective data pertaining to inequities in health, education and economics, and the origin and nature of racial prejudice, will help create the internal disequilibrium necessary to begin looking at things differently. Manifestations of racial prejudice and the relationship of racial prejudice to individual, cultural, and institutional racism must be explored. Progress in changing one's attitudes and beliefs and becoming a social change agent depends to a large extent upon one's ability to recognize White privilege as an ethnocentric force that narrows one's viewpoints and perspectives.

Racism awareness is a lifelong developmental process and will require many years of hard work, considerable frustration, and constant introspection and reassessment. Feeling comfortable and secure with one's own identity, while simultaneously appreciating other racial and ethnic groups, takes considerable time. The multiculturally sensitive and effective physical therapist should recognize a duty to become a change agent within the larger health care system. Physical therapists need to use their power and position to work at the organizational level to address change and eliminate institutional policies and procedures that may be discriminatory and create barriers for others, and work at the patient care level to be culturally competent. This includes an awareness of the dynamics of difference as well as adaptations of our ways in order to be culturally competent.

REFLECTION QUESTIONS

✔ *What stereotypes do you hold about people of a different ethnic group?*

✔ *What prejudices/biases do you hold toward individuals from a different ethnic group?*

✔ *Are you aware of stereotypes and prejudice toward other people based on religion? Sexuality? Age? Gender?*

✔ *Why do you think stereotypes exist?*

✔ *Are you willing to admit to your stereotypes and biases?*

✔ *How are people of color portrayed in the media?*

✔ *Can you identify recent examples of individual, cultural, or institutional racism impacting your personal life? The American society?*

✔ *What are your beliefs about "affirmative action?"*

REFERENCES

Adorno, T. W., Frenkel-Grunswick, E., Levinson, D. J., & Sanford, R. N. (1950). *The authoritarian personality.* New York, NY: Harper.

Allport, G. W. (1954). *The nature of prejudice.* Reading, MA: Addison-Wesley.

Allport, G. W. (1979). *The nature of prejudice* (25th anniversary ed.). New York, NY: Perseus Books.

Allport, G. W., & Kramer, B. M. (1946). Some roots of prejudice. *Journal of Psychology, 22*, 9-39.

American Medical Association. (1995). Board of Trustees Report 50-1-95. Selected AMA Reports, Section 10, Racial and Ethnic Disparities in Health Care.

American Medical Association. (2002). Report 1 of the Council on Scientific Affairs: Racial and ethnic disparities in health care. Retrieved September 28, 2009, from http://www.ama-assn.org/ama/no-index/about-ama/13602.shtml

American Psychological Association. (2003). Guidelines on multicultural education, training, research, practice, and organizational change for psychologists. *American Psychologist, 58*(5), 377-402.

Arredondo, P., & Perez, P. (2003). Expanding multicultural competence through social justice leadership. *Counseling Psychologist, 31*(3), 282-289.

Arredondo, P., Toporek, R., Brown, S. P., Jones, J., Locke, D. C., Sanchez, J., et al. (1996). Operationalization of the multicultural counseling competencies. *Journal of Multicultural Counseling and Development, 24*(1), 42-78.

Bach, P. B., Cramer, L. D., Warren, J. L., & Begg, C. B. (1999). Racial differences in the treatment of early-stage lung cancer. *New England Journal of Medicine, 341*(16), 1198-1205.

Bell, L. A. (1997). Theoretical foundations for social justice education. In M. Adams, L. A. Bell, & P. Griffin (Eds.), *Teaching for diversity and social justice: A sourcebook* (pp. 3-15). New York, NY: Routledge.

Bennet, C. L., Horner, R. D., Weinstein, R. A., Dickinson, G. M., DeHovitz, J. A., Cohn, S. E., et al. (1995). Racial differences in care among hospitalized patients with Pneumocystis carinii pneumonia in Chicago, New York, Los Angeles, Miami, and Raleigh-Durham. *Archives of Internal Medicine, 155*(15), 1586-1592.

Blendon, R. J., Buhr, T., Cassidy, E. F., Perez, D. J., Hunt, K. A., Fleischfresser, C., et al. (2007). Disparities in health: Perspectives of a multi-ethnic, multi-racial America. *Health Affairs, 26*(5), 1437-1447.

Bonilla-Silva, E. (2003). "New racism," color-blind racism, and the future of whiteness in America. In A. W. Doane & E. Bonilla-Silva (Eds.), *White out: The continuing significance of racism* (pp. 271-284). New York, NY: Routledge.

Boonstra, H. (2002). Teen pregnancy: Trends and lessons learned. *Issues in Brief, 1,* 1-4.

Brighman, J. C., Woodmansee, J. J., & Cook, S. W. (1976). Dimensions of verbal racial attitudes: Interracial marriage and approaches to racial equality. *Journal of Social Issues, 32*(2), 9-22.

Brothers, T. E., Robison, J. G., Sutherland, S. E., & Elliott, B. M. (1997). Racial differences in operation for peripheral vascular disease: Results of a population-based study. *Cardiovascular Surgery, 5*(1), 26-31.

Brown, M. K., Carnoy, M., Currie, E., Duster, T., Oppenheimer, D. B., Shultz, M., et al. (2003). *Whitewashing race: The myth of a color-blind society.* Berkeley, CA: University of California Press.

Bruhn, J. G. (1996). Creating an organizational climate for multiculturalism. *Health Care Supervisor, 14*(4), 11-18.

Buck, R. (2007, June 30). The great race divide: Supreme court decision on schools troubles experts on segregation. *The Hartford Courant,* pp. A1, A7.

Charlton, J. I. (2000). *Nothing about us without us: Disability oppression and empowerment.* Berkeley, CA: University of California Press.

Civil Rights Act of 1964. (1964). 78 Stat. Public Law 88-352. Retrieved September 28, 2009, from http://clerk.house.gov/library/reference-files/PPL_CivilRightsAct_1964.pdf

Conigliaro, J., Whittle, J., Good, C. B., Hanusa, B. H., Passman, L. J., Lofgren, R. P., et al. (2000). Understanding racial variation in the use of coronary revascularization procedures: The role of clinical factors. *Archives of Internal Medicine, 160*(9), 1329-1335.

Cose, E. (2007). Sanity and sentencing: The 'get tough' policies of the 1980s don't work; they undermine faith in the fairness of the justice system. *Newsweek, 150*(26), 53.

Cross, T., Bazron, B., Dennis, K., & Isaacs, M. (1989). *Towards a culturally competent system of care* (Vol. 1). Washington, DC: Georgetown University.

Cunningham, W. E., Mosen, D. M., Morales, L. S., Anderson, R. M., Shapiro, M. F., & Hays, R. D. (2000). Ethnic and racial differences in long-term survival from hospitalizations for HIV infection. *Journal of Health Care for the Poor and Underserved, 11*(2), 163-178.

Ehrlich, H. J. (1973). *The social psychology of prejudice: A systematic theoretical review and propositional inventory of the American social psychological study of prejudice.* New York, NY: Wiley.

Escarce, J. J., Epstein, K. R., Colby, D. C., & Schwartz, J. C. (1993). Health care reform and minorities: Why universal insurance won't equalize access. *Leonard Davis Institute of Health Policy Research Quarterly, 3,* 1-2.

Feagin, J. R. (2000). *Racist America: Roots, current realities, and future reparations.* New York, NY: Routledge.

Fordham, S., & Ogbu, J. U. (1986). Black student's school success: Coping with the burden of "acting White." *Urban Review, 18*(3), 176-206.

Fullinwider, R. (2009). Stanford Encyclopedia of Philosophy: Affirmative action. Retrieved October 17, 2008, from http://plato.stanford.edu/entries/affirmative-action

Glater, J. D. (2006). Colleges open minority aid to all comers. *The New York Times.* Retrieved March 15, 2006, from http://www.nytimes.com/2006/03/14/education/14minority.html?_r=1

Goodman, D. J. (2000). *Promoting diversity and social justice: Educating people from privileged groups.* Thousand Oaks, CA: Sage Publications.

Gornick, M. E., Eggers, P. W., Reilly, T. W., Mentnech, R. M., Fitterman, L. K., Kucken, L. E., et al. (1996). Effects of race and income on mortality and use of services among Medicare beneficiaries. *New England Journal of Medicine, 335*(11), 791-799.

Guadagnoli, E., Ayanian, J. Z., Gibbons, G., McNeil, B. J., & LoGerfo, F. W. (1995). The influence of race on the use of surgical procedures for treatment of peripheral vascular disease of the lower extremities. *Archives of Surgery, 130*(4), 381-386.

Halstead, M. (1988). *Education, justice, and cultural diversity: An examination of the Honeyford Affair, 1984-85.* London, England: Falmer Press.

Hardiman, R. (1982). *White identity development: A process-oriented model for describing the racial consciousness of White Americans.* Electronic Doctoral Dissertations for UMass Amherst. Paper AA18210330.

Harding, J. B., Proshansky, H., Kutner, B., & Chein, I. (1968). Prejudice and ethnic relations. In G. Lindzey & E. Aronson (Eds.), *The handbook of social psychology* (Vol. 5, 2nd ed., pp. 1-176). Reading, MA: Addison-Wesley.

Harvey, C. P. (2004). Introduction to understanding and managing diversity—For the student. In C. P. Harvey & M. J. Allard (Eds.), *Understanding and managing diversity: Readings, cases, and exercises* (3rd ed., pp. 1-11). Upper Saddle River, NJ: Prentice Hall.

Helms, J. E. (2006). An update of Helms' White and people of color racial identity models. In J. G. Ponterotto, S. O. Utsey, & P. B. Pederson. *Preventing prejudice: A guidebook for counselors, educators, and parents* (2nd ed., pp. 81-198). Thousand Oaks, CA: Sage Publications.

Henry, W. H. (1990, April 9). Beyond the melting pot. *Time Magazine,* 28-31.

Hodgkinson, H. C. (1985). *All one system: Demographics of education: Kindergarten through graduate school.* Washington, DC: Institute for Educational Leadership.

Hunt, K. A., Gaba, A., & Lavizzo-Mourey, R. (2005). Racial and ethnic disparities and perceptions of health care: Does health plan type matter? *Health Services Research, 40*(2), 551-576.

Ibrahim, S. A., Whittle, J., Bean-Mayberry, B., Kelley, M. E., Good, C., & Conigliaro, J. (2003). Racial/ethnic variations in physician recommendations for cardiac revascularization. *American Journal of Public Health, 93*(10), 1689-1693.

Jones, J. M. (1972). *Prejudice and racism.* Reading, MA: Addison-Wesley.

Jones, J. M. (1981). The concept of racism and its changing reality. In B. P. Bower & R. G. Hunt (Eds.), *Impacts of racism on White Americans* (pp. 27-49). Thousand Oaks, CA: Sage Publications.

Jones, J. M. (1986). Racism: A cultural analysis of the problem. In J. F. Dovidio & S. L. Gaertner (Eds.), *Prejudice, discrimination, and racism* (pp. 279-314). Orlando, FL: Academic Press.

Jones, J. M. (1988). Racism in black and white: A bicultural model of reaction and evolution. In P. A. Katz & D. A. Taylor (Eds.), *Eliminating racism: Profiles in controversy* (pp. 17-135). New York, NY: Plenum Press.

Katz, D., & Allport, F. H. (1931). *Students' attitudes.* Syracuse, NY: Craftsman Press.

Katz, D., & Stotland, E. D. (1959). A preliminary statement to theory of attitude structure and change. In S. Koch (Ed.), *Psychology: A study of science. Volume 3: Formulation of the person and the social context* (pp. 423-475). New York, NY: McGraw Hill.

Kinney, D. G. (1990). Reopening the gateway to America. *Life,* September, 26-38.

Kramer, B. (1949). Dimensions of prejudice. *Journal of Psychology, 27,* 389-451.

Lefebvre, K., & Lattanzi, J. B. (2007). Health disparities and physical therapy: A literature review and recommendations. *HPA Resource/HPA Journal, 7*(1), J1-J10.

Lewin, K. (1951). *Field theory in social science: Selected theoretical papers.* New York, NY: Harper & Brothers.

Lopez, I. F. H. (2006, November 3). Colorblind to the reality of Race in America. *The Chronicle Review,* pp. B6-B9.

McDonald, M. (1970). *Not by the color of their skin: The impact of racial differences on the child's development.* New York, NY: International Universities Press.

McIntosh, P. (1989). White privilege: Unpacking the invisible knapsack. *Peace and Freedom,* July/Aug, 10-12.

McIntosh, P. (2004). White privilege and male privilege: A personal account of coming to see correspondence through work in women's studies. In C. P. Harvey & M. J. Allard (Eds.), *Understanding and managing diversity: Readings, cases, and exercises* (3rd ed., pp. 83-93). Upper Saddle River, NJ: Prentice Hall.

Merriam-Webster. (1983). Discrimination. In *Webster's Ninth New Collegiate Dictionary* (p. 362). Springfield, MA: Author.

Merriam-Webster Online Dictionary. (2009). Discrimination. Retrieved September 28, 2009, from http://www.merriam-webster.com/dictionary/discrimination

Migration Policy Institute. (2008). United States: Top ten sending countries by country of birth, 1986 to 2006 [table available by menu selection]. Retrieved December 29, 2008, from http://migrationinformation.org/datahub/countrydata/data.cfm

National Institute of Neurological Disorders and Stroke. (2003). Five-year plan on minority health disparities. Retrieved August 14, 2008, from http://www.ninds.nih.gov/about_ninds/plans/disparities.htm

Orlando, R. (2000). Racial diversity, business strategy and firm performance: A resource based view. *Academy of Management Journal, 43*(2), 164-177.

Parker, C. G. (2004). The emotional connection of distinguishing differences and conflict. In C. P. Harvey & M. J. Allard (Eds.), *Understanding and managing diversity: Readings, cases, and exercises* (3rd ed., pp. 42-44). Upper Saddle River, NJ: Prentice Hall.

Peterson, E. D., Shaw, L. K., DeLong, E. R., Pryor, D. B., Califf, R. M., & Mark, D. B. (1997). Racial variation in the use of coronary-revascularization procedures: Are the differences real? Do they matter? *New England Journal of Medicine, 336*(7), 480-486.

Ponterotto, J. G., Utsey, S. O., & Pederson, P. B. (2006). *Preventing prejudice: A guidebook for counselors, educators, and parents* (2nd ed.). Thousand Oaks, CA: Sage Publications.

Rokeach, M. (Ed.). (1968). *Beliefs, attitudes and values.* San Francisco, CA: Jossey-Bass.

Rucker-Whitaker, C., Feinglass, J., & Pearce, W. H. (2003). Explaining racial variation in lower extremity amputation: A 5-year retrospective claims data and medical record review of an urban teaching hospital. *Archives of Surgery, 138*(12), 1347-1351.

Schmidt, S. L. (2005). More than men in white sheets: Seven concepts critical to the teaching of racism as systemic inequality. *Equity and Excellence in Education, 38*(2), 110-122.

Schmidt, P. (2008). "Bakke" set a new path to diversity for colleges. *The Chronicle of Higher Education,* p. A1.

Schroeder, S. A. (1996, November 1). Doctors and diversity: Improving the health of poor and minority people. *The Chronicle of Higher Education,* p. B5.

Secord, P. F., & Backman, C. W. (1964). *Social psychology.* New York, NY: McGraw-Hill.

Shavers, V. L., & Brown, M. L. (2002). Racial and ethnic disparities in the receipt of cancer treatment. *Journal of the National Cancer Institute, 94*(5), 334-357.

Shirts, R. G. (1969). Simulation Training Systems: Starpower. Retrieved September 29, 2009, from http://www.stsintl.com/schools-charities/star_power.html

Smedley, B. D., Stith, A. Y., & Nelson, A. R. (2002). *Unequal treatment: Confronting racial and ethnic disparities in health care.* Washington, DC: National Academies Press.

Stepanikova, I., Mollborn, S., Cook, K. S., Thom, D. H., & Kramer, R. M. (2006). Patients' race, ethnicity, language, and trust in a physician. *Journal of Health and Social Behavior, 47*(4), 390-405.

Tatum, B. D. (1997). *Why are all the Black kids sitting together in the cafeteria?* New York, NY: Basic Books.

U.S. Census Bureau. (2007). Income, poverty, and health insurance coverage in the United States: 2006. *Current Population Reports.* Retrieved March 23, 2008, from http://www.census.gov/prod/2007pubs/p60-233.pdf

U.S. Census Bureau. (2008). U.S. Hispanic population surpasses 45 million: Now 15 percent of total. *U.S. Census Bureau News.* Retrieved August 11, 2008, from http://www.census.gov/Press-Release/www/releases/archives/population/011910.html

U.S. Department of Health and Human Services, Centers for Disease Control and Prevention, National Center for Health Statistics. (2007). *Health, United States, 2007 with chartbook of trends in the health of Americans.* Retrieved August 14, 2008, from http://www.cdc.gov/nchs/data/hus/hus07.pdf

U.S. Department of Health and Human Services, Office of the Assistant Secretary for Planning and Evaluation. (2008). Indicators of child, family, and community connections: Family structure. Retrieved August 15, 2008, from http://aspe.dhhs.gov/hsp/connections-charts04/ch1.htm

U.S. Department of Health and Human Services, Office of Minority Health. (2001). "Closing the health gap": Reducing health disparities affecting African-Americans. Retrieved August 14, 2008, from http://hhs.gov/news/press/2001pres/20011119a.html

U.S. Department of Health and Human Services, Office of Minority Health. (2008a). Data/statistics 2008. Retrieved January 14, 2009, from http://minorityhealth.hhs.gov/templates/browse.aspx?lvl=1&lvlid=2

U.S. Department of Health and Human Services, Office of Minority Health. (2008b). Health topics 2008. Retrieved January 14, 2009, from http://minorityhealth.hhs.gov/templates/browse.aspx?lvl=1&lvlid=4

U.S. Department of Health and Human Services, Office of Minority Health. (2009). African American profile. Retrieved August 14, 2008, from http://minorityhealth.hhs.gov/templates/browse.aspx?lvl=2&lvlid=51

U.S. Department of Justice, Office of Justice Programs, Bureau of Justice Statistics. (2007). Homicide trends in the U.S.: Trends by race. Retrieved August 15, 2008, from http://www.ojp.usdoj.gov/bjs/homicide/race.htm

U.S. Department of Justice, Office of Justice Programs, Bureau of Justice Statistics. (2009a). Victim characteristics. Retrieved August 15, 2008, from http://www.ojp.usdoj.gov/bjs/cvict_v.htm

U.S. Department of Justice, Office of Justice Programs, Bureau of Justice Statistics. (2009b). Prison statistics. Retrieved August 15, 2008, from http://www.ojp.usdoj.gov/bjs/prisons.htm

U.S. Department of Labor, Bureau of Labor Statistics. (2008). Labor force statistics from the current population survey. Retrieved August 12, 2008, from http://www.bls.gov/cps

Varnon, R. (2008, August 15). Minorities to outnumber whites in state by 2042. *The Chronicle,* p. 7.

Ventura, S. J., Abma, J. C., Mosher, W. D., & Henshaw, S. K. (2008). Recent trends in teenage pregnancy in the United States, 1990-2002. Retrieved September 29, 2009, from http://www.csctulsa.org/images/Teenage%20Pregnancy%20Trends%20in%20US%201990-2002.pdf

Virginia Historical Society. (2004). The Green decision of 1968. Retrieved May 20, 2009, from http://www.vahistorical.org/civilrights/green.htm

Wijeyesinghe, C. S., Griffin, P., & Love, B. (1997). Racism curriculum design. In M. Adams, L. A. Bell, & P. Griffin (Eds.), *Teaching for diversity and social justice: A sourcebook* (pp. 82-109). New York, NY: Routledge.

Wikipedia. (2009). Jena Six. Retrieved May 20, 2009, from http://en.wikipedia.org/wiki/Jena_Six

9

Cross-Cultural Communication

Helen L. Masin, PhD, PT

"Culture is communication and communication is culture"—Edward T. Hall

Physical therapists work with individuals from all walks of life, often encountering people from cultures and backgrounds different than their own. In the broadest sense, cross-cultural communication occurs when a rehabilitation professional is communicating with anyone who comes from a different cultural status (Kreps & Kunimoto, 1994). This may include different racial, ethnic, gender, sexual orientation, generational, socio-economic, religious or spiritual, technological, or ability status than that of the therapist. When a physical therapist communicates effectively in cross-cultural interactions, the other individual in the interaction feels at ease and a trusting relationship can be built. When a physical therapist communicates poorly, comfort and trust may be jeopardized. As a result, there may be less than optimal outcomes. These principles are relevant when a physical therapist interacts with a patient/client, research subject, student, or colleague who may come from a different culture than their own. This chapter will provide theoretical and practical information on cross-cultural communication, including differing styles of communication and ways to minimize miscommunication.

TECHNICAL AND ADAPTIVE CHANGE IN CROSS-CULTURAL COMMUNICATION

The model of technical and adaptive challenges described by Heifetz and Linsky (2002) provides a helpful template for understanding the multi-factorial issues that should be considered when one is promoting optimal interaction in cross-cultural encounters. Within the context of communication, they define technical challenges as the work of applying current cross-cultural communication knowledge to manage effectively in a particular setting (e.g., health care). The authorities in that setting do the technical work (e.g., a hospital [the authority] provides language assistance services to consumers with limited English proficiency at no cost to the consumer during all hours of operation). This represents technical work related to provision of language assistance services, one of multiple mandates from the Office of Minority Health (OMH) (U.S. Department of Health and Human Services [HHS], OMH, 2001). Adaptive challenges (continuing with using cross-cultural communication as an example) are defined as the work of leadership to

R. L. Leavitt (Ed.).
Cultural Competence: A Lifelong Journey to Cultural Proficiency (pp. 159-186).
© 2010 SLACK Incorporated

create new ways for effectively providing these language assistance services. The adaptive work is done by the physical therapist who is trying to improve the utilization of language assistance services in his or her PT clinic. The therapist may need to educate staff about the National Standards on Culturally and Linguistically Appropriate Services (CLAS) regulations related to language assistance services, and then motivate the staff to recognize and utilize language assistance services for their patients who have limited English proficiency. Although the CLAS guidelines are clear, the adaptive work of implementing the guidelines may be difficult because it involves teaching therapists and students new ways of communicating with patients (Heifetz & Linsky, 2002).

Technical challenges may be considered easier to address than adaptive challenges because they involve concrete knowledge and prescribe specific behaviors. Adaptive challenges are often considered more complex because they involve abstract concepts and changes in the affective domain of values and feelings (May, Morgan, Lemke, Karst, & Stone, 1995). They also typically involve different attitudes and behaviors than one is used to from their past history or professional training (Masin, 2000, 2002, 2004, 2007).

ADAPTIVE CHANGES IN CROSS-CULTURAL COMMUNICATION FOR PHYSICAL THERAPISTS

As an experienced pediatric physical therapist who moved from metropolitan Washington, DC to Miami, FL in 1980, I realized that I needed to find new ways of communicating with the Miami children and families in my care. These challenges introduced me to the adaptive work of cross-cultural communication in ways that I had not previously imagined. I continue this work to this day!

When therapists (like me) are faced with adaptive pressures for effective cross-cultural communication, we may not want to hear that we must change our "old way" of communicating. Additionally, we may not realize how important it is to change. When faced with patients who demonstrate different worldviews or communication styles, we should ask, "What is the meaning of this behavior within the context of culture?" and "How will I behave now that I am aware of this new information?" (Murphy, Censullo, Cameron, & Baigis, 2007). Open-ended questions like these can help the clinician gain an awareness of the worldview of the clients given their different cultural perspectives.

The process of making adaptive changes in cross-cultural communication requires time for reflection and the development of artful communication skills. This chapter will provide both the technical knowledge to address the challenges and provide suggestions for making the adaptive changes. These adaptive changes occur through acquisition of knowledge, attitudes, and behaviors specific to culture, language, and communication. One of the fundamental elements in this process is affective—valuing effective communication between the patient and the therapist in delivery of culturally competent care (American Physical Therapy Association [APTA], 2008).

In the final analysis, the adaptive work will be done by you; you will reflect on pertinent questions and adapt your professional behavior to demonstrate effective cross-cultural communication with your clients, students, research subjects, and colleagues. You will assume responsibility for going beyond the technical work to develop your own resourcefulness in cross-cultural interactions. Hopefully, this chapter will provide you with helpful tools to motivate and inspire you. Throughout this chapter, "critical incidents" from my career are related. In addition, questions are posed for the reader to ponder from his or her own experiences. These questions are designed to facilitate self-assessment regarding adaptive changes that you may choose to pursue for yourself. They are also intended to encourage reflection *in* action and reflection *on* action to promote your personal development in cross-cultural communications from both a social and language perspective.

REFLECTIVE THINKING IN PROFESSIONAL COMMUNICATION ACROSS CULTURES

Reflective thinking is an important tool in developing good communication across cultures. Reflective courses in professional education are designed to help practitioners critically and thoughtfully think about their behaviors, beliefs, and ideas and consider how they relate to their professional practices.

Nursing and medical educators utilize self-reflection in multicultural education as a means to develop self-awareness and promote more equitable service delivery to diverse populations. Self-reflection is cultivated when students are given the opportunity to cognitively and emotionally process (i.e., "reflect on") the social, cultural, and personal meaning of life events and experiences (Hargreaves, 1997; Koehn & Swick, 2006; Murray-García, Harrell, García, Gizzi, & Simms-Mackey, 2005). In occupational therapy, Odawara (2005) describes reflective thinking as an important part of developing general cultural competency. This reflective thinking helps practitioners identify assumptions underlying their practice based on their own cultural community and the culture of occupational therapy. In addition, it can encourage practitioners to evaluate the validity of these assumptions and compare them to the cultural variables from the worldview of the patient. According to physical therapists Shepard and Jensen (2002), reflection is the educational component that turns experience into learning. Reflection *in* action occurs while the experience is happening, reflection *on* action occurs after the experience is ended and the therapist or student is thinking back on what happened. Reflecting on the experiences provides insights into understanding the meaning of the experiences themselves.

As professionals, reflection can be useful in recognizing and refraining from acting on one's own social, cultural, gender, and sexual biases. Although it is human nature to have biases and stereotypes, it is our professional responsibility to make adaptive changes in order to better serve our clients. One of these adaptive changes is moving from ethnocentrism to cultural pluralism in order to provide effective communication with our patients in a multi-cultural world. Ethnocentric communication reflects a belief that one's own cultural way of life is the norm and the standard by which one judges other cultures. Cultural pluralism reflects a belief that cultures are different, but one is not better or worse than another. To practice cultural pluralism and effective communication, one must self-assess and make a commitment to minimize misperception, misjudgment, and misinterpretation in both verbal and nonverbal communication.

"Critical incidents" can be used to guide our reflective thinking. With analysis, they can enable clinicians to see alternative assumptions, values, and beliefs from the perspective of another culture and, most importantly, lead to changes in behavior. Critical incidents are important social dramas that enable one to reflect and problem solve (Odawara, 2005). In this chapter, critical incidents related to physical therapy from the author's clinical experiences in Miami, Florida will be cited. They are designed to provide the reader with an opportunity for reflection *on* action. Hopefully, they will provide insight into the complexities of cross-cultural communication and methods for effectively resolving the issues.

CRITICAL INCIDENT IN CLINICAL RESEARCH/ COLLEAGUE COMMUNICATION

A faculty colleague recently asked if I could suggest a tool to address cultural issues in a research study involving patients in a cardiac rehabilitation program at a major teaching hospital in Miami. She stated that the patients came from a variety of cultures and that she was planning to use the SF-36, a commonly used tool to measure quality of life issues with patients.

Nursing researchers have theorized that assessment models used to study the health-seeking behaviors of mainstream Anglo groups in the U.S. may not be appropriate for patients from other ethnic groups (Poss, 2001). Since Anglo groups tend to be individualistic, the models are based on individualistic assumptions. Because Hispanic groups tend to be more collectivistic, understanding those beliefs and modifying the research model to assess more collectivistic beliefs may help to explain the health intentions and behaviors in that group (Poss). Modifying a research tool, however, is not a simple task. In order for tests to be used cross-culturally without qualification, the validation sample in the new group should be comparable in size and characteristics to the group used for developing the instrument. The new group must also be clinically and statistically similar to those in the original sample (Stuart, 2004). With the increasing recognition of the unique cultural views of research subjects and the context of communities being studied, trans-cultural researchers need to consider controlling bias in data collection and interpretation. This remains a big challenge. Recognizing the importance of these unique cultural views, however, is especially important in Miami because of its diversity.

Miami-Dade County is the largest county in Florida and has over 2 million residents. More than 60% identify themselves as Hispanics, and 20% identify themselves as Black. They come from North, Central, and South America and the Caribbean. Over 50% of the population in Miami was born outside of the U.S., and 70% of the residents speak a language other than English. In the 2005 census, residents described themselves as coming from more than 25 ethnic groups. In addition to the three major languages of English, Spanish, and Haitian Creole, immigrants from other areas including Eastern Europe, Asia, and Africa bring their unique languages and dialects into the Miami community. Even when looking at one cultural group, there is significant diversity. For example, feedback from Haitian Creole community leaders indicates that translation into Creole is often problematic because more affluent older Haitians speak French rather than Creole (Friedemann, Pagan-Coss, & Mayorga, 2008). In addition, many who speak Creole cannot read Creole.

Socio-economic status (SES) is another variable with a profound impact on culture that needs to be taken into account when doing research in Miami-Dade County. This county is one of the poorest in the U.S. (Friedemann et al., 2008). The 2005 census reported that approximately 32% of the residents have not completed high school, and 18.4% live below the poverty level. SES will impact the ability of research subjects to participate in a study because they may have problems with transportation and may be unlikely to attend multiple sessions for data collection. They may also be difficult to locate for follow-up because the subjects may not have a phone and/or may have changed their address. These considerations must be taken into account (Friedemann et al., 2008).

I suggested to my colleague that using the SF-36 with diverse clients in Miami, even if translated into the language of the research participant, may not address the multiple cultural issues that exist. Indeed, using the SF-36 in this situation illustrates the mismatch between a measurement tool best used in an individualistic culture and a subject pool from a collectivistic culture. The SF-36 falls short of addressing the adaptive challenge of being sensitive to the diversity of perspectives so characteristic of Miami. I suggested that she might also consider using the qualitative methodology of Arthur Kleinman (1978) that employs open-ended questions to learn the perspective of the patients from their world-view (see Chapter 3 for specific considerations for cross-cultural assessments).

CROSS-CULTURAL COMMUNICATION AND PHYSICAL THERAPY

Communication is defined in the dictionary as "the exchange of thoughts, messages, or information as by speech, signal, or writing such that one is readily and clearly understood" (American Heritage Dictionary, 1992). Communication and culture have a reciprocal relationship and cannot be separated (Hall, 1959; E. T. Hall & M. R. Hall, 1990).

Each person in the communicative interaction brings a unique set of meanings, communication styles (including verbal and nonverbal norms), generational expectations, gender-specific expectations, socioeconomic levels, sexual orientation expectations, religious and/or spiritual beliefs, ability levels, technological experience or lack thereof, and environmental experiences. Put in a different way, Agar (1994) stated that:

> *"communication in today's world requires culture. Problems in communication are rooted in who you are, in encounters with a different mentality, different meanings, a different tie between language and consciousness. Solving the problems inspired by such encounters inspires culture…When people learn culture, when they burst out of their former unconscious ways and gaze at the new landscape of possibilities, they can change in positive ways" (pp. 23-24).*

Physical therapists need "extensive knowledge" of communication techniques and should be "skilled" in their use in the clinical environment (Lopopolo, Schafer, & Nosse, 2004). Furthermore, the development of effective communication skills is closely linked to both effective service delivery and student supervision. These issues were apparent in Lopopolo et al.'s research even though they addressed communication in settings where the speakers and listeners spoke and understood the same language. When one adds the additional dimension of speakers and listeners having different languages and cultures, it is clear that communication becomes even more challenging.

Given the increasing diversity and the changing demographics in the U.S. (see Chapter 1) and that there are 6,170 languages and 10,000 cultures in the world (Triandis, 1995), effective cross-cultural communication is becoming increasingly important in our professional physical therapy practice. Indeed, effective cross-cultural communication is considered one essential part of the knowledge, attitudes, and skills essential for physical therapy patient-practitioner interaction. The APTA has included this concept in the APTA Core Values (2003), the APTA-adopted Generic Abilities (May et al., 1995), and the APTA Vision Statement 2020 (APTA, 2005) (see Chapter 1). Mandates for cultural competence and effective communication are affirmed in Federal laws such as the Individuals with Disabilities Education Act of 1991 and Title VI of the Civil Rights Act of 1964.

The APTA House of Delegates adopted *Professionalism in Physical Therapy: Core Values* in 2003 as a way to elucidate the central tenets of professionalism in physical therapy practice, education, and research (APTA, 2003). The core value of compassion/caring includes communicating effectively both verbally and nonverbally, with patients taking into consideration individual differences in learning styles, language, and cognitive abilities. It also includes recognizing and refraining from acting on one's social, cultural, gender, and sexual biases. This document also defines social responsibility as a core value—that is, the promotion of a mutual trust between the profession and the larger public that necessitates responding to societal needs for health and wellness, in part by effective communication.

Another document used in the physical therapy profession to define and facilitate professional behavior is the Generic Abilities (GA). May et al. (1995) identified 10 abilities (or in the language of Heifitz and Linsky, "adaptive skills") that are essential to success as a physical therapist that are not directly linked to the technical skills of the physical therapy profession. They include commitment to learning, interpersonal skills, communication skills, effective use of time and resources, use of constructive feedback, problem solving, professionalism, responsibility, critical thinking, and stress management.

Each of these 10 abilities can relate to the development of cross-cultural communication. A commitment to learning is demonstrated when the PT continually seeks new knowledge related to learning about the cultures and communication styles of the clients they are serving. Interpersonal and communication skills are demonstrated when the PT communicates effectively both verbally and/or nonverbally with a wide diversity of clients, learns essential PT phrases in the client's language, or communicates via an interpreter as appropriate. In addition to facilitating cross-cultural communication, appropriate use of an interpreter leads to effective utilization of time and resources, another GA. Use of constructive feedback is demonstrated when the PT utilizes information from cultural informants to enhance their interaction with clients. Problem solving and critical thinking are demonstrated when the PT recognizes that language may be a barrier to effective treatment and then adapts by using a medical interpreter. Professionalism is demonstrated when the PT learns to demonstrate culturally appropriate greetings and salutations from the client's culture. Responsibility is demonstrated when the PT realizes that it is part of the job to learn more about the language and culture of the clients being served. Finally, stress management is demonstrated when the PT recognizes the stressors of not understanding the culture and/or language of clients being served and takes action to learn the basic culture and language of those clients (Lattanzi, Masin, & Phillips, 2006; Masin, 1995; Masin & Tischenko, 2007).

Finally, the *APTA Vision Statement for Physical Therapy 2020* (APTA, 2005) offers a third platform from which the importance of culturally competent communication is recognized as critical to the future of the profession. This document specifically states that physical therapists "will provide culturally sensitive care distinguished by trust, respect, and an appreciation for individual differences" (APTA, 2005). In order for therapists to demonstrate culturally sensitive care, they need to be able to effectively communicate verbally and nonverbally with the patients in their care.

Together, these three documents—the Profession's Core Values, GA, and the Vision Statement—indicate that the provision of professional physical therapy services requires the ability to communicate effectively with respect for differences in race/ethnicity, gender, sexual orientation, socio-economic status, generation, language, technological skill, physical ability, cognition, and learning styles of the clients being served.

CRITICAL INCIDENT

Learning Spanish has been one of my goals since moving to Miami. I have studied Spanish with Spanish-speaking teachers from the Caribbean in Miami. They advised me that certain words in Caribbean Spanish are considered rude in South American Spanish. While teaching about a physical therapy handling technique with a nine-month-old infant in Montevideo, Uruguay, I made that error. I was demonstrating on the stage at the Montevideo Children's Hospital with about 300 clinicians in the auditorium. I said to the infant, "Coje el juguete" ("take" the toy in Caribbean Spanish; "screw" the toy in Uruguayan Spanish). A great hush filled the auditorium. The translator came running onto the stage and said, "No Helen, no Helen—toma el juguete, toma el juguete!"("take the toy" in Uruguayan Spanish). I quickly realized that I had just used one of those words that my teachers had warned me about in front of an audience of 300 people! Although my mistake was unintentional (and very embarrassing), it made me aware that speaking the language was not enough. I realized that knowing the culture as well as the language was necessary in order to communicate effectively.

This incident is used to demonstrate that the process of communication relies on more than words. Each variety of the language has its unique regional and social dialects and reflects a unique social experience. This social experience makes the vocabulary a productive source of cultural information. Words are complex linguistic structures that are also cultural emblems and symbols with social meaning that preserve the experience of human activity. For each cultural group, the language of that group contains the social meaning that describes human activity in that culture (Pederson, 1989). Indeed, according to Anderson, (1997), cross-cultural communication is both a social and a language phenomenon. For therapists, knowing one without the other gives an incomplete picture. Both the social and language aspects must be understood to have effective cross-cultural communication.

EVIDENCE BASE FOR CULTURAL AND LINGUISTIC COMPETENCE IN HEALTH CARE

Goode, Dunne, and Bronheim (2006) completed an extensive review of the literature on the impact of cultural and linguistic competence in health and mental health care on health outcomes and well-being, and the costs and benefits to the system. The authors reviewed 561 publications from January 1995 to March 2006 on Medline related to this topic. Their meta-analysis indicated that the health outcomes' literature related to cultural and linguistic competence is in the early stages of development. Like any new area of research, there is a developmental progression to the research. When it involves a complex area such as cultural and linguistic competence, the research first focuses on reviews to identify issues for investigation and better define the core concepts. Consistently, many of the early studies reviewed in this meta-analysis were qualitative and the majority focused on defining the concepts and developing research questions. The research is now progressing toward pilot and controlled studies designed to test the impact of cultural and linguistic competence on cost to the health care delivery system, and quality and effective care in relation to health outcomes and well-being. More research needs to be conducted in all of these areas.

CRITICAL ELEMENTS OF EFFECTIVE CROSS-CULTURAL COMMUNICATION

CROSS-CULTURAL COMMUNICATION AND CULTURAL BELIEFS, ATTITUDES, AND BEHAVIORS

The first step in enhancing cross-cultural communication in health care is recognizing your own cultural beliefs, attitudes, and behaviors as well as the beliefs, attitudes, and behaviors of the physical therapy profession. Beliefs are what one holds as true, attitudes are how you feel about those beliefs, and behavior is how you act on those beliefs (Dillman, 1978). For example, you may believe that the health care professionals will communicate their caring and compassion toward you by how they interact with you verbally and nonverbally. If they demonstrate caring and compassion by actively listening and verbally and nonverbally acknowledging your concerns, you will probably develop a positive attitude toward those professionals. On the other hand, if you feel you are not listened to or acknowledged, you may develop a negative attitude toward them and be unlikely to utilize those providers in the future.

As a physical therapist, you likely share a common belief in the effectiveness of biomedical Western medicine with the other providers. However, many of the clients served in physical therapy may or may not share these same beliefs. They may believe in a traditional healing system from their country of origin. Their expectations, beliefs, and behaviors toward health professionals may be different from the expectations, beliefs, and behaviors of the biomedical Western model. These different expectations can lead to miscommunication.

CRITICAL INCIDENTS: CASE EXAMPLES

The following critical incidents from my professional life and one highly publicized account demonstrate communication mishaps based on different cultural points of view.

Critical Incident in Clinician-Patient Interaction 1

A critical incident at the Early Intervention Program (EIP) where I worked in Miami involved a two-year-old boy with epilepsy whose family was Haitian Creole. The pediatric neurology team at the local teaching hospital was treating him. His mother was very dedicated to him; she regularly brought him to the clinic and gave him the prescribed Phenobarbital. However, he still had breakthrough seizures and the staff was extremely concerned about him. The EIP team had a Haitian Creole interpreter speak with his mother and express our concern. The interpreter did not discover anything verbally that might explain the seizures.

One of the staff suggested that we have the mother show us how she was giving her son the seizure medication. The mom asked us for a tub of water. She then placed her son in the tub of water, added the medicine to the water and bathed him in the water. Her behavior was congruent with her belief. We, however, were stunned and would never have thought this to be the problem. This experience had a profound impact on me and began my journey of studying cross-cultural communication. I wondered what other beliefs, attitudes, and behaviors might be miscommunicated in health care settings, and how these misinterpretations might be negatively impacting patient care.

This example dramatically demonstrates that having the technical knowledge related to typical medication administration was not enough. We had to go beyond our technical skills related to our own culture and learn adaptive skills to work effectively with individuals from other cultures. In order to understand what was happening with this child, we had to learn new skills in interviewing in order to recognize other ways that medication might be administered.

Critical Incident in Clinician-Patient Interaction 2

Another incident in the EIP involved a one-year-old girl from Haiti who was referred for physical therapy due to developmental delays associated with her premature delivery. Her mother brought her faithfully to the therapy appointments. I communicated with her mother in French and we appeared to have good rapport in our interactions. When I asked her mother to observe the therapy so that she could follow-up at home, she politely refused. After several sessions in which I asked her to participate, she no longer brought her daughter for PT. I was confused because I thought we had a good relationship. Unfortunately, I did not realize the mother's expectations about me as a "healer." After consulting with a medical anthropologist, I learned that one reason why the mother may have stopped coming for PT is that in Haiti, the family brings the child to the healer (called a mambo) and the healer provides the needed care and returns the child to the family. When I asked the mother to participate in the PT session, I did not realize that I was violating her expectations of what the healer would do. Although we spoke in French, I did not have the cultural knowledge to be able to recognize the difference in the health care expectations. I was operating from the biomedical Western model focusing on change and progress through parent education. The mother may have expected that I would treat her daughter like a traditional healer. Since I did not follow her unspoken expectations, she may have been discouraged from returning to PT for her daughter.

The situation described above demonstrates the importance of effectively integrating knowledge of both language and culture to enhance patient care. Although I knew the language of the family (the technical challenge), I had to dig deeper to understand the cultural expectations (the adaptive challenge) regarding my role as the "healer." Without exploring the life ways of the family and their expectations of my role, I did not understand the mother's reluctance to participate in the home program. She did not have a context in which to frame the experience of the home program because she did not understand the assumptions of biomedical Western medicine for patient and family education.

Critical Incident in Clinician-Patient Interaction 3

A third critical incident at the EIP program where I worked involved a one-year-old girl whose parents were Cuban American and were very concerned about her refusal to be spoon fed by them. The family came to our EIP program and stated that their daughter had a "fit" whenever they attempted to spoon feed her. After speaking with the parents and hearing their descriptions of the problem, I asked them to show me how they were spoon-feeding her. They fed her one spoonful and then wiped the excess from around her mouth with a napkin. The little girl started crying and waving her hands in protest after each spoonful. I asked the parents if I could feed her. Instead of wiping her mouth after each spoonful, I let the food drip down her chin and proceeded with the next spoonful. She ate the whole bowl of food! Her parents were delighted and wanted to know what I had done that enabled her to eat without becoming upset. I explained that she appeared to be tactile defensive around her mouth. She became upset because wiping her mouth after each spoonful was giving her a noxious sensation. By letting the food remain on her chin until the meal was finished, she was able to eat comfortably.

After this experience, I began my research related to maternal views of child rearing and physical therapy in our Miami EIP programs (Masin, 1995). My findings made me aware of cultural beliefs related to feeding and eating in some Cuban American families. One belief is that having a messy baby made you appear to be a "bad mother." Therefore, wiping the child's mouth after every spoonful would prevent looking like a "bad mother." However, if the child was tactile defensive around the mouth, this belief could result in the mealtime problems described above. This family's belief related to feeding was congruent with their attitudes and behaviors with their daughter. There was no language barrier in this case because her parents were fluent in English. However, knowledge of the cultural issues around feeding enabled me to make suggestions to the parents that helped them manage their daughter's spoon-feeding. In summary, the technical challenge was knowing that the child was tactile defensive around her mouth. The adaptive challenge was recognizing the cultural value that was impacting the parent's style of feeding her.

WHEN THE SPIRIT CATCHES YOU, YOU FALL DOWN

A tragic example of cross-cultural miscommunication was reported by an investigative journalist and medical anthropologist, Anne Fadiman in *The Spirit Catches You and You Fall Down* (1998). This book, which received critical acclaim and was read by many lay people as well as health professionals, detailed the case history of a young girl, Lia Lee, from a Hmong family who immigrated from Laos. Lia was treated medically for seizures by the medical staff at Merced Hospital in California. The family held strong beliefs regarding the spiritual meaning of their daughter's illness, which was described as "soul loss" in Hmong culture. Although Hmong interpreters were utilized in communications with the family, the medical staff at the hospital did not understand the cultural norms and expectations of the family. As a result, they misinterpreted the behavior of the family's caring for their daughter's seizure disorder as non-compliant. "The language problem was the most obvious problem, but not the most important. The biggest problem was the cultural barrier" (Fadiman, p. 69). American medicine both preserved her life and compromised it. The child developed severe neurological damage secondary to multiple miscommunications including those related to the anticonvulsant regimen.

In her book, Fadiman suggested that this miscommunication may have been managed more successfully if Arthur Kleinman's concept (1978) of Explanatory Models (EMs) and qualitative interview questions were used to better understand the cultural assumptions held by patients that may impact communication (see Chapter 3). When the EM of the health professional is different than the EM of the client, miscommunication can result. When both parties are operating from different belief systems, their communications reflect those different belief systems. Although they may think they are communicating with each other, the questions and answers they exchange may not be based on similar assumptions (Mullavey-O'Bryne, 1993).

Kleinman, who is both an MD and a medical anthropologist, developed eight interview questions to evaluate illness from the perspective of the patient. These questions help one to understand the EM of patients with regard to their health condition. The EM is the individual's explanation for the etiology, onset of symptoms, pathophysiology, course of sickness, and treatment for the particular problem being addressed (Kleinman, 1978). The interview questions reflect a concern for the psychosocial and cultural facets that give meaning to illness and provide a foundation for developing a mini-ethnography. The questions can be incorporated in an initial interview to assist in understanding the cultural perspective of the patient related to the disorder.

Fadiman contacted Kleinman personally and told him Lia's story. She then gave him the "answers" that Fadiman thought the parents might have given if they had been asked the Kleinman's eight questions at the initial intake at Merced Hospital. Fadiman's "answers" to Kleinman's questions were based on her extensive research in the Hmong community in order to write her book. The eight questions and Fadiman's answers are cited below:

1. *What do you call the problem? Qaug dab peg.* That means the spirit catches you and you fall down

2. *What do you think has caused the problem?* Soul loss

3. *Why do you think it started when it did?* Lia's sister Yer slammed the door and Lia's soul was frightened out of her body.

4. *What do you think the sickness does?* It makes Lia shake and fall down. It is because a spirit called a *dab* is catching her.

5. *How severe is the sickness? Will it have a short or long course?* Why are you asking us those questions. If you are a good doctor, you should know the answers yourself.

6. *What kind of treatment do you think the patient should receive?* You should give Lia medicine to take for a week but no longer. After she is well, she should stop taking the medicine. You should not treat her by taking her blood or the fluid from her backbone. Lia should also be treated at home with our Hmong medicines and by sacrificing pigs and chickens. We hope Lia will be healthy, but we are not sure we want her to stop shaking forever because it makes her noble in our culture, and when she grows up she might become a shaman.

7. *What are the chief problems the sickness has caused?* It has made us sad to see Lia hurt, and it has made us angry at Yer.

8. *What do you fear most about the sickness?* That Lia's soul will never return.

Kleinman validated that Fadiman's proposed "answers" were correct based on her study of Hmong culture. Fadiman then asked Kleinman for suggestions to prevent such miscommunications in the future. When Fadiman explained to Kleinman that Lia's family had been perceived as non-compliant, that she had been removed from her home, and subsequently sustained severe neurological damage, he offered three specifics for Lia's physicians. First, get rid of the term *non-compliance* because "it is a lousy term—it implies moral hegemony. You don't want a command from a general, you want a colloquy" (Fadiman, p. 261). Second, instead of a model of coercion with the family, develop a model of mediation by finding a member of the Hmong community or a medical anthropologist to help with negotiations. Remember that mediation requires compromise on *both* sides. Third, recognize that the culture of the patient and the culture of biomedicine are equally powerful. He stated "If you can't see that your own culture has its own set of interests, emotions, and biases, how can you expect to deal successfully with someone else's culture?" (Fadiman, p. 261).

In this case, the technical challenge was related to the administration of Phenobarbital for the seizure disorder. The adaptive challenge was recognizing and modifying care based on the differing EMs between the biomedical Western model and the spiritual model of the Hmong community. Each of the critical incidents described above have led me to utilize the EM framework in working as a physical therapist in cross-cultural settings.

CROSS-CULTURAL COMMUNICATION AND CULTURAL VALUES

Many cultural value systems have a direct or indirect relationship to cross-cultural communication (see Chapters 2 and 4 for more detail). Two examples that are themselves interrelated are considered here: high/low context communications and monochronic/polychronic time orientation.

HIGH CONTEXT AND LOW CONTEXT COMMUNICATION

Basic cultural, and often geographic, differences are sometimes associated with communication style. Although each individual is different, certain geographic regions may demonstrate similar assumptions related to communication. In general, people from North America, Northern and Western Europe, Australia, and New Zealand tend to focus on transactions, value competition, communicate directly, emphasize content, utilize linear logic, prefer flat organizational structures, and rely on litigation. In contrast, people from Mediterranean countries, Asia, Africa, the Middle East, and Central and South America tend to focus on relationships, value collaboration, communicate indirectly, use circular reasoning, prefer hierarchical structures, trust silence, and rely on mediation (Goldman & Schmale, 2005).

Another way of framing these differences has been described by Hall (1976). He describes high context and low context cultural assumptions and communication. The context is the information that surrounds an event and gives it meaning. These meanings vary from culture to culture.

Hall describes a continuum of communication from low (LC) to middle to high context (HC). He describes low context communication as a message in which the majority of information is included in the message itself (e.g., "what you say is what you mean," "just the facts, please," or "just the bottom line"). This type of communication is usually associated with the culture of biomedical Western medicine. Western medical communication utilizes a direct question/answer mode to give and receive information in clinical settings. Low context communication relies on explicit communication: it is sender-focused; separates tasks from relationships; idealizes business as a well-oiled machine with replaceable parts; relies on facts, statistics, and details; prefers direct writing and speaking; prefers straight line reasoning; adheres to the letter of the law and requires contracts; and establishes trust through specifically stating and writing the agreement (Goldman & Schmale, 2005). Individualist cultures tend to use low context communication.

High context communication is at the opposite end of the continuum. High context communication styles rely on implicit communication: it subordinates tasks to relationships, promotes group initiative and decision making, uses an indirect style in writing and speaking, prefers circular or indirect reasoning, adheres to the spirit of the law, utilizes trust and/or silence to enhance communication, and views agreements as dynamic depending on changing situations or circumstances (Goldman and Schmale, 2005). Most of the information is in the physical context or internalized in the person with a small amount in the spoken message itself. Nuances in communication are considered important and the communication is listener-focused. People from high context cultures have extensive information networks among family, friends, colleagues, and clients and are involved in close personal relationships. Indeed, high context cultures tend to be collectivistic cultures.

The film *Crouching Tiger, Hidden Dragon* (Hsu, Kong, & Lee, 2000) is an example of high context communication. There is minimal dialogue among the protagonists but the meaning is conveyed in nonverbal cues such as body posture, gaze aversion, physical setting, and status in the social hierarchy. Much of what is communicated in the film is understood from inference and nonverbal communication.

Active Listening for Contextual Cues When Communicating With Clients

When working with clients, the physical therapist can listen to what the client says to gain insight into the client's context. Individualistic values in conversation will be oriented toward competition, informality, directness, practicality, materialism, valuing youth, relative equality of the sexes, individualism/privacy, personal control over the environment, time dominance, precise time reckoning, future orientation, "doing" state of personal qualities, human equality, and self help (Leavitt, 2002). These values are typically associated with low context communication.

In patient interactions, clients from places with predominate individualistic communication styles may expect the PT to be on time (time dominance), discuss the importance of making progress with their PT (personal control), have an expected timetable for recovery (time dominance and personal time reckoning), and will ask to be informed directly about their diagnosis (directness, practicality) and prognosis (future orientation, self help, and "doing" orientation).

In contrast, collectivistic values in conversation will be oriented toward group welfare, fate, dominance of human interaction, loose time reckoning, past orientation, a "being" state of personal qualities, hierarchical status or rank, birthright inheritance, cooperation, formality, indirectness or "saving face," idealism, spiritualism, valuing elders, and relative inequality of the sexes (Leavitt, 2002; Odawara, 2005). These characteristics are associated with high context communication. In patient interactions with clients who hold these collectivist values, they may not directly discuss their diagnosis (formality, hierarchical status of therapist, saving face) or prognosis (fate). They may wish to establish a more personal relationship with the therapist (dominance of human interaction, cooperation, and a "being" state), and may not be concerned about keeping a strict appointment time (loose reckoning of time). In the Hispanic cultures, this is known as *personalismo*.

People with high context communication styles may get frustrated when individuals with a low context communication style don't provide them with enough information or do not seem personally invested in them. On the other hand, people with low context communication styles get impatient and irritated when individuals with high context communication styles give them too much information or seem to get too "personal." An example of how high context communication may come to the forefront in a physical therapy encounter is when a client may greet the therapist by asking, "How was your weekend?" or "How is your family?" From the client's perspective, this kind of personal communication is helpful in building trust in the personal as well as the professional relationship. Hall theorizes that this is because people from a collectivist culture keep themselves informed about everything related to the people who are important in their lives (Hall, 1976; E. T. Hall & M. R. Hall, 1990). The physical therapist, on the other hand, may be surprised at what is perceived as an inappropriately personal greeting in a professional setting.

MONOCHRONIC AND POLYCHRONIC TIME ORIENTATION

In physical therapy practice, time-related concerns often impact communication. Time measurement is a man-made construct, and different cultures relate to time in different ways. Traditional agrarian cultures orient to time based on growing seasons, sunrise, and sunset. Time is perceived as flowing and the perception of time is based on the rhythms of the natural environment. Events happen concurrently and fixed schedules are not important. There is more focus on personal interaction and less concern about completion of the task at hand (Leavitt, 2002). This is referred to as *polychromic time*.

In communication, individuals from Mediterranean and South American cultures often view time as polychromic. They view time with a flexible perception, tend to hesitate to strictly measure or control time, welcome interruptions, multitask, put human feelings before schedules, and value the past as well as the present. For example, multiple conversations may occur simultaneously with multiple people. Conversations are oriented toward people and the focus is on human relations. Conversation is valued, so you would not end a conversation because you have a schedule to keep. The lines between business life and social life are blurred. Time is not a commodity; it flows and passes (Hall, 1984).

In contrast, industrial cultures have divided time into units for measurement of production. Time is perceived as linear and the perception of time is based on hours and minutes. Time is an important concept and events occur in chronological order. There is a separation of work tasks and socializing, and schedules are important (Leavitt, 2002). This is referred to as *monochronic time* and is often associated with low context cultures.

People who view time from a monochromic, linear perspective (the typical physical therapist) view time as a commodity to be saved, spent, or wasted. They complete tasks in order, focus on tasks at hand with a timetable for completion, separate work from family and social life, attempt to control time with schedules, and focus on the future. Monochronic time is oriented to tasks, schedules, and procedures. It is arbitrary and imposed. Schedules prescribe everything from social life to business life to sex life. Conversations occur one-on-one, and each speaker speaks in turn. Time is seen as a commodity to be managed. However, this view of time is not inherent in man's biological rhythms or his creative drives (Hall, 1984).

CULTURAL VALUES WITHIN THE FAMILY AND ACROSS THE GENERATIONS

CROSS-CULTURAL COMMUNICATION WITHIN THE FAMILY

Cultural values within collectivist and individualist societies typically relate to communication style within the family. In most communities with collectivistic orientation, respect for elders is considered paramount. Children and young adults should speak and act respectfully toward elders. There is a sense of duty or obligation to family and people from older generations. Also, anything done by a family member is a reflection on the whole family. It is important for family members to maintain "face" or dignity in all communications. If the behavior is positive, the whole family is validated. If the behavior is negative, the whole family is shamed and the dignity of the family is compromised. Therefore, the actions of one individual have an impact on all other members of the extended family as well as the perception of the family in the community. In contrast, individualist cultures tend to be more associated with a value for youth, with less attention paid to respect of elders.

CROSS-CULTURAL COMMUNICATION ACROSS THE GENERATIONS

Communication differences have also been studied with regard to the generations. Although relevant to all people in everyday and professional lives, it is informative to look specifically at generational differences between physical therapist faculty and students, or therapists and patients who are frequently separated by one or two generations. To communicate effectively across generations, one must have knowledge of and appreciation for the characteristics, rewards, and preferred feedback for each generational group (Gleeson, 2007). The four primary generational groups commonly identified in Western culture are Traditionalists, Baby Boomers, Generation X, and Millenials. The characteristics of each group and the preferred style of rewards and feedback are summarized in Table 9-1.

Boomer or Traditionalist faculty members may have differing expectations of students based on their generational culture. Pellegrino (1983), from the generation of traditionalists, stated that the professional must put his or her patient's needs ahead of his or her own self-interest. This may be a challenge for those of a different mindset. Younger students or faculty may perceive a need for more "balance" between their personal and their professional lives. This may lead to conflict and miscommunication in both the classroom and the clinic.

The spoken preferences among Traditionalists are for formal, linear thinking; polite, direct, respectful communication with no slang or foul language; and a preference for following the chain of command. For example, patients and faculty from this generation may expect that students will address them with formal titles (e.g., Mr., Ms., or Dr.) followed by their surname.

The spoken preferences for Baby Boomers are for small talk to build camaraderie and connection, valuing team building and consensus building. Baby boomers may call each other by first names but expect students to address them by their titles.

In contrast, the Gen Xers prefer spoken communication to be informal, very direct, getting to the point quickly, and wanting to know how this affects them directly. They may think that following the chain of command is a waste of time. Students may address each other informally and may use first names when addressing patients or faculty members.

Millenials prefer spoken communication to be informal, needing to see how things are important now, wanting to know why things matter right now. They may need help in seeing the big picture and may not see the need for following the chain of command. They need to be taught how to resolve conflict. They may also use first names when addressing patients or faculty members.

Given these differences in characteristics, rewards, preferred feedback, and spoken preferences, physical therapists need to consider the generational culture when working with their clients, colleagues, faculty members, and students.

CRITICAL INCIDENT WITH CLINICIAN-STUDENT COMMUNICATION

One student from the Gen X generation in our DPT program experienced anxiety in her clinical internship with a clinical instructor (CI) who was a Baby Boomer. The Gen Xer was fearful that she was failing her clinical internship because her CI had not given her much feedback on her performance. The CI was pleased with the student's performance and did not expect to give the student feedback unless something went wrong. Each party misinterpreted and misunderstood the generational communication expectations. As the supervisor in this situation, I had to educate both the student and the clinician about how different generational expectations resulted in miscommunication. The student, the CI, and I met to discuss more effective ways to convey feedback between them. The CI agreed to meet weekly with the student to give the student more regular feedback on her performance. The student was relieved to learn that she was not failing her clinical. She also recognized that she needed to ask for additional feedback from her CI if she wanted more information about her performance.

The technical challenge in this case was negotiating constructive feedback in the clinical setting. The adaptive challenge was learning that different generations have differing expectations regarding feedback and then adapting the communication to effectively address those differing expectations.

TABLE 9-1

GENERATIONAL GROUP	YEARS BORN	CHARACTERISTICS	REWARDS	PREFERRED FEEDBACK
Traditionalists	Before 1946	Conservative, have faith in institutions, patriotic, loyal, fiscally conservative	Satisfaction of a job well done	No news is good news
Baby Boomers	1946-1964	Competitive, question authority, idealistic, the "me" generation	Money, title, recognition	Once a year whether you need it or not
Generation X	1965-1981	Distrustful of institutions, resourceful, eclectic, highly adaptive to change and technology, self reliant	Freedom is the ultimate reward	"So how am I doing?"
Millenials	1982-2000	Realistic, pragmatic, cyber literate, media savvy, globally concerned, environmentally conscious	Work that has meaninge	From a virtual coach with the push of a button

Adapted from Lancaster, L., & Stillman, D. (2002). *Why generations collide: Who they are, why they crash, how to solve the generational puzzle at work.* New York, NY: Harper Collins.

VERBAL AND NONVERBAL COMMUNICATION STYLES

Different cultural groups, in part based on their cultural value systems, have developed different verbal and nonverbal styles of communicating (see Table 9-2). Verbal characteristics include language, pacing, tonality, intent, speed, and use of silence. Nonverbal communication includes visual, auditory, olfactory, tactile, and vestibular signals and is multi-channel communication. These channels work together to convey a specific message, and nonverbal components include gesture, facial expression, proxemics (distance), haptics (touch), and oculesics (eye movements). For example, tone of voice, facial expression, and body posture may combine to convey a message of happiness or sadness. Nonverbal communication skills are developed as infants, long before mastery of verbal communication skills. According to Mehrabian & Wiener (1967), 60% to 90% of communication is nonverbal, and 10% to 40% is verbal. When participating in any communication, it is important to recognize and interpret both verbal and nonverbal characteristics of the communication.

CROSS-CULTURAL VERBAL COMMUNICATION

Verbal communication is characterized by language per se, speed and pacing, tonality, and intent. In the U.S., regional differences in the English language can be seen in pacing, speed, and tonality (e.g., the fast, clipped pace of New York speech versus the slow, rhythmical pace of the deep South). Similar verbal variations occur in speakers of other languages. For example, in Miami, where 58% of the population speaks Spanish as a first language, the pacing, tonality, intent, and speed of communication can vary dramatically. The Cuban-American Spanish is more fast-paced and louder than the more slow and soft-spoken Nicaraguan Spanish. The individualistic/collectivistic orientation of the speaker may also influence communication. For example, the client from a more individualistic culture may be very direct in speaking with the physical therapist about their concerns. In contrast, the client from a more collectivistic culture may be more indirect and be more concerned about maintaining "face" in interactions with the physical therapist. Recognizing these variations in verbal communication can assist the therapist in developing a better understanding of verbal communication with clients whose language is different than that of the therapist.

TABLE 9-2

DIFFERENCES IN COMMUNICATION STYLES

LATINO-HISPANIC

Communication:

- Hissing may be used to gain another's attention.
- Official or business conversations are preceded by social greetings. Conversations may switch between official and social language.
- Interruption during conversations is usually tolerated.
- Raising one's voice is used to gain the conversation floor.

Touching:

- Touching between two people in conversation is common.

Eye contact:

- Avoidance of eye contact is a sign of attentiveness, respect; sustained eye contact may be perceived as a sign of threat or challenge to authority.

Distance:

- Distance between two speakers is relatively close.

AFRICAN AMERICAN

Communication:

- Distinction between "arguing" and "fighting." Arguing can involve verbal abuse, while fighting can be physical.
- Asking personal questions of someone one has just met is perceived as inappropriate.
- Indirect questions are sometimes seen as harassing.
- Interruption during conversations is usually tolerated.
- Conversations are considered to be private between participants.

Touching:

- Touching another's hair may be perceived as offensive.

Eye contact:

- Preference for indirect eye contact during listening; direct eye contact during speaking.

ASIAN AMERICAN

Communication:

- It is considered impolite for children to interrupt in conversation.
- Addressing others is regulated by hierarchies as seen in language and behaviors.
- Social status is established by one's age, sex, job status, and marital status. Therefore, it is common to ask questions related to these factors.
- Kinship terms are very important in establishing the relationship between two family members. These terms may extend beyond the family to include community members.
- Facial expressions are composed.
- Giggling when embarrassed may occur.
- Finger beckoning is used for small children and not adults.

Touching:

- Touching and hand holding between members of the same sex is acceptable.
- Hand holding and kissing between members of the opposite sex in public is unacceptable.

Eye contact:

- Avoidance of eye contact is a sign of attentiveness, respect; sustained eye contact may be perceived as a sign of threat or challenge to authority.

NATIVE-AMERICAN

Communication:

- Personal questions may be considered snooping or prying.
- It may be acceptable to ask the same question several times.

Eye contact:

- Avoidance of eye contact is a sign of attentiveness, respect; sustained eye contact may be perceived as a sign of threat or challenge to authority. Prolonged and continued direct eye contact is undesirable.

Reprinted from Brice, A., & Campbell, L. R. (1999). Cross-cultural communication. In R. L. Leavitt (Ed.), *Cross-cultural rehabilitation: An international perspective* (pp. 91). London, England: Harcourt Brace and Company.

Ladyshewsky (1999) reports examples of communication difficulties between Australian clinical educators (CI) and students of Southeast Asian origin. These examples represent the challenges that can occur when two people come from different cultural backgrounds and have different communication styles. The two interactions described below demonstrate the technical and adaptive challenges across both cultures and generations. In each scenario, the technical challenge is effective communication between the student and the CI. The adaptive challenge is recognizing that in Asian cultures, students are not socialized to challenge their instructors (elders) because to do so would bring shame on the instructor (elder). Therefore, the adaptive challenge becomes modifying the supervisor's communication so that the student can understand that Australian teaching/learning styles are different. In Australia, students are expected to be active problem solvers and it is acceptable to challenge the professor. Meeting this adaptive challenge requires significant change in both the supervisors and the students.

Scenario One

Supervisor: The students' problem solving abilities seem very poor. We teach Australian students to be very independent whereas this doesn't appear to be the case with these students.

Southeast Asian student: One's own ideas are not as important as what the actual facts are or what is accurate. Rather than take the wrong course of action, it is more appropriate to hear the information from an expert so that the course of action is correct.

Scenario Two

Supervisor: The students don't appear to personalize the problems as their own—they throw it back to you. Since you identified the problem, you must solve it for them. It is not your typical adult learning situation—you are here to tell them what to do.

Southeast Asian student: It is impolite to be assertive or aggressive with your supervisor. You are taught in school [in southeast Asia] not to talk to your teacher directly. You can disagree but only to a certain level. Because professional behavior is such an important part of your evaluation, if you act in a bad manner you will get low marks.

The use of silence is also part of verbal communication. For example, a North American therapist may interpret the silence of an Asian American patient as a lack of interest in the therapy. However, the patient may be silent as an indication of respect for the therapist.

CROSS-CULTURAL NONVERBAL COMMUNICATION

It is impossible to *not* communicate nonverbally (Singelis, 1993). Once you enter the room, you are communicating nonverbally via your appearance, gestures, and facial expression. While nonverbal communication is important when the therapist and the client come from the same culture, it is even more important and potentially more challenging when the therapist and client come from different cultural and/or language backgrounds. Nonverbal communication incorporates proxemics (distance between speakers), haptics (touch between speakers), oculesics (eye movement between speakers), vocalics (loudness and speed between speakers), facial expressions, and gestures. Different cultures attach different expectations to each of these areas. Social skill requires that nonverbal messages are correctly produced and received.

As indicated above, some nonverbal messages are sent automatically without any volitional action. For example, when someone winces in pain, the receiver interprets the meaning immediately without words. It is conveyed directly and emotionally from observing the image itself. However, the nature of nonverbal communication can also be ambiguous because the meaning of the nonverbal communication may vary from culture to culture. For example, laughter indicates humor in some cultures and embarrassment in others.

There is evidence that nonverbal communication is both a biologically determined behavior that is consistent across cultures (i.e., culture-general behaviors) (Ekman, 1971; Izard, 1971) and a learned behavior governed by cultural norms (i.e., culture-specific behaviors) (Hall, 1959). Culture-general characteristics refer to aspects of nonverbal communication that span different cultural groups. Ekman and Izard found six facial expressions that were recognizable in all cultures: anger, fear, happiness, sadness, surprise, and disgust. Nevertheless, environmental context and individual personality may lead to variation in how, when, and to what degree these expressions are used.

CRITICAL INCIDENT IN CLINICIAN-PATIENT COMMUNICATION

As a therapist from a North American background working in Miami, I quickly appreciated that nonverbal communication profoundly impacts rapport in intercultural interactions with clients and their families. For example, the parents of many of the children I saw greeted me by kissing me on the cheek when they arrived for therapy. Initially, I was confused by their behavior until I realized that a kiss on the cheek was a traditional Cuban-American cultural greeting once a professional and personal relationship was established. Indeed, not to use this greeting would be considered rude on my part.

Proxemics in Cross-Cultural Communication

Proxemics is the physical space involved in communication patterns. The preferred distances for formal communication vary across cultures. Some people prefer to be closer together and others prefer to remain more apart. For some Anglo-Europeans, an arm's length is optimal for patient-professional communication. For some Latin Americans, less than an arm's length is appropriate for patient-professional communication. For example, as a student studying Spanish, my teacher recommended watching the Spanish TV *novellas* (Spanish language soap operas) to help me learn the language. When watching, my gut reaction of discomfort indicated that I might be experiencing a cultural snafu. I recognized that the distance between the speaker and the listener in some Latin American cultures is closer than the distance between speaker and listener in Euro-American cultures. Therefore, the distance between the person operating the camera and the actors in the novellas was closer than that in Euro American soap operas. I was experiencing the discomfort of having my space invaded by actors and actresses on the TV!

Haptics in Cross-Cultural Communication

Haptics is the use of touch in communication patterns, and this varies across cultures as well. For example, when having a conversation with friends, I may touch them occasionally when speaking to them. However, in conversing with my Latin American friends, they touch me more frequently to make a point or emphasize what they are saying. This type of non-sexual touch may be appropriate between an unrelated man and woman in North American culture, but it is strictly forbidden in certain Middle Eastern cultures. Non-sexual touch between same-sex people in some Asian and African cultures can be misinterpreted by people from Euro American backgrounds where same-sex hand holding or affection may be perceived as sexual in nature. Thus, the intention of the person touching may be different than the message received by an observer from a different culture.

The film, *The Doctor* (Ziskin & Haines, 1991), based on a true story, depicts how miscommunication can occur when the physician is communicating in a low context style and his patient is communicating in a high context style with different preferences with regard to proxemics and haptics. When the physician is talking with his patient from a Mexican background about preparation for his impending heart transplant, the patient hugs the doctor. The doctor becomes visibly distressed and lets out an audible sigh of relief when the patient lets go. In the biomedical Western culture (with its associated low context communication style), when the patient hugged the physician, the doctor perceived it as an uncomfortable violation of his personal and professional space. On the other hand, the use of touch by the patient was a high context communication style indicating his trust in the doctor.

Oculesics in Cross-Cultural Communication

Oculesics is the utilization of eye movements in communication patterns. These also vary across cultures. In Anglo-European cultures, the use of direct eye contact is considered a sign of attention. It may also signify trust and respect between people communicating with each other. However, in certain Native American groups, for example, downcast eyes are a sign of respect and attention. The same physical behavior has totally different meaning depending on the specific cultural context in which it is used.

Facial Expression and Gestures in Cross-Cultural Communication

The use or lack of facial expression also varies across cultures. Facial expression can vary from minimal to maximal affect. Minimal affect has been associated with some Asian American cultures, which has given rise to the Western description of the "inscrutable Oriental." Minimal affect and the use of silence have also been associated with some members of the Native American cultures. Maximal affect has been ascribed to some members of the African American culture (Project Craft Video, 1997).

The use or lack of gestures similarly varies across cultures. People from Hispanic or Middle Eastern backgrounds tend to be more expansive in their use of gestures. People from Northern Europe are likely to demonstrate fewer expressive gestures. The teaching video *Communicating Across Cultures* (Project Craft Video, 1997) demonstrates the potential for gestures to be misinterpreted. A Kuwaiti student utilizes a gesture of an outstretched arm with the palm facing down and moving the fingers together toward the body to beckon a person to come to him. He describes an encounter with an Anglo-American student on his campus in which the student outstretched his arm with his palm facing up and beckoned him with his index finger. For the Kuwaiti man, this gesture was extremely offensive. He stated that in Kuwait, beckoning with the index finger is done for dogs, not for people. Alternatively, when the therapist uses the "A-okay sign" in North America, this means that you are doing a good job. However, in certain Latin American cultures, this same sign may be perceived as an obscene gesture. Without a working knowledge of nonverbal communication, a therapist could inadvertently use a nonverbal communication pattern that might be offensive to clients. Misattribution is when the incorrect meaning is attributed to a nonverbal communication.

In addition to misattribution, nonverbal communication can be impaired through missing signals. This occurs when signals are unfamiliar to the therapist or too subtle to be recognized by someone outside of the culture of the patient. For example, a North American therapist may not recognize the subtle use of a slight sucking of air and tilt to the head by a Japanese patient to indicate a negative response (Singelis, 1993).

It is important to also remember that individual personality characteristics or the environmental context may also impact verbal and nonverbal communication styles. Context confusion can occur when one party expects a certain behavior but the behavior is not carried over into another environment. For example, a North American therapist may notice the patient who is of Hispanic descent joking and laughing with other Hispanic patients in the waiting room. The therapist may assume that that patient will demonstrate the same lighthearted behavior in the clinic. However, the patient believes it is appropriate to act more formally when interacting with the professional therapist. Or, one client may use a lot of gestures and movement when communicating with friends but be more reserved with fewer gestures when in a medical setting. A client may speak loudly in the PT gym to be heard, but that same client may be very soft-spoken in a private treatment room.

Enhancing Cross-Cultural Communication

Physical therapists need to learn the knowledge, attitudes, and skills to diplomatically and effectively navigate different communicative interactions while demonstrating respect and openness toward the other person(s) involved in an interaction. Research indicates that good interpersonal communication between patients and their health care practitioners often determines patient perceptions: good communication can lead to trust in the provider, patient loyalty, adherence to treatment schedules, and overall positive health outcomes (AMA, 2006).

There are numerous ways to demonstrate that we value our clients and put their needs ahead of our own. First we must recognize and appreciate how our own culture and the culture of biomedical Western medicine impact us, our values, and our communication style. According to Hall (1984), "one of the many paths to enlightenment is the discovery of ourselves, and this can be achieved whenever one truly knows others who are different" (p. 8).

Once we understand our personal and professional cultural lenses, we can begin to appreciate the cultures and languages of the clients we serve. We can recognize that broad categories may be acceptable for descriptive purposes but they can also be used to perpetuate racial or ethnic stereotyping or prejudice by what we say. We also recognize that differences within groups (i.e., intra-group variation) can be equal to or greater than between group variations (i.e., inter-group variation). We can work to eliminate assumptions about any group just as we would not make assumptions about all children with a diagnosis like Down Syndrome. Next are specific suggestions for ways to enhance communication.

PATIENT-CENTERED COMMUNICATION

In order to enhance patient-practitioner communication in diverse settings, patient-centered care (PCC) using patient-centered communication is recommended. PCC is care that is both respectful of, and responsive to, individual patient preferences, needs, and values. Patient-centered communication is a narrower subset of PCC. According to Lipkin et al. (1984) and AMA (2006), practitioners who are patient-centered have the knowledge, attitudes, and skills necessary to elicit a patient's "story" of their illness, express interest and commitment to patients (or students), and overcome barriers to communication (Lipkin et al.). I have developed an approach called participant-centered problem solving (PCPS) (Masin, 1998a, 1998b, 2000, 2002, 2004). Both PCC and PCPS require:

- Adopting a bio-psychosocial perspective rather than assuming only a biomedical perspective
- Understanding the patient/student as a person in his or her own right
- Sharing power and responsibility for communication with both the patient and the therapist/student
- Building a therapeutic alliance
- Understanding that the clinician/professor is a person and not just a skilled technician

Another patient-centered model of communication is the LEARN model of culturally effective communication (Berlin & Fowkes, 1983). It has five elements:

1. Listen
2. Elicit
3. Assess
4. Recommend
5. Negotiate

Listening involves identifying and greeting the family or friends of the patient and, if appropriate, asking if they would prefer an interpreter. The interview starts with open-ended questions and the therapist does not interrupt the patient when he or she is speaking. *Eliciting* involves learning the patient's health beliefs as they pertain to the health condition and the reason for the visit as well as expectations. Eliciting can be enhanced with Kleinman's EM and its related questions. *Assessing* involves identifying potential attributes and problems in the life of the client that may impact their health and health behaviors. *Recommending* involves developing a plan of action and explaining the reasons for the plan of action. Finally, *negotiating* involves discussing the plan of action after having made your recommendations (Berlin & Fowkes, 1983).

Through adopting these or similar patient-centered perspectives, the practitioner enhances the communication process and helps to develop a trusting relationship with the patient or the student. We can enhance our effectiveness in cross-cultural communication if we are open to exploring the possibilities presented by our own worldview and the worldview of each patient/client that we encounter.

ENHANCING RAPPORT IN CROSS-CULTURAL INTERACTIONS

The concept of rapport is frequently referred to as an essential element in patient care by a variety of health professionals. Rapport is a therapeutic alliance based on trust and cooperation and established through a shared understanding of the patient's perspective. It is reinforced by interpersonal communication skills such as an open question style and checking for patient agreement (Norfolk, Birdi, & Walsh, 2007). Mental health counselors have long recognized that rapport is a basic building block of the therapeutic alliance. The development of rapport may be supported by the appropriate use of facial expressions that indicate interest and involvement from the counselor to the client (Sharpley, Jeffrey, & McMah, 2006). Qualitative researchers must develop rapport in ethnographic research. It is essential to develop good relationships in order to get in-depth intimate interviews with the subjects and get robust data. Rapport is essential in order to establish the process of give and take between the researcher and the subjects (Gaglio, Nelson, & King, 2006). Similarly, improved patient outcomes are expected if a physical therapist develops rapport with each patient.

One tool available to facilitate rapport is Neurolinguistic Psychology (NLP). NLP is the establishment of a cooperative communication mode in which the individuals are aware of and responsive to one another. It is marked by harmony but does not necessarily indicate agreement. When people are in rapport, they have behavioral patterns that match. These include breathing rates, postures, tempo of speech, and language patterns that become similar in nature. To build rapport, a therapist can match or pace the other person in the communication dyad. To break rapport, a therapist can mismatch or change the pace as it relates to the other person in the interaction (Konefal, 2002; O'Connor & Seymour, 1993).

According to NLP, there are three primary types of rapport. The first is cultural in which the form of dress and greeting are similar to the people you are meeting. For example, in working with Latino families in early intervention in Miami, it is culturally appropriate to touch the person with your cheek while blowing a kiss with your mouth.

The second rapport is verbal, which is demonstrated when the therapist uses the same or similar descriptive phrases and conversation content as the client or student. For example, the client may state that they cannot "see" what the therapist wants them to do. The therapist might respond by saying, "When you *look* at your legs, be sure to keep them parallel." The therapist is using the visual terminology of the patient to build verbal rapport. Another example would be the student who says I am not "grasping" the material. The clinical educator might reply by saying, "*Hold* the client's wrist while you sweep tap here and feel for the activation of the forearm." The therapist is using the kinesthetic terminology of the student to build verbal rapport. In this way, the learning style of the client or the student is acknowledged and utilized to assist in the learning process.

Behavioral rapport, the third type, is demonstrated when the posture and body movements, vocal tonality and tempo, and breathing rate and position of the therapist are similar to the client or the student (Bernieri & Rosenthal, 1991; Masin, 2000, 2002). For example, the client may be sitting back in the chair opposite the therapist with hands folded gently in the lap. The therapist can assume a similar posture before beginning verbal discussion of the client's history. At the unconscious level, matching the posture of the client indicates to the client that the therapist recognizes the client's perspective. When working with students, a therapist may sit next to the student at a desk when going over plans of care. At the unconscious level, the clinical instructor is indicating to the student that the student's position is valued and understood.

Another example is when the therapist matches the body language of the client while listening to an interpreter. By matching the client's body posture, the therapist is creating behavioral rapport at the nonverbal level with the client. This can help to build behavioral rapport with the client even though the therapist does not speak the same language as the client. Since nonverbal communication is such a large part of every communication, behavioral rapport can provide a mechanism for tapping into this important aspect of the communication with the client.

Ladyshewsky (1999) reported examples of students from Southeast Asia having difficulty building rapport with patients in Australia, secondary to both language and cultural barriers. The following are quotes from clinical educators:

> "It takes longer to develop rapport with patients, this relates to the communication difficulties...the students are spending so much time listening, thinking, translating, etc... It becomes difficult for the patients to develop rapport. The students, because they are anxious and busy thinking, often come across as very blunt—this further cuts off rapport" (p. 168)

> "The [Southeast Asian] student's language sounds clipped, the accent sounds brusque or rude and this puts the patient off—even though the student is trying hard. Statements are too brusque and staccato" (p. 168)

Both of these quotes reflect the technical challenges faced by Asian students related to developing verbal rapport since English is their second language. The adaptive challenges in both cases involve educating the clinical instructors on how to teach the students to be more effective and for the students to actually make the changes. The clinical faculty might suggest that the students utilize behavioral rapport (i.e., having the students match the body language of the patients).

CRITICAL INCIDENT IN CLINICIAN-PATIENT COMMUNICATION

While working with preschool children in Miami who are hard of hearing, I was asked by the classroom teacher if I could assist her in communicating with one of her students named Jorge. She reported that he was profoundly deaf from birth, had minimal vocalizations, and appeared withdrawn in the classroom. She reported that his mother was Columbian, his father was Mexican, and the family spoke Spanish in the home. Because of Jorge's hearing impairment, I decided to utilize matching postures as a means of building behavioral rapport. Jorge and I were alone in a classroom with a therapy ball. Initially, Jorge covered his eyes and turned his body away from me. I matched his posture for several minutes until I noticed that he was peeking through his fingers to see what I was doing. Once I saw that he was spending more time looking at me rather than looking away, I tapped the therapy ball several times and waited to see if he would do the same. When he did not, I matched his posture of covering his eyes and turned away again. When I noticed him peeking at me again, I tapped the ball again. This time, he tapped the ball too. We continued tapping the ball and repeating each other's tapping rhythms with the ball while I repeated the word "ball." He began smiling and laughing and I began smiling and laughing. After several minutes, I demonstrated sitting on the ball to see if Jorge would sit on the ball. He sat on the ball briefly, but then decided to lie down on his tummy on the ball. I continued to repeat the word "ball" while he rolled back and forth. After several repetitions, he repeated the word "ball" after I said it. It was a joyous moment for both of us! I had spent extra time building behavioral rapport nonverbally by matching Jorge's posture and initial gaze aversion. Once we had rapport behaviorally, he felt comfortable enough to follow my lead and say the word "ball" for the first time. Jorge, his teacher, and I were all delighted. We had discovered that by allowing Jorge the additional time to develop rapport nonverbally, he was able to process auditory input and formulate simple words that he had not previously been able to say. By matching his nonverbal cues, I was able to create the mutual trust and collaboration that was foundational for cross-cultural communication between a preschooler with profound hearing loss and myself. This experience validated my belief in the use of behavioral rapport as a method of enhancing cross-cultural communication even when verbal communication is minimal.

In summary, the use of cultural, verbal, and behavioral rapport enables physical therapists to develop a repertoire of skills to assist them in working effectively with clients when they speak different languages or have impairments (e.g., hard of hearing) which make communication challenging. The technical challenge is building rapport in difficult situations. The adaptive challenge is modifying one's own behavior to ensure that the communication is as effective as possible.

CULTURALLY AND LINGUISTICALLY APPROPRIATE SERVICES

Therapists can also demonstrate commitment to diversity, cultural pluralism, and effective cross-cultural communication by implementing culturally and linguistically appropriate services (CLAS) standards at work. "Because culture and language are vital factors in how health care services are delivered and received, it is important that health care organizations and their staff understand and respond with sensitivity to the needs and preferences that culturally and linguistically diverse patient/consumers bring to the health encounter. Providing CLAS to these patients has the potential to improve access to care, quality of care, and ultimately, health outcomes" (HHS, OMH, 2001).

CLAS enumerates 14 standards to ensure that all people entering the health care system receive equitable and effective treatment in a culturally and linguistically appropriate manner. They specifically address the needs of racial, ethnic, and linguistic population groups that experience unequal access to health services. The ultimate aim is to eliminate racial and ethnic health disparities and improve the health of all Americans (see Chapter 6 for a full discussion of health disparities).

The 14 Standards are organized by themes. Standards 1 through 3 address culturally competent care, Standards 4 through 7 address language access services, and Standards 8 through 14 address organizational supports for cultural competence. Standards 4 through 7 will be addressed here as they directly relate to language and communication. They also hold another distinction: CLAS Standards 4 through 7 are current Federal requirements for all recipients of Federal funds, unlike the other standards that are either recommendations or guidelines. Standard 4 is a mandate for qualified language assistance services. It states: *Health care organizations must offer and provide language assistance services including bilingual staff and interpreter services at no cost to each patient/consumer with limited English proficiency (LEP) at all points of contact in a timely manner during all hours of operation.*

"Language services" refers to having available bilingual (or preferably, bi-cultural) staff who can communicate directly with the patients in their preferred language. Language services must be available to anyone with LEP who seeks services no matter how small their language group in the community. This also includes services in American Sign Language for individuals who are deaf or hard of hearing. Face-to-face interpretation should be provided by trained staff or contract or volunteer interpreters. If unavailable, telephone interpreter services should be used. The National Health Law Program (NHeLP) addresses using telephone interpreter services as a supplemental system since interpreters who are familiar with medical terminology or concepts may not be readily available.

Although reimbursement for interpreter services varies from state to state, providers agree that the costs for not providing interpreter services puts them at risk for both ethical and malpractice litigation. Additional information regarding reimbursement for interpreter services is available at http://www.healthlaw.org.

CLAS Standard 5 provides notices to patients/consumers of the right to language assistance services. It states: *Health care organizations must provide to patients/consumers in their preferred language both verbal offers and written notices informing them of their right to receive language assistance services.*

This mandate requires that all individuals with LEP should be informed (in a language that they can understand) that they have a right to free language services and that those services are available to them. Health care organizations are required to inquire about the preferred language of each patient/consumer and to record this information in all records. Although the hospital or agency must offer the language services, the availability of services does not guarantee that they will be utilized when needed. Facilities must develop effective ways to publicize the availability of bilingual interpreter services.

CLAS Standard 6 mandates the qualifications for bilingual and interpreter services. It states: *Health care organizations must assure the competence of language assistance provided to limited English proficient patients/consumer by interpreters and bilingual staff. Family and friends should not be used to provide interpretation services (except on request by the patient/consumer).*

This mandate addresses the critical importance of having accurate and effective communication between patients/consumers and clinicians as an essential component of any health care encounter. Lack of trained interpreters frequently leads to misunderstanding, dissatisfaction, omission of vital information, misdiagnoses, inappropriate treatment, and lack of compliance. Prospective and working interpreters must demonstrate knowledge and facility with the terms and concepts relevant to the health care encounter. A person with LEP may choose a family member or friend as an interpreter after being informed of the availability of free interpreter services. However, CLAS notes that the error rate of untrained "interpreters" (including family members and friends) is high enough to make their use more dangerous in some circumstances than no interpreter at all. Some health care institutions have been sued for malpractice when family members were used for interpretation. Minors should not be used for interpretation on behalf of other patients at any time.

Health care organizations must use clear and consistent role definitions and practice standards to facilitate seamless integration of interpreters into clinical or administrative interactions. Standard tools for assessing interpreter skills need to be developed to implement certification. The following are some essential tools:

- Interpretation skills and techniques
- Ethics of interpreting in a health care encounter
- A review of key medical terminology
- Basic clinical concepts
- The workings of the American medical system
- An overview of the role of culture
- How to manage cultural issues and professional interpretation issues

Although many health care institutions offer "medical" classes in target languages, the idea of teaching health professionals another language for the purposes of diagnosis and treatment is controversial. Because of the potential for errors, health care organizations are advised not to suggest these courses as adequate to communicate with patients who have LEP.

CLAS Standard 7 states: *Health care organizations must make available easily understood patient-related materials and post signage in the languages of the commonly encountered groups and/or groups represented in the service area.*

This mandate requires that written materials be routinely provided to consumers with LEP in their own language. These materials should include information that is essential for making educated decisions about health care. These include applications for benefits, consent forms, and medical or treatment instructions. Signage in commonly encountered languages should include patient rights, the process for conflict and grievance resolution, and direction to facility services. Guidelines for determining which documents must be translated because they are vital are available at http://www.hhs.gov/ocr/civilrights/resources/specialtopics/lep.

Materials should be responsive to the cultures and the literacy of the target audiences. The translated written materials should reflect the cultural nuances as well as the differences in dialects for the target population. The materials should be appropriate for the acculturation, literacy, and educational levels of community members. Special recommendations are made by using audiotapes for individuals who cannot read or have visual impairments, large print or Braille for persons with visual impairments, and use of American Sign Language for persons who are deaf or hard of hearing.

Although these four mandates are required for all institutions receiving Federal funds, their interpretation and implementation varies.

UTILIZING INTERPRETERS IN PHYSICAL THERAPY

Physical therapists need to abide by CLAS standards as well. Whenever possible, interpreters rather than translators should be utilized. Translators merely restate the words from one language to another, but interpreters decode the words and provide the meaning behind the message. Optimally, the interpreter should be bilingual, bicultural, and have some understanding of physical therapy and rehabilitation (Lattanzi et al., 2006). As previously mentioned, it is ideal while listening to the interpreter to create rapport by matching the body language of the client.

Speech and language pathology researchers report that although interpreters are used to enhance communication, the question still remains as to how familiar health professionals are with the complexities of the interpretation process and the risks of utilizing an untrained interpreter. Cross-linguistic interactions run a great risk of breakdown because they involve different cultures as well as different languages (Isaac, 2001). For example, professional jargon can be misinterpreted even when an interpreter is involved. Haffner (1992, in Isaac, 2001) describes an incident in which the physician recommended sitz baths for his patient who was being seen post-partum. The patient understood "sitz" as "sits" and she reported fatigue from standing up and sitting down in her bathtub for 20 minutes each day. In this case, failure to explain technical terms resulted in misunderstanding and a literal (and incorrect) interpretation of the term *sitz*. This is a clear example of why interpreters should be both bilingual and bicultural. When utilizing interpreters, clinicians should work to create a partnership with the interpreter, respect the skills each brings to the interaction, and understand what needs to be done so that the patient achieves the most appropriate outcome.

Even when interpreters are involved, medical errors can occur. Flores et al. (2003) found that medical/interpretation errors are common even when medical interpreters are utilized. An average of 31 errors per clinical encounter were documented, and many of these had potential negative clinical consequences. However, more errors occurred when ad hoc interpreters were used. Flores et al. suggest improved medical interpreter training and third party reimbursement for such interpreter services.

In summary, it is recommended that health professionals be aware of the complex aspects of interpretation; the skill the interpreter brings to the interaction; and the need to develop a flexible working style so that control can be shared between the health professional, the interpreter, and the patient, taking into account the patient's cultural background, aims, and goals (Isaacs, 2001).

Conclusion

Hopefully, the tools described in this chapter will assist you in understanding technical and adaptive challenges and in developing effective cross-cultural communication skills in interactions with individuals and groups that you work with as a physical therapist. Developing cultural competence and cultural proficiency is a lifelong process. As you begin to develop your knowledge, attitudes, and skills, remember that every communication is a cross-cultural communication. If you acknowledge your cultural heritage and then seek to enhance your knowledge about the cultural heritage of others, you will be both a teacher and a learner. Through demonstrating cultural pluralism and effective cross-cultural communication, you will be promoting professionalism in physical therapy for people of all backgrounds.

Reflection Questions

✔ *Write down how you describe yourself culturally. Notice what verbal descriptors you have used. Have you included gender, race, ethnicity, religion, geographic region, or other descriptors? What do your verbal descriptors tell you about what you value? How do your words reflect your values?*

✔ *Remember a time when you made an assumption about someone based on his or her language and appearance and later found out it was inaccurate. How did the assumption affect your communication with that person? Was your communication effective? If so, what made it so? If not, what could you have done differently?*

✔ *Remember a time when you needed the assistance of another health care professional. What expectations did you have regarding their communication with you? Was it what you expected? Why or why not? Was your experience congruent with the expectations for the professional communication of physical therapists? Why or why not?*

✔ *Which communication style is most like yours? Which communication style is most like that of your clients? Which communication style is most like that of your colleagues? How do these differing communication styles impact your cross-cultural interactions?*

✔ *Think of a situation in which you have had a miscommunication with a professional or student from a generation different than yours. What do you think caused the miscommunication? How did you resolve it?*

✔ *Can you think of a time when you felt you had positive rapport in your interactions with a client from a culture different than your own? What made you feel that you had rapport? Can you think of a time when you felt you did not have rapport with a client from a culture different than your own? What made you feel that you did not have rapport?*

References

Agar, M. (1994). *Language shock: Understanding the culture of conversation.* New York, NY: William Morrow.

American Heritage Dictionary of the English Language (3rd ed.). (1992). Boston, MA: Houghton Mifflin.

American Medical Association. (2006). *Ethical force program consensus report: Improving communication— Improving care.* Chicago, IL: Author.

American Physical Therapy Association. (2003). Professionalism in physical therapy: Core values. Alexandria, VA: Author. Retrieved September 29, 2009, from http://www.apta.org/AM/Template. cfm?Section=Policies_and_Bylaws&TEMPLATE=/CM/ContentDisplay.cfm&CONTENTID=36073

American Physical Therapy Association. (2005). APTA Vision Sentence for Physical Therapy 2020 and APTA Vision Statement for Physical Therapy 2020. Retrieved September 29, 2009, from http://www.apta.org/AM/Template.cfm?Section=Policies_and_Bylaws&TEMPLATE=/CM/ContentDisplay. cfm&CONTENTID=33814

American Physical Therapy Association. (2008). Blueprint for teaching cultural competence in physical therapy education. Retrieved September 29, 2009, from http://www.apta.org/AM/Template.cfm?Section=Policies_and_Bylaws&CONTENTID=49349&TEMPLATE=/CM/ContentDisplay.cfm

Anderson, R. (1997). Examining language loss in bilingual children. *Communication Disorders and Sciences in Culturally and Linguistically Diverse Population Newsletter, 3*(1): 2-5.

Berlin, E. A., & Fowkes, W. C., Jr. (1983). Teaching framework for cross-cultural care. Application in family practice. *Western Journal of Medicine, 139*(6), 934-938.

Bernieri, F. J., & Rosenthal, R. (1991). Interpersonal coordination: Behavior matching and interactional synchrony in fundamentals of nonverbal behavior. In R. S. Feldman & B. Rime (Eds.), *Fundamentals of nonverbal behavior* (pp. 401-432). New York, NY: Cambridge University Press.

Brice, A., & Campbell, L. R. (1999). Cross-cultural communication. In R. L. Leavitt (Ed.), *Cross-cultural rehabilitation: An international perspective* (pp. 83-94). London, England: Harcourt Brice and Company.

Civil Rights Act of 1964. (1964). 78 Stat. Public Law 88-352. Retrieved September 28, 2009, from http://clerk.house.gov/library/reference-files/PPL_CivilRightsAct_1964.pdf

Dillman, D. A. (1978). *Mail and telephone surveys: The total design method.* Hoboken, NJ: John Wiley & Sons.

Ekman, P. (1971). Universal and cultural differences in facial expressions of emotion. In J. Cole (Ed.), *Nebraska symposium on motivation 1971* (vol. 19, pp. 207-283). Lincoln, NE: University of Nebraska Press.

Fadiman, A. (1998). *The spirit catches you and you fall down.* New York, NY: Farrar, Straus and Giroux.

Flores, G., Laws, M. B., Mayo, S. J., Zuckerman, B., Abreu, M., Medina, L., et al. (2003). Errors in medical interpretation and their potential clinical consequences in pediatric encounters. *Pediatrics, 111*(1), 6-14.

Friedemann, M. L., Pagan-Coss, H., & Mayorga, C. (2008). The workings of a multicultural research team. *Journal of Transcultural Nursing, 19*(3), 266-273.

Gaglio, B., Nelson, C. C., & King, D. (2006). The role of rapport: Lessons learned from conducting research in a primary care setting. *Qualitative Health Research, 16*(5), 723-724.

Gleeson, P. B. (2007). Understanding generational competence related to professionalism: Misunderstandings that lead to a perception of unprofessional behavior. *Journal of Physical Therapy Education, 21*(3), 23-28.

Goldman, K. D., & Schmale, K. J. (2005). E=MC^2: Effective multicultural competence. *Health Promotion Practice, 6*(3), 237-239.

Goode, T. D., Dunne, M. C., & Bronheim, S. M. (2006). *The evidence base for cultural and linguistic competence in health care.* New York, NY: The Commonwealth Fund.

Hall, E. T. (1959). *The silent language.* New York, NY: Doubleday.

Hall, E. T. (1976). *Beyond culture.* New York, NY: Anchor Books.

Hall, E. T. (1984). *The dance of life: The other dimension of time.* New York, NY: Anchor Books.

Hall, E. T., & Hall, M. R. (1990). *Understanding cultural differences: Germans, French, and Americans.* Boston, MA: Intercultural Press.

Hargreaves, J. (1997). Using patients: Exploring the ethical dimension of reflective practice in nurse education. *Journal of Advanced Nursing, 25*(2), 223-228.

Heifetz, R. L., & Linsky, M. (2002). *Leadership on the line: Staying alive through the dangers of leading.* Boston, MA: Harvard Business Press.

Hsu, L. K., Kong, W. (Producers), & Lee, A. (Director). (2000). *Crouching tiger, hidden dragon* [Motion Picture]. United States: Sony Pictures Classic.

Individuals With Disabilities Education Act Amendments of 1991. (1991). Public Law No 102-119, 105 Stat. 587.

Isaac, K. M. (2001). What about linguistic diversity? A different look at multicultural health care. *Communication Disorders Quarterly, 22*(2), 110-113.

Izard, C. E. (1971). *The face of emotion.* New York, NY: Appleton-Century-Crofts.

Kleinman, A. (1978). Concepts and a model for the comparison of medical system as cultural systems. *Social Science & Medicine, 12*(2B), 85-95.

Koehn, P. H., & Swick, H. M. (2006). Medical education for a changing world: Moving beyond cultural competence into transnational competence. *Academic Medicine, 81*(6), 548-556.

Konefal, J. (2002). *Neurolinguistic psychology practitioner manual.* Coral Gables, FL: University of Miami.

Kreps, G. L., & Kunimoto, E. N. (1994). *Effective communication in multicultural health care settings.* Thousand Oaks, CA: Sage Publications.

Ladyshewsky, R. (1999). Cross-cultural supervision of students. In R. L. Leavitt (Ed.), *Cross-cultural rehabilitation: An international perspective* (163-172). London, England: Harcourt Brice and Company.

Lancaster, L. C., & Stillman, D. (2002). *When generations collide: Who they are, why they crash, how to solve the generational puzzle at work.* New York, NY: HarperBusiness.

Lattanzi, J. B., Masin, H. L., & Phillips, A. (2006). Translation and interpretation services for the physical therapist. *HPA Resource, 6*(4), 1, 3-5.

Leavitt, R. L. (2002). Developing cultural competence in a multicultural world: Part I. *PT Magazine, 10*(12), 36-48.

Lipkin, M., Jr., Quill, T. R., & Napodana, R. J. (1984). The medical interview: A core curriculum for residencies in internal medicine. *Ann Intern Med, 100*(2), 277-284.

Lopopolo, R. B., Schafer, D. S., & Nosse, L. J. (2004). Leadership, administration, management and professionalism (LAMP) in physical therapy: A Delphi study. *Physical Therapy, 84*(2), 137-150.

Masin, H. L. (1995). Perceived maternal knowledge and attitudes toward physical therapy during early intervention in Cuban American and African American Families. *Pediatric Physical Therapy, 7*, 118-123.

Masin, H. L. (1998a). Communicating with cultural sensitivity. In C. M. Davis (Ed.), *Patient practitioner interaction* (pp. 159-178). Thorofare, NJ: SLACK Incorporated.

Masin, H. L. (1998b). Developing rapport and reducing negativity in communication using Neurolinguistic Psychology. In C. M. Davis (Ed.), *Patient practitioner interaction* (pp. 139-159). Thorofare, NJ: SLACK Incorporated.

Masin, H. L. (2000). Integrating the use of the Generic Abiilities, Clinical Performance Instrument, and Neurolinguistic Psychology Processes for clinical education intervention. *Physical Therapy Case Reports, 3*(6), 258-266.

Masin, H. L. (2002). Education in the affective domain: A method/model for teaching professional behaviors in the classroom and during advisory sessions. *Journal of Physical Therapy Education, 16*(1), 37-45.

Masin, H. L. (2004). Affective education and participant centered problem solving for educators. In M. M. Edmonds, C. M. Davis, B. Whitehead, J. L. Echternach, & H. L. Masin. *Educating physical therapists as primary care practitioners: Competencies for the learner and faculty development* (pp. 65-75). Baton Rouge , LA: Darbonne and Bartolett Publishers.

Masin, H. L. (2006). Communications in physical therapy. In M. A. Pagliarulo (Ed.), *Introduction to Physical Therapy* (pp. 79-105). St Louis, MO: Mosby.

Masin, H. L., & Tischenko, A. K. (2007). Professionalism, attitudes, beliefs and transformation of the learning experience: Cross-cultural implication for developing a Spanish elective for non-Spanish speaking physical therapy students. *Journal of Physical Therapy Education, 21*(3), 40-46.

May, W. W., Morgan, B. J., Lemke, J. C., Karst, G. M., & Stone, H. L. (1995). Model for ability based assessment in physical therapy education. *Journal of Physical Therapy Education, 9*(1), 3-6.

Mehrabian, A., & Wiener, M. (1967). Decoding of inconsistent communications. *Journal of Personality and Social Psychology, 6*(1), 109-114.

Mullavey-O'Byrne, C. (1993). Intercultural communication for health care professionals. In R. W. Brislin & T. Yoshida (Eds.), *Improving intercultural interactions: Modules for cross-cultural training programs* (pp. 171-196). Thousand Oaks, CA: Sage Publications.

Murphy, S. T., Censullo, M., Cameron, D. D., & Baigis, J. A. (2007). Improving cross-cultural communication in health professions education. *Journal of Nursing Education, 46*(8), 367-372.

Murray-García, J. L., Harrell, S., García, J., Gizzi, E., & Simms-Mackey, P. (2005). Self reflection in multicultural training: Be careful what you ask for. *Academic Medicine, 80*(7), 694-701.

Norfolk, T., Birdi, K., & Walsh, D. (2007). The role of empathy in establishing rapport in the consultation: A new model. *Medical Education, 41*(7), 690-697.

O'Connor, J., & Seymour, J. (1993). *Introducing NLP: Psychological skills for understanding and influencing people.* London, England: Thorsons.

Odawara, E. (2005). Cultural competency in occupational therapy: Beyond a cross-cultural view of practice. *American Journal of Occupational Therapy, 59*(3), 325-334.

Pedersen, L. (1992). A natural history of English: Language, culture and the American heritage. *American heritage dictionary of the English language* (3rd ed., pp. xv-xxiii). Boston, MA: Houghton Mifflin.

Pellegrino, E. D. (1983). What is a profession? *Journal of Allied Health, 12*(3), 168-176.

Poss, J. E. (2001). Developing a new model for cross-cultural research synthesizing the health belief model and the theory of reasoned action. *Advances in Nursing Science, 23*(4), 1-15.

Project Craft Video. (1997). *Communicating across cultures.* Northridge, CA: University of California.

Sharpley, C. F., Jeffrey A. M., & McMah, T. (2006). Counsellor facial expression and client perceived rapport. *Counselling Psychology Quarterly, 19*(4), 343-356.

Shepard, K. F., & Jensen, G. M. (2002). *Handbook of teaching for physical therapists* (2nd ed.). Boston, MA: Butterworth-Heinemann.

Singelis, T. (1993). Nonverbal communication in intercultural interactions. In R. W. Brislin & T. Yoshida (Eds.), *Improving intercultural interactions: Modules for cross-cultural training programs* (pp. 268-194). Thousand Oaks, CA: Sage Publications.

Stuart, R. B. (2004). Twelve practical suggestions for achieving multicultural competence. *Professional Psychology Research and Practice, 35*(1), 3-9.

Triandis, H. (1995). A theoretical framework for the study of diversity. In M. M. Chemers, S. Oskamp, & M. Costanzo (Eds.), *Diversity in organizations: New perspectives for a changing workforce.* (pp 11-36). Thousand Oaks, CA: Sage Publications.

U.S. Department of Health and Human Services, Office of Minority Health. (2001). *National standards on culturally and linguistically appropriate services in health care—Final report.* Washington, DC: Author.

Ziskin, L. (Producer), & Haines, R. (Director). (1991). *The doctor* [Motion picture]. United States: Silver Screen Partners IV.

10

Developing Cultural Competence Through Service Learning

Pamela J. Reynolds, EdD, PT

I believe this project increased my professional development exponentially; however, it pales in comparison to the amount of personal growth that I attained during this project. It was extreme culture shock to me the first day of volunteering. I grew up in a town where everyone came from the same race, religion, and socio-economic status. At college, I was, and still am, considered to be part of the majority. Now suddenly I was the minority and it was strange to me, I did not feel as though I should be there. However, by the end of the first day, I felt at home with the kids. By the last day, I understood that it was not about differences, but rather about people, and I felt not only that I should be there, but it also was a privilege to be there.

Experts generally agree that the development of cultural competence begins with an awareness of one's own values and biases and becoming more sensitive to differences in diverse individuals or groups (Campinha-Bacote, 1999; Lattanzi & Purnell, 2005; Leavitt, 2003). Developing cultural awareness, sensitivities, and competence have been detailed thoroughly by other chapter authors in this text. The quotation from one student's written reflection after a service learning experience vividly describes culture shock leading to cultural awareness and finally understanding of the other. During the first of seven semesters in a Master of Physical Therapy Program, this student provided services at an after-school mentoring and activities program. It was in a neighborhood where a large majority of the children came from families that were socially and economically disadvantaged, and they qualified for federally funded breakfast and lunch programs. This student expresses having "extreme cultural shock." Culture shock is the "pronounced reactions to the psychological disorientation most people experience when immersed in culture markedly different from their own" (Leavitt, p. 18). Culture shock does raise awareness.

In an early study looking at the benefits of service learning in the professional preparation of physical therapists by this author, understanding individual and cultural differences was the most frequently identified outcome. Students repeatedly reflected on their increased cultural sensitivity and understanding and respect for individual

R. L. Leavitt (Ed.).
Cultural Competence: A Lifelong Journey to Cultural Proficiency (pp. 187-202).
© 2010 SLACK Incorporated

differences. One of the student participants wrote: "As a health care professional, one should look at patients as an individual and take into consideration how his or her lifestyle will impact their potential and desire to heal. Most of all, this experience has taught me not to judge someone based on their lifestyle or economical state" (Reynolds, 2005, p. 46).

Culture is much broader than just a person's ethnicity, genetics, or environmental background. Any individual or group whose norms, beliefs, values, lifestyles, etc. differ from our own can be considered culturally different. Listening to and understanding others are all important steps in the development of cultural competence. Students working on an interdisciplinary service learning project in a homeless shelter expressed it this way: "I need to kill all the stereotypes I possess. Everyone has a story. Homelessness results from a variety of reasons. It is not my job to judge" (Gupta, 2006, p. 59). Examples in this chapter will acknowledge and honor broadly defined individual and group cultural diversities. The objectives for this chapter are to:

- Describe the pedagogy of service learning and how it can be utilized to develop student health professionals' cultural competence. Most of the examples cited are related to the academic environment and student activities. However, it should be recognized that practicing health care professionals can utilize the educational strategies of service learning as well as in developing cultural competency.

- Appreciate the importance of building principles-based community partnerships that are sensitively built on mutual respect, trust, and commitment.

- Explain how to design an educational service learning experience that facilitates development of cultural competence, social responsibility, and professional citizenship skills.

- Provide strategies for implementing the reflective component of service learning that will make the connection between theory and practice and promote cultural competence.

SERVICE LEARNING PEDAGOGY

Service learning is a structured learning experience that meets identified needs in the community "with explicit learning objectives, preparation, and reflection. Students engaged in service learning are expected not only to provide direct community service but also to learn about the context in which the service is provided, the connection between the service and their academic coursework, and their roles as citizens" (Seifer, 1998, p. 274). Also, "unlike practica and internships, the experiential activity in a service-learning course is not necessarily skill-based within the context of professional education" (Bringle & Hatcher, 1996, p. 222).

The ideological perspectives that underlie service learning have been further detailed by Kahne and Westheimer (1996). They differentiated charity- versus change-oriented goals and distinguished three domains: moral, political, and intellectual. However, the domains of each category are by no means discrete. The distinction between charity and change goals in each domain should be viewed as a continuum of service learning goals from good to best (Figure 10-1).

	Charity Goal		**Change Goal**
MORAL:	Giving	→	Caring
POLITICAL:	Civic Duty	→	Social Reconstruction
INTELLECTUAL:	Additive Experience	→	Transformative Experience

FIGURE 10-1. Charity to change-oriented goals. Adapted from Kahne, J., & Westheimer, J. (1996). In service of what? The politics of service learning. *Phi Delta Kappan, 77*(9), 592-599.

Initially, providing or giving service to a community organization usually emphasizes charity, not change. Giving does develop the students' sense of altruism, which can be easily expressed and quite powerful. However, in many service experience activities, students view the individuals they serve as clients instead of a resource. Caring is the primary moral change-oriented goal of service learning. The aim of caring is to extend relationships and develop new connections. In other words, "to create opportunities for changing our understanding of the other and the context within which he or she lives" (Kahne & Westheimer, 1996, p. 596). Also, in the caring dimension, "the distance between the one caring and the one cared for diminishes" (Kahne & Westheimer, p. 596). Development of cultural competence is closely related to the caring or moral change-oriented goal as described here.

Within the political charity goal and civic duty domain, volunteerism and compassion for the underprivileged are the fundamental concepts (Kahne & Westheimer, 1996). Service learning goals oriented toward political change require students to critically reflect on social policies and conditions. These experiences are expected to facilitate acquisition of skills for political participation and the formation of social bonds (Kahne & Westheimer).

In the intellectual domain, the service learning change goal provides a powerful learning environment with authentic, experience-based opportunities. Experiences should serve to motivate students, engage and stimulate them toward higher order thinking in varied surroundings, and promote interdisciplinary studies. Critical inquiry and reflective action are necessary to elicit the full power of service learning activities in this domain (Kahne & Westheimer, 1996). The following student quote expresses one of the more transformational reflections that this author has received. This student, along with five other classmates, traveled from an eastern state to the west coast to work with Habitat for Humanity.

> "Personally, this trip helped me change my outlook on certain aspects of life. One was culture shock. We lived in a mostly Black neighborhood—not including the Habitat staff, the six of us were the majority of the white people in the neighborhood. We were afraid to go outside at first, afraid to look at people the wrong way, and afraid to leave our belongings unattended. By the time we left, we were saying hello to everyone, talking horsepower on mowers with a stranger on the street, and even making small talk with the chefs of the best barbecue ribs I ever tasted.

> "Professionally, I'll take what I learned from my experience with culture shock into my practice. I'll never see a person just as the color of their skin. In addition, I'll understand that a person of a minority may have apprehensions toward the majority population. Just as I was scared to walk among a majority population, others may feel that same way when they walk into a physical therapy clinic. I'm more compassionate to these feelings, since I have now had them myself" (Reynolds, 2005, p. 52).

Both the political and intellectual change goals could become strategies in our life-long journey toward cultural proficiency, described by Cross, Bazron, Dennis, and Isaacs (1989) as the continuing need to develop new approaches that will increase culturally competent practice. Approaches may include but are not limited to community-based research, which involves a collaborative approach to research that equitably involves community members, organizational representatives, and academic researchers in the design and accomplishment of research projects aimed at meeting community-identified needs and objectives. The research is conducted *with* rather than *on* a community partner. Community-based research includes a critical action component such that the knowledge gained is combined with action to enhance the well-being of the community and its constituents (Israel, Schultz, Parker, Becker, & Community-Campus Partnerships for Health [CCPH], 2001; Strand, Marullo, Cutforth, Stoecker, & Donohue, 2003).

Community-based research may also be referred to by the terms *community based particpatory research* or *community-based action research* (Strand et al., 2003). *Participatory* is added to the term *community-based research* to honor and indicate that the community partner is an equal participant in research. *Action* is sometimes found in the term because of the aforementioned critical action component associated with community-based research. In the health professions, the preferred term for this form of research is community-based participatory research (CBPR).

A fundamental belief of CBPR is that through active and meaningful community participation, community benefits are maximized and risks to its members are prevented or minimized (Grignon, Wong, & Seifer, 2008). Thus, CBPR is a shift to engaging community members as research partners as opposed to the traditional research process that would view community members as subjects. Each partner brings his or her expertise to the inquiry process. They share ownership and responsibility in all steps of the research process, which ultimately improves understanding of the problem or issue being studied. The knowledge gained combined with action then improves the health and well-being of community members (Reynolds, 2005). Ethical considerations differ as well in CBPR from those found in more traditional research approaches. "Human protections concerns in community-based participatory research are not just about the individual, but also inherently concern the respect, beneficence, and justice for the community as well" (Grignon et al., pp. 2-3).

Outcomes and products of CBPR are varied and can be divided into three categories (Maurana, Wolff, Beck, Simpson, & CCPH, 2001):

1. Peer-reviewed articles

2. Applied products such as training materials and resource guides to improve community health, technical assistance, and program development grants

3. Dissemination products such as community forums, Web sites, and presentations or written briefs to legislative bodies and policymakers

How does service learning differ from volunteerism, community service, traditional practica, clinical rotations, field experiences, and internships (Furco, 1996)? Volunteerism and community service benefit the recipient of the service, not the learner. Traditional practica, clinical rotations, internships, and field experiences include specific course or instructional objectives and focus on the development of students' skills essential to their profession and education. In contrast, service learning emphasizes an equal balance between the service and the learning components, and the instructional learning objectives are matched with community-identified needs (Furco). Although implementation of service learning into coursework can be discipline-specific and skill-based, it can also include advocacy and policy-level work on such issues as access to health care, housing, poverty, the environment, education, and the human services (Bringle & Hatcher, 1996).

Gelmon, Holland, and Shinnamon (1999) note that the effect of service learning experiences on students was much more evident at sites that did not involve an exclusive focus on community-based clinical skill development. Students were strongly influenced when they worked with individuals in non-clinical settings and when they learned about the context of patients' daily lives within the complex and delicate network of support services on which they depended (Gelmon et al.). Although service learning in a clinical setting can be valuable, issues of clinical skill development and application usually impede realization and recognition of potential service experience benefits. Volunteering as a teacher's assistant, this student reflects learning a lot about the school setting and how this experience will be utilized in future clinical practice:

> *"Being involved with a population of children that had backgrounds that were both culturally and socio-economically different than my own childhood experience was*

extremely enlightening. It provided me with a greater awareness of the variations of backgrounds present within our society. I feel that by being involved with these children, I have learned how difficult it can be for many children to grow up in today's society. Many of these children come from families that have very little money, gang relations, drug involvement, and association with various other types of crime. The challenge for these children to overcome these adversities is immense without external support. Many of these children were extremely appreciative of the attention that they received from me, and allowing these children the opportunity to learn was extremely rewarding... I feel professionally that this experience will give me a better comprehension of the diverse backgrounds that my patients may come from. It will increase my compassion and understanding when dealing with patients that have been brought up under different circumstances than I have" (Reynolds, 2005, pp. 51-52).

Reciprocal learning is the second factor that distinguishes service-learning programs from other community-service programs (Furco, 1996). The student and the patient are both the teacher and the learners. Community organizational partners play a crucial role in designing the service-learning experiences in accord with community interests and priorities. Thus, both parties help to determine what is learned and provide input on program development (Bringle & Hatcher, 1996; Furco, 1996; Seifer, 1998). It is this element of reciprocity that moves service learning to the level of a philosophy. Reciprocity, as a philosophy in service learning, implies a meticulous effort to "move from charity to justice, from service to elimination of need" (Jacoby, 2003, p. 5).

Reflection is the third and crucial component of service learning. Reflection activities are active-learning processes that facilitate students' connection between their service in the community and instructional objectives (Furco, 1996; Gelmon et al., 1999; Reynolds, 2005). Reflection is the mechanism for moving students toward recognition of achieving specific academic objectives. It is asking the student to step back and be thoughtful about the experience. As students discuss their experience, the facilitator, through questions about what they learned, leads them toward recognition of academic objectives they have met.

DESIGNING EDUCATIONAL SERVICE LEARNING EXPERIENCES

There are basically three components required in designing an academic course-based service learning experience. Preparation is first, which involves the establishment of principles-based community partnerships and the development of learning and service objectives. Developing a plan of action and performing the actual service is the second step. The third component is reflection or the analysis of the experience through which the participant not only connects the service experience to the instructional or learning objective, but also draws new meaning from it (Campus Compact, 2003).

DEVELOPING CULTURALLY COMPETENT COMMUNITY PARTNERSHIPS

Developing culturally competent community partnerships is vital to successful service learning experiences in the community setting. Too often in the past, academic institutions have treated communities as their laboratory. They have gone into the community, provided service to meet their academic need or to collect data, and then retreated behind their academic walls without consideration of community needs. Results were neither shared with nor used to benefit the community (SenGupta, 2000; Strand et al., 2003) Thus, the community sometimes hesitates or even refuses when approached by an academic institution to "work with" them. Building culturally competent partnerships with the community involves a sensitive exchange of ideas across the cultural boundaries of community organizations and academic institutions. Partnerships must be developed and nurtured in a manner that honors and respects the depth of the educational resources that communities offer.

Establishment of community partnerships for service learning experience requires clear, open, and accessible communications that are built on mutual trust, respect, genuineness, and commitment (CCPH, n.d.; Seifer & Maurana, 2000). Collaborating with a community partner is a two-way street. Understanding the community partner's mission and service needs is important, but the community partner also needs information about the academic institution and its culture, policies, procedures, services, and resources (SenGupta, 2000). The community's service needs are 24 hours a day, seven days a week, whereas most academic institutions work in semester blocks. Information and resource sharing need to be negotiated so that the voices of all partners can be heard equally. CCPH has identified nine principles for the development of sustainable community-academic institution partnerships (Seifer & Maurana, 2000). However, practicing health care professionals can also utilize the following principles in developing partnerships with community organizations as part of their professional social responsibilities and ongoing journey toward cultural proficiency:

1. *Agree upon values, goals, and measurable outcomes.* The mission, goals, and/or objectives for the project should be written and agreed upon by all members of the partnership (Bell-Elkins, 2002).

2. *Develop relationships of mutual trust, respect, genuineness, and commitment.* Partnering is often challenged by biases and expectations that stakeholders bring to the table on behalf of their respective constituencies. While these preconceptions have historical precedent, they are not healthy for a developing partnership. A community-campus partnership must grow and mature in such a way to diminish and eliminate preconceived biases (Freyder & O'Toole, 2000).

3. *Build upon strengths and assets, and also address needs.* Reporting problem-oriented data is important, but it only conveys a partial truth in a negative manner. Recognizing the capacity and skills of people and their neighborhoods, however, builds on assets instead of only recognizing deficiencies. In bringing together the community and campus, the gifts and capacities of individuals, citizen associations, and local institutions need to be recognized (Connors & Prelip, 2000).

4. *Balance power and share resources.* Development of collaborative agendas needs to include the interests of all partners. The work of achieving a balance of power begins with acknowledging and respecting the importance of each partner's value and unique resources (Connolly, 2000).

5. *Have clear, open, and accessible communication.* Each partner needs to be aware of each other's viewpoints and diversity in values, beliefs, practices, lifestyles, and problem-solving strategies. Just being aware of differences, however, is not enough. Partners must also learn about what affects each other's worldview, including historical, societal, political, and/or religious influences. Partners must be able to identify their own culture and cultural blind spots, prejudices, and biases. Knowledge bases and resources are shared in successful partnerships. It is critical to involve the community in the initial planning phase. Whenever possible, recruiting trusted advocates from within the community is the best way to build bridges and minimize distrust and misinformation (SenGupta, 2000).

6. *Agree upon roles, norms, and processes.* Like academic institutions, each community organization has its own norms of operation. Working with the community requires a long-term investment, not an episodic relationship based on when one course is in need of a service dimension. The quantity and quality of communication between partners is a sure sign of the health of the relationship (SenGupta, 2000). Members of the partnership group create the leadership and together form group norms about the patterns of communication, processes, and decision making (Bell-Elkins, 2002; Huppert, 2000).

7. *Ensure feedback to, among, and from all stakeholders.* All stakeholders should be included in the feedback process including service users, organizational members, and policy-makers. Multiple and diverse approaches to seek and use feedback need to be developed. Differences and conflicts must be managed so they become positive aspects of the communication feedback loop (Sebastian, Skelton, & West, 2000).

8. *Share the credit for accomplishments.* When sharing the credit for accomplishments, the community partner should be involved in development of the publicity. Often, university public relations offices that are not involved with the partner organization publicize programs and accomplishments without sensitivity to the community partner's perspective (Blake & Moore, 2000).

9. *Take time to develop and evolve.* Partnerships are formed by an ongoing group and, like most relationships, they develop and mature through a series of continuous stages that broaden and deepen over time. During the first stage, partners defined their common ground and common passions. Infrastructure building is the next stage. Performance of mission work defines the third stage. Partners celebrate and share their successes during the fourth stage, as well as reflect on their challenges and lessons learned. In the final stage, the partnership recognizes future opportunities that push the partnership to a higher level, applying lessons learned to other social change agendas (Heady, 2000).

DEFINING THE SERVICE LEARNING EXPERIENCE

The complexity of a service-learning experience will require more explanation to the neophyte participants. Both learning and service objectives should be clearly identified. The requirements for qualitative assessment by means of written reflections/journals needs to be understood (Seifer & Connors, 2007).

Learning and service objectives are usually derived from educational goals or outcomes, which are comprehensive and very broad-based (Campus Compact, 2003). Goals and outcomes represent what the student (health care professional) is expected to achieve by the end of the course (experience). Objectives specify what the student is to learn by the end of the experience (Shepard & Jensen, 2002). One goal or outcome can have multiple objectives leading toward its achievement.

Learning and service objectives should be written in behavioral terms, which have three components. First is the condition or situation in which the student is to perform. The second and most critical part is to describe an observable behavior. The third part is the criterion or what is considered acceptable and unacceptable performance. Shepard and Jensen (2002) state that "even partial behavioral objectives, which identify at least the content area of knowledge to be acquired and the level of mastery (behavior) but not the grading criterion, are useful in identifying for the student what is to be achieved by her or his efforts" (Shepard & Jensen, p. 61).

Table 10-1 provides an example of a broad educational goal/outcome, followed by several learning objectives, identified community partner need or goal, and service objective designed to meet the community organization's identified need. The community organization represents the situation in which the student will perform. The behaviors are specified in both the learning and service objectives. The learning objective is the academic or instructional objective. The service objective represents the behavior that will meet the community organization's expressed need or some aspect of their mission. When the service has been completed, the reflection process facilitates the connection from the service objective back to the learning objective.

Implementing and assessing the service experiences are far more complex than a traditional lecture or clinical skills laboratory. For one thing, there are more people to

TABLE 10-1

EXAMPLES OF LEARNING AND SERVICE OBJECTIVES BASE ON ONE BROAD-BASED GOAL/OUTCOME

Goal/Outcome: Promote exercise, health, fitness, wellness, and education programs in the community with consideration to special populations including but not limited to women (pregnant or diagnosed with osteoporosis), children and adolescents, the elderly, recreational and elite athletes, individuals with obesity, and persons of different cultures and ethnicities.

Learning Objectives *Student will:*	Community Organizational *Partner's goal/need:*	Service Objectives *Student will:*
Develop health promotion and wellness educational materials and/or activities for adults (or children), which utilize evidenced-based age, gender, impairment, and population-specific information.	An agency providing services for children and adults who are legally blind is concerned with the increasing rates of obesity among their adolescent and young adult clients.	Explore the literature and seek out the expertise of multidisciplinary clinicians who work with the visually impaired to develop, implement, and evaluate physical activities for this population.
Recognize the minimal resources that new refugees have when resettling in the United States, and teach them to maximize those resources.	The mission of the community's international institute is to help foreign-born residents and citizens learn the skills that will be important for their successful adjustment to American life.	Promote overall healthy lifestyle for the refugee family by educating them about good nutrition and facilitating economical, nutritional choices when grocery shopping.
Design, organize, deliver, and evaluate a public health education presentation.	Resident manager of a public housing Seniors' high-rise apartment building expressed concern about the increased incidence of falls and injuries as a result of falls among the residents.	Develop, implement, and evaluate the effectiveness of community-based fall risk screening and education program for balance assessment, fall prevention, and utilization of ambulatory assistive devices.
Recognize and contrast natural ("normal") aging process and pathologic ("abnormal") aging, and describe the difference between usual and successful aging.	Retired nuns residing at a local convent are requesting assistance in setting up exercise programs to improve or maintain their general fitness level, wellness, and functional abilities. Most sisters who will participate in this project reside are considered "well elderly."	Examine, evaluate, and develop an individualized wellness plan for each participating client.

involve. Also, the activity does not take place on the college or university campus, but in the community. As part of the plan of action, it is helpful if a couple of students and their faculty visit the community organization's site well ahead of the service event(s). Another option is to invite a member of the community organization to come to campus and provide an orientation for all of the students. The two-way communication should remain open.

Providing the service requires a plan of action that defines how the service will be carried out to meet established service objectives. Organizing that plan of action can be facilitated or guided by the faculty member but should remain primarily the work of the student. Putting this component in the hands of the student can promote leadership development, communication, and problem-solving skills. It strengthens ownership of the service project(s).

Assessment of the service itself is multi-factorial because of the number of people involved. Gelmon, Holland, Driscoll, Spring, and Kerrigan (2001) detail the principles and strategies of assessing the impact of service learning not only on students, but also faculty, community organizations, service users, and the academic institution. As part of their reflection, students are asked to describe how they will recognize that they have achieved their objective(s) and whether they were in fact met.

STRATEGIES FOR IMPLEMENTING REFLECTION

The work of John Dewey (1938) and David Kolb (1983) are at the heart of reflection strategies for most service learning practitioners. Dewey, recognized as one of the greatest American educational philosophers, established the theoretical foundation for experience-based education. He believed that "all genuine education comes about through experience" (Dewey, p. 25). However, not all experiences are equally educative and genuine. He summarizes: "Wholly independent of desire or intent, every experience lives on in future experiences. Hence the central problem of an education based upon experience is to select the kind of present experiences that live fruitfully and creatively in subsequent experiences" (Dewey, pp. 27-28). In concert with Dewey's statements, Kahne and Westheimer (1996) affirm that the goal of service learning is to construct a learning experience that positively shapes the "students' understandings of both disciplinary knowledge and the particular social issues with which they are engaged" (Kahne & Westheimer, p. 595).

Kolb's (1983) model for the learning cycle has also been embraced by service learning practitioners. He believes that experiential learning stimulates development of students' knowledge and gives relevance to classroom teaching. Kolb's learning cycle begins with a *concrete experience.* Usually these experiences involve other people. The person next steps back to think about this concrete experience observing his or her own behavior during the experience. This is the second stage of *reflective observation.* The third stage is *abstract conceptualization.* At this point, the individual endeavors to draw meaning from the experience and integrating theories or explanations to derive understanding of the experience. It is during this stage that one may develop ideas or action strategies that can be tested. This then leads to the fourth stage of *active experimentation.* In this stage, learning is gained through testing different approaches from the ideas formed during the third stage (Eyler & Giles, 1999; Kolb).

Health care practitioners "use this cycle constantly in clinical practice when treating patients (concrete experience), observing and reflecting on what happened to the patient as a result of that treatment (reflective observation), thinking about how a successful intervention with one patient may work on similar patients and theorizing why (abstract conceptualization), and then trying the intervention on other patients (active experimentation)" (Shepard & Jensen, 2002, p. 60).

This model could be applied to the development of an individual's cultural competence. After meeting and interacting with an individual or group of people who are very different from oneself, the learner would step back to analyze this *concrete experience.* Through *reflective observation,* the learner could become aware of their bias and different value systems. A quote from a student who is working in a homeless shelter demonstrates this. "Realizing that I am part of the dominant culture has been the biggest eye-opener...I used to think that everything I did was normal and what everyone else (minorities) did was abnormal or wrong. It's been so important for me to realize this" (Gupta, 2006, p. 59). *Abstract conceptualization* could result in what Campinha-Bacote (1999) defines as cultural knowledge or the process of increasing one's understanding of different cultural groups including their values, beliefs, lifestyle traditions, and ways of solving problems in their worldview. *Active experimentation* in Kolb learning cycle reflects Cross et al.'s (1989) cultural competence phase on the journey to cultural proficiency. That is, cultural differences are accepted and respected; there is continuous expansion of cultural knowledge and resources, adaptation of services, as well as self-assessment about culture; and there is vigilance toward the dynamics of cultural differences. The following reflection from a student who was working at a center caring for people in the end stage of their HIV-AIDS disease process represents this phase of the cycle:

"I have grown as a person in the short time I have spent with the people at CCR. I listen to their stories and shared hugs, tears, and laughter. A lot of them have had a rough life and others have created their own tragedies, but I have learned that I'm not in this life to judge or be judged. I am sharing this life with them and trying to do the best I can. I am more aware of my own judgment of people and thankful I recognize it now and tell myself to let go. It takes all kinds to fill this big world and I am especially thankful that I have created this opportunity for myself to experience a wider range of mankind [sic]" (Reynolds, 2000, p. 187)

Service learning activities are also consistent with Newmann and Wehlage's (1993) model of authentic learning experiences. They use the word *authentic* to differentiate between educational outcomes that are significant and meaningful and those that are trivial and useless. Three criteria more precisely define authentic learning outcomes. First, the activity should allow the student to construct meaning and synthesize knowledge. Dewey's (1938) experiential educational learning philosophy would compare favorably to this criterion. Second, the student needs to use disciplined methods of inquiry to construct meaning. Kahne and Westheimer's (1996) intellectual change-oriented goal would also support this second parameter. They believe that as critical inquiry combines with action, students' understanding is transformed in both disciplinary knowledge and the particular social issues with which they are involved (Kahne & Westheimer). Third, students' benefit should have value or meaning beyond that of success in an academic course (Newmann & Wehlage). An objective of most educational programs preparing future health care practitioners is to prepare them for practice beyond that of their daily role, including social responsibility and citizenship. Dewey would agree and notes that it is the "problematic" that leads and organizes the learning. The learning and problem-solving activities that occur within a context of social interactions can have far greater consequence than a course grade (Dewey). This "authentic" learning experience can foster cultural competence.

Elyer and Giles (1999) are two leading service learning practitioners who have simplified Kolb's model of learning into three easily remembered questions to initiate reflection on the service experience. They are: What? So what? and Now what? Table 10-2 gives examples of questions that can be asked under each of these questions (Midwest Health Professions Service Learning Consortium, 2003).

These three questions can also guide written journal entries. Under "What," the student might state what they expected before beginning their service. The "So what" could be a description of what really happened, including unexpected challenges and their solutions. "Now what" should reflect the interpretation and new meaning they have drawn from the experience. It should also identify new approaches and how they might do things differently in the future.

Table 10-3 is an example of the learning contract and guidelines for written reflection that I use with my students. Evaluating and grading written reflections and journals can be challenging. There are no right or wrong answers. I am usually looking for depth and breadth of the meaning the student has derived from the experience. Developing a grading rubric (Table 10-4) for assessment of students writing can be very beneficial both for the student and instructor. First decide on the primary traits you are looking for, such as clarity of purpose, organization, creativity or risk taking, use of evidence from the literature and so forth (Shepard & Jensen, 2002).

CONCLUSION

This chapter has emphasized the use of service learning to develop cultural competence. However, the utilization of service learning experience should not be limited to

TABLE 10-2

SUB-QUESTIONS—WHAT? SO WHAT? NOW WHAT?

WHAT?

What was the service learning experience?

What happened? What did you do?

What did you expect?

What was the difference between your pre and post experience?

SO WHAT?

So what are your feelings regarding the experience or the situation or the circumstance?

So what did you do about it?

So what did you do as a result?

So what might you do later?

So what polices or procedures might result in a better _____?

NOW WHAT?

Now what will you do with this knowledge?

Now what will you do differently if confronted with this situation again?

Now what will you suggest that could prove useful?

What effect, if any, did that have long term?

Adapted from Midwest Health Professions Service Learning Consortium. (2003). *Reflection in service learning: Strengthening the connection.* Dayton, OH: Center for Healthy Communities.

this single purpose. The depth of educational resources that our communities offer us is boundless. Respectfully mining this resource with cultural sensitivity is mandatory. Service for the greater good of humankind is everyone's responsibility. Albert Schweitzer (1990) believed that there is a vast untapped reservoir of idealism in individuals and communities, which, if nurtured, honored, and given specific opportunities, can become a powerful resource for combating the tragic problems of those who are in the greatest need. Schweitzer writes:

> "One can save one's life as a human being, along with one's professional existence, if one seizes every opportunity, however unassuming, to act humanly toward those who need another human being. In this way we serve both the spiritual and the good. Nothing can keep us from this second job of direct human service… Everyone in his [sic] own environment must strive to practice true humanity toward others. The future of the world depends on it" (Schweitzer, 1990, pp. 90-91).

ADDITIONAL WEB-BASED RESOURCES FOR DEVELOPING SERVICE LEARNING EXPERIENCES

- Campus Compact: http://www.compact.org
- Community-Campus Partnerships for Health: http://www.ccph.info
- Corporation for National and Community Service: http://www.nationalservice.gov
- Learn and Serve America's National Service-Learning Clearinghouse: http://www.servicelearning.org

TABLE 10-3

TWENTY HOURS OF SERVICE: LEARNING CONTRACT AND GUIDELINES FOR WRITTEN REFLECTION LEARNING CONTRACT (25 POINTS)

- **Learning Objectives (Create 2 to 3 Objectives)** (10 points)
  - o What is it you hope to learn from this service experience? About the challenges and assets of the community where you are attending school? About yourself? About your community?
  - o The learning objective should be based on the needs of agency, the student's learning goals, and the course's learning objectives.
  - o Example: Discuss two examples of how my understanding has changed about the impact poverty has on the lives of children 5 to 12 years old.

- **Service Objectives (Create 1 to 2 Objectives)** (5 points)
  - o Identify and describe the nature of the service in which you will be engaged.
  - o The service objectives should indicate your role in helping to achieve the service organization's goal or need.
  - o Example: Develop and implement a 10-week physical exercise activity and nutritional education program at an after-school mentoring and activity program.

- **Plan of Action** (5 points)
  - o What is your plan to accomplish your learning and service objectives?
  - o The "WHEN" and "HOW."

- **Assessment – Criteria – Outcome** (5 points)
  - o How will you know if you have met your objectives?
  - o How will you measure/observe it?
  - o What is an acceptable outcome?

Written Reflection Paper related to community experience. All written papers will be organized as follows:

A. Cover Page

B. Body of Text

    1. WHAT? Describe the community agency for which you contributed your volunteer hours:

        i. Community agency's mission, vision, goals, needs, etc.

        ii. Review learning and service objectives from your Learning Contract: What did you do?

    2. SO WHAT?

        i. Evaluation: What went well? What was problematic? What did you do about it? What were your solutions?

        ii. What improvements could be made in the future?

        iii. How have you grown personally?

        iv. How have your grown professionally?

    3. NOW WHAT?

        i. Identify and discuss a potential future project that could be completed with this agency as a capstone project requiring 100 service hours.

        ii. Reflect on the potential role a health care professional could engage in with your particular community agency.

C. References should be placed at the end of the body of the paper and before the Appendix.

D. Appendix

    1. Copy of Learning Contract

    2. Log documenting dates and hours of service to a community agency or agencies

E. Follow the program's "Guidelines for Preparation of Manuscripts and Written Projects" in the *Student Handbook*.

TABLE 10-4	
BASIC RUBRIC FOR ASSESSING STUDENTS' WRITTEN REPORTS AND REFLECTIONS	
GUIDE TO ACCEPTABLE PROPOSAL, WRITTEN, AND ORAL REPORTS	
Unacceptable Quality	Incomplete proposal, written, and oral reports or contains incomplete required elements or lacks sufficient clarity to afford judgments of the completeness.
Acceptable Quality	All elements of the proposal, written, and oral reports are complete.
High Quality	All elements of the proposal, written, and oral reports are complete AND finished in a timely manner AND specific examples of how objectives/reflections were met/gained through project AND visual aids are used to enhance oral presentation.
Highest Quality	All elements of the proposal, written, and oral reports are complete AND finished in a timely manner AND visual aids are used to enhanced oral presentation AND specific examples of how service project objectives were met are explained in depth AND reflections on personal/professional growth gained by service project experiences include recognition of the context of the larger social issues.

REFLECTION QUESTIONS

✔ *Do you believe all physical therapy students should be required to do service learning?*

✔ *Do you believe practicing physical therapists have a professional responsibility to do service learning or volunteer work?*

✔ *Can you identify a specific service learning project that you might enjoy exploring?*

REFERENCES

Bell-Elkins, J. (2002). *Assessing the CCPH Principles of a partnership in a community-campus partnership.* Seattle, WA: Community-Campus Partnerships for Health.

Blake, J. M., & Moore, E. (2000). Principle 8: Partners share the credit for the partnership's accomplishments. *Partnership Perspectives, 1*(2):65-69.

Bringle, R. G., & Hatcher, J. A. (1996). Implementing service learning in higher education. *Journal of Higher Education, 67*(2), 221-239.

Campinha-Bacote, J. (1999). A model and instrument for addressing cultural competence in health care. *Journal of Nursing Education, 38*(5), 203-207.

Campus Compact. (2003). Service-learning definitions and principles of good practice. In *Introduction to service-learning toolkit: Readings and resources for faculty* (2nd ed., pp. 5-10). Providence, RI: Author.

Community-Campus Partnerships for Health. (n.d.). About us. Retrieved December 15, 2006, from http://www.ccph.info

Connolly, C. (2000). Principle 4: The partnership balances the power among partners and enables resources among partners to be shared. *Partnership Perspectives, 1*(2), 33-40.

Connors, K., & Prelip, M. (2000). Principle 3: The partnership builds upon identified strengths and assets, but also addresses areas the need improvement. *Partnership Perspectives, 1*(2), 27-32.

Cross, T. L., Bazron, B. J., Dennis, K. W., & Isaacs, M. R. (1989). *Towards a culturally competent system of care: A monograph on effective services for minority children who are severely emotionally disturbed.* Washington, DC: CASSP Technical Assistance Center, Georgetown University Child Development Center.

Dewey, J. (1938). *Experience and education.* New York, NY: Collier Books.

Eyler, J., & Giles, D. E., Jr. (1999). *Where's the learning in service-learning?* San Francisco, CA: Jossey-Bass.

Freyder, P. J., & O'Toole, T. P. (2000). Principle 2: The relationship between partners is characterized by mutual trust, respect, genuineness and commitment. *Partnership Perspectives, 1*(2), 19-25.

Furco, A. (1996). Service-learning: A balanced approach to experiential education. *Expanding Boundaries: Service and Learning* (pp. 2-6). Washington, DC: Corporation for National Service.

Gelmon, S. B., Holland, B. A., Driscoll, A., Spring, A., & Kerrigan, S. (2001). *Assessing service-learning and civic engagement: Principles and technique* (3rd ed.). Providence, RI: Campus Compact.

Gelmon, S. B., Holland, B. A., & Shinnamon, A. F. (1999). *Health professions schools in service to the nation: 1996-1998 final evaluation report.* San Francisco, CA: Community-Campus Partnerships for Health.

Grignon, J., Wong, K. A., & Seifer, S. D. (2008). *Ensuring community-level research protections: Proceedings of the 2007 educational conference call series on institutional review boards and ethical issues in research.* Seattle, WA: Community-Campus Partnerships for Health.

Gupta, J. (2006). A model for interdisciplinary service-learning experience for social change. *Journal of Physical Therapy Education, 20*(3), 55-60.

Heady, H. R. (2000). Principle 9: Partnerships take time to develop and evolve over time. *Partnership Perspectives, 1*(2), 71-78.

Huppert, M. E. (2000). Principle 6: Roles, norms, and processes for the partnership are established with the input and agreement of all partners. *Partnership Perspectives, 1*(2), 47-56.

Israel, B. A., Schulz, A. J., Parker, E. A., Becker, A. B., & Community-Campus Partnerships for Health. (2001). Community-based participatory research: Policy recommendations for promoting a partnership approach in health research. *Education for Health, 14*(2), 182-197.

Jacoby, B. (2003). Fundamentals of service-learning partnerships. In B. Jacoby (Ed.), *Building partnerships for service-learning* (pp. 1-19). San Francisco, CA: Jossey-Bass.

Kahne, J., & Westheimer, J. (1996). In service of what? The politics of service learning. *Phi Delta Kappan, 77*(9), 592-599.

Kolb, D. A. (1983). *Experiential learning: Experiences as a source of learning and development.* Englewood Cliffs, NJ: Prentice Hall.

Lattanzi, J. B., & Purnell, L. D. (2005). *Developing cultural competence in physical therapy practice.* Philadelphia, PA: F.A. Davis.

Leavitt, R. L. (2003). Developing cultural competence: Working with older adults of Hispanic origin (monograph). In M. Thompson & J. Okubo (Eds.), *Cultural diversity of older Americans: An independent home study course for individual continuing education.* La Crosse, WI: American Physical Therapy Association Section on Geriatrics.

Maurana, C. A., Wolff, M., Beck, B. J., Simpson, D. E., & Community-Campus Partnerships for Health. (2001). Working with our communities: Moving from service to scholarship in the health professions research. *Education for Health, 14*(2), 207-220.

Midwest Health Professions Service Learning Consortium. (2003). Reflection in service learning: Strengthening the connection. Dayton, OH: Center for Healthy Communities.

Newmann, F. M., & Wehlage, G. G. (1993). Five standards of authentic instruction. *Educational Leadership, 50*(7), 8-12.

Reynolds, P. J. (2000). *How service learning experiences benefit physical therapist students' professional development: A grounded theory study.* Unpublished Dissertation. Pittsburgh, PA: Duquesne University.

Reynolds, P. J. (2005). How service learning experiences benefit physical therapist students' professional development: A grounded theory study. *Journal of Physical Therapy Education, 19*(1), 41-51.

Schweitzer, A. (1990). *Out of my life and thought.* New York, NY: Henry Holt & Company.

Sebastian, J. G., Skelton, J., & West, K. P. (2000). Principle 7: There is feedback to, among and from all stakeholders in the partnership, with the goal of continuously improving the partnership and its outcomes. *Partnership Perspectives, 1*(2), 57-64.

Seifer, S. D. (1998). Service-learning: Community-campus partnerships for health professions education. *Academic Medicine, 73*(3), 273-277.

Seifer, S. D., & Connors, K. (Eds.). (2007). *Faculty toolkit for service-learning in higher education.* Scotts Valley, CA: National Service-Learning Clearinghouse.

Seifer, S. D., & Maurana, C. A. (2000). Developing and sustaining community-campus partnerships: Putting principles into practice. *Partnership Perspectives, 1*(2), 7-11.

SenGupta, I. (2000). Principle 5: There is a clear, open and accessible communication between partners, making it an ongoing priority to listen to each need, develop a common language, and validate/clarify the meaning of terms. *Partnership Perspectives, 1*(2), 41-46.

Shepard, K. F., & Jensen, G. M. (2002). Preparation for teaching students in academic settings. In K. Shepard & G. Jensen (Eds.), *Handbook of teaching physical therapists* (2nd ed., pp. 39-69). Boston, MA: Butterworth Heineman.

Strand, K., Marullo, S., Cutforth, N., Stoecker, R., & Donohue, P. (2003). *Community-based research and higher education: Principles and practices.* San Fransico, CA: Jossey-Bass.

11

Physical Therapy and Cultural Competence in the Global Community

MOVING FROM A BIO-MEDICAL TO A SOCIAL JUSTICE MODEL

Ronnie Leavitt, PhD, MPH, PT

Despite a range of estimates and some disagreement on the exact numbers of disabled people, it is generally estimated that there are about 650 million persons with a disability (PWD) in the world (approximately 200 million of which are children), or around 10% of the population (World Health Organization [WHO], 2005a, n.d.a). Definitions and prevalence indicators of disability vary. The prevalence rate of moderate and severe disability (i.e., those people who are more likely to need rehabilitation) is estimated at 5.2% (Helander, 1999; Parnes, 2008). Disability is not evenly distributed among socio-economic groups. It is estimated that 70% to 80% of PWD live in Third World countries (Elwan, 1999; World Confederation for Physical Therapy [WCPT], 2003). WHO and The Pan American Health Organization (PAHO) estimate that rehabilitation services for individuals with disabilities in the Third World serve a minute fraction (1% to 3%) of the total number of those in need (PAHO, 1994a; WHO, 2001a) and that 1% to 2% of children with disabilities in developing countries receive an education (United Nations [UN] Educational, Scientific and Cultural Organization [UNESCO], 1998). Women with disabilities generally face a double disadvantage in that they are stigmatized by both gender and disability status.

Without improved programs of disability prevention, the absolute numbers and relative proportions of the PWD will grow in the next decades as the world's population increases and medical advances allow for the survival of increased numbers of children under 5 and elderly above the age of 65 who are in a marginal state of health. The most common disabilities are associated with chronic conditions (cardiovascular and respiratory diseases, cancer, diabetes), injuries (especially road accidents, landmine explosions, violence), mental illness, malnutrition, infectious diseases (HIV/AIDS), environmental degradation, and other poverty-related impairments (WHO, 2005a, 2008a). By the year 2035, Helander (2000) estimates that about 150 million people would benefit from some rehabilitation.

R. L. Leavitt (Ed.).
Cultural Competence: A Lifelong Journey to Cultural Proficiency (pp. 203-226).
© 2010 SLACK Incorporated

The situation for PWD can be improved in the 21st century. International activities continue to expand as evidenced by key developments in disability legislation and action plans by the WHO. New models of care, with a far greater emphasis on the existing cultural ways of the people and their environment, are developing. These models are intended to enhance the quality of life for the PWD by improving service delivery, providing more equitable opportunities, and promoting and protecting human rights. There is a move away from Western, bio-medical style models to social models of disability.

The purpose of this chapter is to present an overview of the culture of disability and the culture of rehabilitation services throughout the world, with emphasis on the present situation in developing nations and the concept of community-based rehabilitation (CBR). In reviewing the literature, I have focused on an array of descriptive, personal experiences as well as the accessible quantitative and qualitative research to summarize a range of concrete examples and viewpoints (see Chapter 5). These selective illustrations of practice point to the need to understand how each culture (family, neighborhood, society at large) specifically addresses PWD and how each situation must be addressed within its own unique cultural context.

Most physical therapists have little or no knowledge of the social construction of disability outside of the industrialized world or alternative models of rehabilitation, yet we, individually and the American Physical Therapy Association (APTA), are increasingly interested in global health and international physical therapy and rehabilitation. There is no doubt that the world is constantly becoming more intertwined, that we are all affected by the health of people throughout the world, and that we are increasingly traveling and working internationally. Our ability to be culturally competent will have a great impact on our capacity to be involved.

HISTORICAL OVERVIEW OF HEALTH POLICY AND REHABILITATION INTERVENTIONS

Health care systems have historically existed in some form in all societies. Forms of rehabilitation, in contrast to mechanisms of curing or healing (restoring a sense of normalcy), also have a long history and allow individuals with disability to be maintained within societies (Ackerknect, 1971; Benton, Baker, Bowman, & Waters, 1981; Granger, 1976; Leavitt, 1992; Sanders, 1986; Tappen, 1961). J. R. Hanks and L. M. Hanks (1948) hypothesized that the degree to which a society is willing or able to bear the costs incurred in caring for PWD depends upon several interrelating materialistic and cultural factors. Some of these determinants are the relative socioeconomic status of the society (which includes such factors as the number and type of productive units, the need for labor, the amount of economic surplus, and its mode of distribution), the social structure of the society (including whether the society is egalitarian or hierarchical, how it defines achievement, and how it values age and sex), the cultural definition of the meaning of the disability (does the symptom of the disability require magical, religious, medical, legal, or other measures?), and the position of the society in relation to the rest of the world.

Although there are significant differences in health status and health care systems, including rehabilitation, among contemporary societies, the differences are most extreme between the developed or industrialized societies and the so-called developing or Third World societies. These differences, although influenced by socio-cultural practices, primarily reflect the wide economic gap between the two groups—a gap that is widening (United Nations Children's Fund [UNICEF], 1995).

A major impediment to the process of public policy development regarding individuals with disabilities is the fact that general health care and rehabilitation for PWD has historically been a very low priority throughout the world (Groce, 1987, 1992; Kaufman & Becker, 1986; Leavitt, 1992; PAHO, 1993, 1994b). Reasons include the following:

The term *international health* has framed most of the health work throughout the world during the better part of the last century. International health relates more to health practices, policies, and systems in different countries. It typically focused on foreign aid activities, disease control in poor countries, and medical missionary work. More recently, the term *global health* seems preferred. The term *global* emerged during the 1960s with the green revolution, when the World Bank advocated the slogan "think globally, act locally." It is intended to foster a vision of the possibility of health for the whole planet, going beyond geopolitical boundaries. The term stresses the commonality of health issues that require a collective, partner-based action. Today, the WHO declares "global priorities" such as the eradication of malaria and the efforts toward HIV/AIDS reduction (Tarantola, 2005).

- The cost-benefit ratio of providing rehabilitation to PWD, which has always been considered poor compared to other health programs.

- There has traditionally been an under-estimation of the potential achievements that a disabled person can accomplish.

- The history of negative attitudes toward persons who are disabled (Leavitt, 1992; Westbrook, Legge, & Pennay, 1993). In many societies, PWD have been considered to be deviant from the norm and have been seen to have a social stigma or "attitude that is deeply discrediting…a failing, a shortcoming, a handicap" (Goffman, 1963, p. 5).

- When discrimination limits participation by people with disabilities in various social roles, their plight becomes even more invisible.

- An apparent absence of urgency. Rehabilitation is associated with disease and illness that is, for the most part, neither acute, communicable, nor "exciting." The general public will not be at risk nor will its opposition be mobilized if rehabilitation services are not given to the populations in need.

- On an individual level, mainstream biomedical practitioners tend to reflect a value orientation that stresses mastery of disease and taking personal credit for recovery. In cases in which an individual has a disability, often very little dramatic curing can occur. In some instances, further loss of function is anticipated. Although a wide array of simple and complex technologies are available, the provision of these services does not ensure dramatic results. Thus, many caregivers find rehabilitation frustrating and often not worthwhile.

- Individuals with disabilities are a disadvantaged minority and, accordingly, have little political influence when lobbying for the opportunity to affect public policy.

When this low priority of care is coupled with a scarcity of resources, the result is limited access to rehabilitation. Recent events such as the Asian tsunami, the HIV/AIDS epidemic, the threat of avian flu, and others siphon some of the already limited dollars going toward rehabilitation. Access may be limited by shortages of personnel and facilities. In many countries, geographical impediments and architectural as well as cultural barriers further limit access. Most national development policies stress a concentration of services in urban areas despite the fact that in developing nations, a majority of the population may live in rural or peri-urban communities.

THE INDUSTRIALIZED WORLD

Rehabilitation was originally conceived of in narrow terms, such as giving someone an artificial leg. The U.S. had no comprehensive programs for PWD prior to World War I, although such programs did exist in Europe (Groce, 1992; Hazenhyer, 1946).

The war-injured from World War II and the polio epidemic in the U.S. were instrumental forces in the further development of the art and science of rehabilitation. Modern programs consider many more facets of rehabilitation, including psychological, social, educational, and vocational services for individuals having a broad range of ills. In the U.S., Howard Rusk, MD, is generally recognized as the "father of comprehensive rehabilitation." He developed the first comprehensive medical training program in rehabilitation in the world in 1946 and opened the (Rusk) Institute of Medical Rehabilitation (IMR) in New York in 1951 (Blum & Fee, 2008).

In developed nations, there is presently a great demand for services. Often, however, the most complete set of services exists only in urban areas and only at the hospital or professional level. This system is very expensive and not necessarily conducive to societal integration of PWD. Even community care is based on the premise that services are to be primarily provided by professionals. A mix of inpatient hospital and outpatient and/or home care services is often available, especially in urban areas.

In the last few decades, Western societies have seen an increase in public visibility and empowerment of individuals with a disability, along with a concomitant increase in legislation mandating the rights of the disabled. For example, in the U.S., the Rehabilitation Act of 1973 (calling for civil rights for PWD), Public Law 94-142, the Education for All Handicapped Children Act (1975), and the Americans With Disabilities Act of 1990 are revolutionary in that they are based on the philosophy that in a just society, all individuals (including PWD) must be accorded equal access and opportunity to pursue their individual goals. The relative newness of these laws implies that the non-physical components of the rehabilitation process (such as guaranteeing PWD the opportunity for education or employment) have begun to develop even later in history than the physical components. This mid-to-late 20th century phenomenon indicates that societies have begun to accept the idea that all persons have a right to a certain level of social well-being. Thus, an analysis of the cost-benefit ratio associated with rehabilitation has begun to consider humanitarian benefits as well as associated economic costs to society. Nevertheless, even in the most developed societies, an analysis of the literature (Bogdan & Biklen, 1977; Goerdt, 1984; Nagler, 1993; National Organization on Disability, n.d.; Safilios-Rothschild, 1970; Wright, 1983; Zola, 1982) and personal experience lead to the conclusion that public policy, as it presently exists, often fails to function optimally and integrate PWD into the larger society. Although services are generally available, they are arguably not comprehensive enough. In modern times, nations appear ambivalent and vacillate between doing nothing and doing something for individuals with disabling conditions (see Chapter 5).

THE DEVELOPING WORLD

In the developing world, the delivery of health care services has not completely paralleled that of the more industrialized world. Historically, with the colonization of Asia, Africa, Latin America, and the Caribbean, everything Western (including the medical care systems) received official support. Typically, the health system was centrally controlled at the Ministry of Health. Health services were distributed through urban-based hospitals, with minimal resources left for rural dispensaries. Tertiary and curative care by highly trained personnel was emphasized. National programs were disease-oriented (e.g., malaria, smallpox), without follow-up to ensure further disease prevention and health promotion. Often the hospitals and medical programs were supported by religious or private voluntary organizations. The major human resources were physicians, assisted by nurses and occasional auxiliaries. This system of care is known as the "Western medical model." At the same time, traditional systems of medicine, such as care given to persons by a *shaman*, *obeah*, *espiritisma*, and others, were ignored or consciously suppressed (Bryant, 1970;

Gish, 1979; King, 1966; PAHO, 1993). Nonetheless, in 1951, a UN Rehabilitation Unit was established to facilitate bringing the medical and technological rehabilitation advances from the developed to the developing countries.

During the 1960s and 1970s, developing nations, which were becoming increasingly independent of their colonial ties, prepared national health plans and policies based on the Western medical model while attempting to be less dependent on outside agencies. Paradoxically, these countries experienced relatively few successes in eliminating communicable diseases, controlling rapid population growth, or decreasing food shortages. These factors, along with interrelated environmental realities of Third World nations such as the majority of people living in rural areas, the enormous presence of poverty, and a general decline in the world economy, have reduced the Western medical model's effectiveness.

A realization that the conventional Western medical model was inappropriate and unsuccessful in meeting the health needs of a majority of people in the developing world led to efforts to develop alternative strategies. A new era began within the fields of health and rehabilitation in the Third World in 1977. The World Health Assembly (WHO, 2005b) declared that "the main target of governments and the WHO in the coming decades should be the attainment by all citizens of the world by the year 2000 of a level of health that will permit them to lead a socially and economically productive life" (WHO & UNICEF, 1978, p. 3). In 1978, at the Alma-Ata International Conference on Primary Health Care (PHC), PHC was identified as the means by which this goal could be achieved. The Alma-Ata Declaration defines PHC as "essential health care based on practical, scientifically sound and socially acceptable methods and technology made universally available to individuals and families in the community through their full participation and at a cost that the community and country can afford" (Helander, 1993, p. 38). PHC has as its themes the maximum use of local resources, including trained community health workers and traditional healers; personal and community participation; affordable and accessible care; the integration of prevention, promotion, treatment, and rehabilitation; and coordination between the health sector and other related development sectors such as agriculture, housing, and education. There is an implicit recognition of the influence of culture—both in its broadest sense at the societal level, as well as the more specific cultural ways at the family and individual level.

Since the 1970s, many nations have initiated major shifts in policy and practice and have explicitly stated that health care is a right to which all citizens, including PWD, are entitled. The principles of PHC are purportedly observed and supported yet implementation is where the real challenge lies. Since the initiation of a PHC focus, economic conditions in many nations have worsened, impeding or reversing improvements in the delivery of service. Health for All by the Year 2000 (HFA/2000) has not been attainable (Mesa-Lago, 1992; Tarimo & Creese, 1990; UN, 2006).

Today, the quantity and quality of care and general and rehabilitative medical remain vastly uneven throughout the world (UNICEF, 1995; WHO, 2008a). Presently, vital health statistics confirm striking differences between the developed and less developed worlds. There are increasing inequities in health outcomes, access to care, and cost of care. When comparing the industrialized and developing world, the World Health Report (WHO, 2008a) states that the life expectancy between the richest and poorest countries exceeds 40 years. Annual expenditures on health ranges from $20 to $6000 per person. The epidemiological picture of disease and disability, although becoming more similar over time, is still rather different. Acute and communicable diseases are more prevalent in the developing world, although chronic diseases are increasingly common. Furthermore, the burden of disease related to injuries (road traffic, interpersonal violence, and war), and thus disability, is expected to rise dramatically over the next decade.

Similarly, PWD living in the developing world experience more difficulty receiving care and integrating into society than those who live in the industrialized world. Although some care has historically been provided at the household or community level, it has been minimal. International rehabilitation programs, such as the World Rehabilitation Fund and Rehabilitation International, have helped to provide care. However, these programs have largely depended on charitable and religious organizations for administrative and financial support and have reached only a fraction of those in need (Groce, 1992). At best, only a few services, for a select few, are provided at major teaching hospitals in the capital cities. Comprehensive and timely rehabilitation services are rarely available due to lack of trained personnel and limited private and public resources. Even the most basic adaptive equipment is usually unavailable. Educational and vocational services are even more of a rarity than physical rehabilitation.

Highly technical medical procedures may be available in a capital region, but poor or rural populations cannot readily access this sophisticated tertiary care. Although many developing nations have policies supporting PHC, the capacity to implement this is marginal. Obstacles such as poor physical infrastructure; urban-based allocation of resources; lack of administrative expertise; and scarcity of financial, technical, and human resources are widely found. The disparity in the provision of health care services between lower and upper socioeconomic groups is even more profound in developing countries than in developed countries and worse for PWD than for those without (Wiman, Helander, & Westland, 2002).

COMMUNITY-BASED REHABILITATION

Community-based rehabilitation (CBR) has its roots in the idea of providing rehabilitation services to those who have little or no access to such services. In the environmental context, poverty is the norm, and some degree of ignorance, prejudice, and superstition limit the cultural belief system of people in the community. At the same time, previous efforts at rehabilitation, if they existed, were too often inaccessible to people (especially in rural areas), too capital and technology-intensive, too specialized, and too Western in style.

Specific to disability prevention and rehabilitation within the less developed countries, the WHO has adopted a PHC approach with two main strategies. Because the major causes of impairment in the Third World are considered potentially avoidable, the first strategy is primary prevention. The second strategy is the delivery of rehabilitative community-based services with an appropriate system of supervision and referral. Specifically, the WHO advanced the concept of CBR (Helander, Mendes, & Nelson, 1983; Helander, Mendes, Nelson, & Goerdt, 1989; Smilkstein, Mendis, Sanghavi, Campbell, & Kamwendo, 1984; WHO, 1981, 1984). CBR is a strategy for enhancing the quality of life of PWD by improving service delivery, providing more equitable opportunities, and promoting and protecting their human rights. This policy involves measures taken at the community level to use and build upon the resources of the community. The family of a disabled person is often the most important resource. The supporting personnel in such a program, who are likely to be local persons with minimal traditional or specialized education, are often referred to as community rehabilitation workers (CRWs). Ideally, the CBR system should be multi-level and multi-sectoral. CBR represents one possible solution to meeting the rehabilitation component of PHC. A meaningful working definition of CBR and alternative models continues to evolve from within the WHO and from individuals working in the field (WCPT, 2003; WHO 2001a, 2003, 2005c).

The philosophical principles of the CBR approach are equality of rights, solidarity with others who are denied equality, and integration into the mainstream of community life. These require recognizing the capability of PWD to fulfill their human rights and facilitating participation in the social and economic activities of society while maintaining personal dignity. Personal empowerment is a major component of CBR.

CBR based the provision of rehabilitation services on a three-tier referral system:

1. A basic home and community level

2. Intermediate supports

3. National, specialized services

At the community level, CBR involves PWD, their families, and the community workers. It may be a component of an integrated community development program that bases decisions on the will of the community. At the intermediate level, the sponsor (i.e., the government or non-governmental organization [NGO]), is likely to be involved with the training and technical supervision of community personnel and provide managerial support as well as direct medical interventions when a referral is appropriate. At the national level, it is expected (but certainly not always the case) that the government, in cooperation with the community, will be involved with planning, implementing, coordinating, and evaluating CBR and will provide tertiary care and technical support for some individuals who should then be referred back to the community level as soon as feasible.

Since the development of the CBR concept, its goals have been elaborated on and presented in seminal documents such as the 1982 UN World Program of Action Concerning Disabled Persons. In 2002, the WHO, ILO, and UNESCO repositioned CBR as a strategy within the local community for the development of rehabilitation services, equalization of opportunities and social inclusion of all children and adults with disabilities, and poverty reduction (WHO, 2003). Most recently, at the UN Convention on the Rights of Persons with Disabilities (UN, 2006) the ideals to support community-based services, whether they be formally linked to the WHO model or to an independent government or non-governmental model, were elucidated. In 2008, the WHO noted that CBR had been implemented in more than 90 countries (WHO, 2008a). These documents reflect the consensus that CBR has moved more toward a human rights model and away from a bio-medical model.

Field testing of CBR began in 1979 and continues today (Jonsson, 1994; Periquet, 1984). Numerous community-based programs have been adopted throughout many regions of the world—many use the CBR label but lack some of its critical components. A review of the literature supports the notion that these programs take on a variety of forms based on local conditions, existing resources, and experiences from other development programs, and exist under the auspices of public and private sponsorships. For example, Werner (1986) favors PWD living together in a village setting; Miles (1994) prefers neighborhood centers staffed by community and professional workers; and Thorburn (1994) relies on home visiting by CRWs and the development of parent associations.

As the concepts become more widely spread and better understood, more models develop. Some remain focused on small projects in rural areas while others consider national programs. Although each has its own particular constraints and CBR is not a panacea, programs across a variety of cultures in developing and developed nations are being implemented and appear to be accomplishing some of their goals to a considerable degree (Boutros-Ghali, 1992; Finkenflügel, 1994; Groce & Zola, 1993; Helander, 1993; R. Jaffer & R. Jaffer, 1994; Kay & Dunleavy, 1996; Leavitt, 1992, 1999; Momm & Koenig, 1989; PAHO, 1993; Peat & Shahani, 1989; Thorburn, 1994; Thorburn & Marfo, 1994; Werner, 1986; Zaman & Munir, 1994). However, detailed descriptions and/or evaluations of CBR programs are limited and mostly appear in newsletter publications (Werner, 1983-2008).

THE CHALLENGES CONFRONTING CBR

The evolution of the CBR concept has supported the development of promising rehabilitation programs for PWD. Yet, according to Helander (1993; Leavitt, 2008), too many services remain insufficiently planned and donors or governments abandon many projects during times of economic hardship. There remains significant debate over multiple issues relating to CBR, and barriers to successful care are still plentiful.

The following discusses some of the more broadly defined issues facing CBR, and some suggestions to enhance the likelihood for success in the future. Hopefully, by physical therapists becoming more learned about this field of study, colleagues working in global health will bring this information to the local population who could then be the ultimate determiners of program structure and function.

PUBLIC POLICY

Leaders, both within the disability rights movement and political arena, must foster reasonable and effective public policy and practice given the realities of life in developing nations. Naturally, each nation or community needs to complete its own specific epidemiological and situational analysis before the development of policy. It is also understood that the situation of PWD is an overall function of the fundamental societal processes and current conditions. Significant changes can only occur with modifications of the system as a whole. For example, socioeconomic development (such as a decrease in poverty and/or increase in community development) would, in itself, undoubtedly improve the status of PWD, perhaps even more so than rehabilitation programs per se (Turmusani, Vreede, & Wirz, 2002; WHO, 2003, 2005c; Wirz & Thomas, 2002).

While recognizing the difficult choices regarding the allocation of limited resources, PHC can be viewed as a means to improve the cost-benefit ratio of money spent on PWD. The principles of PHC, such as the importance of early intervention and using low-cost, socially acceptable practices, support the Alma-Ata Declaration of the WHO and provide the foundation for the delivery of rehabilitation services.

Prevention of disability should continue to be stressed. This can only occur in conjunction with other PHC activities, including the provision of clean water, enforced safety regulations, prenatal care, adequate labor and delivery facilities, and staffing and development of universal immunization services. Cost-benefit analyses generally support the concept that preventive services serve society best.

The question of whether a CBR project should stand alone or be associated with other health or development services continues to be debated and poses some ethical questions (Turmusani et al., 2002). Some believe that rehabilitation services are more likely to succeed if CBR clearly exists as its own PHC program, rather than be blended into a more general health care or development program. Most agree that rehabilitation should be "de-medicalized" as much as possible. An argument in favor of keeping CBR separate is that it must be a "special" service because there is simply too much unique information for the CRW to learn and convey to the families of individuals with disabilities. As it is, the CRW must function as a special educator, physical therapist, occupational therapist, speech and language pathologist, etc. If the CRW must share this time and energy with health arenas such as family planning or nutrition, the rehabilitation information may be diluted sufficiently to sacrifice its value. The 3D Project in Jamaica is an example of this type of program (Leavitt, 1992, 1999, 2008).

Alternatively, some argue that CBR should be a component of a full-scale development program that reinforces community participation at all levels and the empowerment of individuals. It is especially prudent for a worker to be multi-skilled in villages that are very isolated or where there is very limited transportation service. Hopeful Steps is a program in Guyana (begun in the mid 1980s) that envisions the development of a CBR program as part of a larger model of community development that would become an empowering process for the community. Hopeful Steps considered the need to place the problems of PWD in the wider context of their environment. It has become part of the village infrastructure, integrated with education, employment, and other sectors (Hopeful Steps, 2007; Stout & O'Toole, 1999). Whether the program stands alone or is integrated, it is critical that all community-level health workers be aware of a broad array of health impairments, and, in addition, should reinforce each other's teaching and support each other's programs.

No matter the structure, it is pitiful to be inefficient in the use of such marginal resources. Ingstad (1999; Instad & Whyte, 2007) in her review of CBR in Botswana, notes that at the national and local level, government and non-government agencies are often attempting to work in parallel without adequate communication or coordination. Even in Jamaica (Leavitt, 2008)—a more middle-income nation—rehabilitation and early intervention agencies do not seem to work together to gain more efficiency.

To enhance the life course for persons who are disabled, a multi-disciplinary commission should be instituted to explore and implement alternative comprehensive policies and programs. All sectors within a nation must be encouraged to work together rather than in isolation, to be advocates, and to continue to educate the public on disability and rehabilitation to improve the prevailing societal attitudes (WHO, 2003). For example, ministries of education could develop and operate more classrooms for children with physical and mental impairments. When possible, attempts should be made to place children in existing classes to provide the most integrated, least restrictive environment. This would also be the most cost-effective. Long-term institutionalization (for children or adults) will further isolate PWD.

Furthermore, governments must address the apparent societal reluctance to employ PWD in meaningful, productive employment positions. Public policy should support vocational training and the public sector should set a good example. In the private sector, incentives can be developed, possibly in the form of tax breaks, for enterprises that hire a PWD. Thorburn (2008) notes, however, the marked difference between what is available for adults as compared to children—especially those with intellectual disability. If they are lucky enough to go to school, they have almost no services once they leave school. Integrating PWD into the workforce becomes both cost-effective and humane by supporting individuals who prefer to become gainfully employed rather than remain non-productive members of society. The ultimate goal of rehabilitation (that is, the ability to play an active role in society with dignity and self-esteem) is thereby more likely to be achieved.

The concept of multi-sectoral collaboration should also apply to cooperation between professionally trained health workers and local indigenous healers. The idea of a physical therapist serving as a "culture broker" enticing each to recognize and respect the other is appealing. Finally, collaboration between and among both government and non-government agencies must be at the forefront if programs are to be efficient.

COMMUNITY PARTICIPATION

Community participation and its concomitant increase in self-reliance are prerequisites for successful community health programs (Leavitt, 1999; WHO, 2003). If a program is initiated from the top down by an outside organization or concerned individuals, the intent should be to turn the program over to the community. In order to make people aware of the benefits of CBR and success stories of individuals, there needs to be awareness training at community events and at the national level by people with a range of disabilities. This requires that groups be targeted by focused strategies using culturally appropriate activities and specific language. However, constraints to this ideal scenario should not be minimized.

Bottom-up initiation of a program or program management is often quite difficult. It may be difficult for people to perceive or accept ownership of a self-serving program. Hopeful Steps has stressed this philosophy throughout their history and specifically believes that rehabilitation is not a product to be dispensed from the top-down, but rather a process in which the villagers are intimately involved. Programs have emerged as a response to the local people's needs rather than a preconceived agenda. The hope has been to diminish the ignorance, prejudice, and superstition about PWD; to "de-Westernize" the rehabilitation process; and to develop self-esteem and self-reliance within the community (Hopeful Steps, 2007; O'Toole, 1994; Stout & O'Toole, 1999).

Dr. Marigold Thorburn (1994, 1999), the founder of CBR in Jamaica and an internationally renowned advocate for CBR and children with disabilities, notes the difficulties in securing local government or private funding and recruiting middle-level managers from the community. She emphasizes the central role of family, particularly primary caregivers to children with disabilities, and the development of parents' groups as key to the development of community participation. However, Jelsma and Zhanje (1999) report that parents do not necessarily want to be responsible for treating their children; rather, they want to play with them without being considered co-therapists. Additionally, Thorburn advocates expanding the roles of PWD to include, for example, decision making and education of others. One must stress the abilities and competence of PWD and increase their responsibilities and rights; that is, CBR should advance a sense of empowerment.

Personal empowerment and community participation are surely linked to improved attitudes among family and community members in order to lessen the degree of stigma toward PWD at the societal level. Thorburn (1994) and others (Thorburn & Marfo, 1990; WHO, 2003) have continually focused on the need for training for parents and the wider community (such as the parent-teacher associations) to begin the process of eliminating bias toward PWD. She believes that "the most critical factor in the development of a program...is the attitude of the parents towards the child. From a positive, caring, educating and advocating stance by parents will come positive community attitudes...and fulfilling role for disabled people in their own communities" (Thorburn, personal communication, January 14, 1995).

An alternative model in which community participation is emphasized is the Independent Living (IL) movement. In the IL movement, activities are primarily consumer-driven (in this case, by PWD). With either CBR or IL, equality and social integration are enhanced through direct participation of PWD in local and national political bodies. Additionally, disabled persons and their families must form their own organizations to gain political clout, access to human rights, and privileges that others in society already have.

HUMAN RESOURCES

The WHO estimates a shortage of over 4 million health workers worldwide, with Africa facing the greatest shortages (WHO, 2008a). The development of human resources is one of the most critical factors facing CBR programs. There has been a tendency to overlook the potential to train community-based individuals. When developing CRWs, local, relatively unskilled members of the community who are themselves disabled or show concern for individuals with disabilities can be the most appropriate people to be trained in rehabilitation and advocacy principles and techniques. Attention should be paid to the type of training and level of skill development, which has often been noted as a central concern in many community-based health programs.

Training models are numerous and must fit with the local culture and resources. CRWs are capable of providing intellectual stimulation, exercise programs, and social interaction. For example, the WHO manual *Training in the Community for People With Disabilities* (Helender et al., 1989) has thus far been translated into over 40 languages. It is directed toward the achievement of independence in mobility, self-care, play and schooling opportunities, income-generating opportunities, and the enjoyment of family and social life through the use of local resources. There are 30 training packages, each focused on a particular subject such as activities for people who have difficulty moving, play activities, prevention of complications, etc. There are four additional guides for community members having special tasks within CBR: local supervisors, the community rehabilitation committee, people with disabilities, and schoolteachers. It is presumed that basic principles can be used globally, but questions remain, such as how a manual can be culturally and socially relevant within a local context and how best to disseminate the technologies in societies with low literacy.

The Center for Promotion of Integral Rehabilitation (CEPRI) in Nicaragua (Schneider & Segovia, 1999) and Project Projimo in Mexico (Werner, 1986) are examples of CBR projects that train PWD themselves (typically people with spinal cord injuries) to be the trainers for other PWD. At CEPRI, many of the trainers were injured in the political turmoil of the 1980s and 1990s and thus may be more likely to be empowered themselves. In addition, CEPRI has paid special attention to reaching women with disabilities since this group is often discriminated against to a greater extent based on gender.

One issue is whether CRWs/trainers are to be paid employees or volunteers. Helander (1993) notes that it is easier to recruit non-salaried volunteers in Asia, whereas in Africa the tendency is to seek financial compensation. Most CBR volunteers are women. It is assumed that volunteers are women with extra time, that they are selected by the community, that it is easy for them to work in the community after being trained in CBR, and that they volunteer solely because they want to help others. These assumptions are often inaccurate (Ingstad, 1999). At times, a program must begin with people willing to volunteer with the intention of salaried positions at a later date. In either case, CBR workers can find compensation through appreciation by other people, training that might prove useful for self-satisfaction or future career prospects, or the knowledge that their efforts diminish the dependency of a family member who is disabled. Also, CRWs are most likely to bridge the gap between the community culture and the medical culture (Leavitt, 2008).

CBR recognizes that PWD will often need services besides those given by community-level workers. In fact, as more people are identified as being disabled, professional, specialized support services, both within and outside of institutions, are likely to increase. To this end, the infrastructure must be developed to educate and provide regional training of rehabilitation professionals and to promote the development of rehabilitation institutions or departments within hospitals. Physical therapists, special educators, and specialists in vocational rehabilitation counselors are paramount. The development of other allied health professionals in occupational therapy and speech and language pathology must follow because services in these areas of expertise are almost universally absent. WCPT (2003) suggests that the physical therapist should have first contact status as a practitioner within a PHC setting.

There is a dilemma about how to advance already existing rehabilitation professions within the developing world while still maintaining an emphasis on meeting the needs of the majority of PWD, primarily in rural areas, and not just those with access to the limited facilities in the major cities. Similarly, what is the most appropriate educational degree for training specialized professionals? How can you advance professional status through university degrees and employment opportunities, yet keep people interested in working in CBR?

Studies in South Africa (Cornielje & Ferrinho, 1999; Futter, 2003) highlight the difficulty in preparing physical therapists to work in disadvantaged communities. For the most part, existing physical therapists (largely white) abdicate their responsibilities to the larger society by primarily practicing in private settings in elite or middle-class urban areas. In part, this is because students are not made aware of the social, political, economic, cultural, or religious differences influencing the health of PWD. The contrast between community settings where low technology, low cost, and adaptation are required and an urban, more highly technological and costly, institutional setting are pronounced, and physical therapists are not trained on how to adapt. Furthermore, they report that professionals have tended to concern themselves with improved physical performance of the PWD, with little attention to what happens to PWD after they return to their home environment. Educational philosophy and content changes needed consideration. As an antidote, the Institute of Urban Primary Health Care (IUPHC) has developed a training program for community rehabilitation facilitators (CRFs). Here, the emphasis is on understanding rehabilitation as part of social and community development and the empowerment of CRFs and PWD (Cornielje & Ferrinho).

A different problem exists in Vietnam, a nation with less history of professional education for rehabilitation therapists. Kay, Huong, and Chau (1999) describe the Vietnam Project, a multidisciplinary effort to improve rehabilitation through up-grading education of local professionals. The authors recognize the challenge, especially for a newly emerging profession in a developing nation, to balance their desire to advance their education and be considered professionals, and yet not mystify the profession, making it more inaccessible to those most in need. Kay et al. remind us of the many obstacles to up-grading, such as almost complete lack of educational materials, mentors, or continuing education. This project involved a series of multi-disciplinary workshops, given mostly by visiting volunteer professionals from the U.S. on the medical, surgical, and rehabilitation management of particular diagnoses as selected by the Vietnamese. The themes running across all of the workshops—including an emphasis on generalizable assessment and problem-solving skills, the use of the multi-disciplinary team approach, a focus on realistic and appropriate functional goals, and application of skills and knowledge to a range of environments from a central or provincial hospital to a community-based project—are all essential, generic skills required of any competent rehabilitation professional. This program continued through the early 2000s.

In most situations, the educational programs for any rehabilitation professionals must be modified to include concepts of PHC and CBR. Medical and allied health educational curricula are usually based on the Western medical model, without consideration of the particular needs of the local population or the alternative strategies that could be implemented to meet these needs. Knowledge of the total national environment should provide health workers with a better understanding of their clients and the need for community-based services. For example, traditional health beliefs and practices should be acknowledged as factors affecting PWD. Although historically little information has been available, culture-specific beliefs and behaviors should be directly addressed as potential confounding variables and, when appropriate, as potential means of effecting positive outcomes. Rehabilitation professionals and CRWs must consciously consider such information and have greater insight into this domain (Leavitt, 1992, 1999). Although it is predominantly practical factors (such as the availability of services and the cost of care) rather than philosophical issues (such as beliefs about the efficacy of a treatment) that govern the acceptance or rejection of community health programs, cultural-specific models may be highly influential (Fabrega, 1974; Helander et al., 1983; Kay & Salzman, 1994; Leavitt, 1992; Young & Garro, 1982). There is huge inter- and intra-cultural variation all over the world. Cultural competence in developing countries is not necessarily present.

The concepts of "team," interdisciplinary communication and action, and collaboration must be strengthened. When health personnel resources are severely limited, it is even more important for professionals and community workers at every level to understand that all individuals are working for the benefit of PWD—they are all members of the same team. Organizations and professionals should be encouraged to have a more reciprocal relationship at the local level with community-based projects. In addition, the relationship between any service provider and those who are the recipients of those services must be based on mutual power and mutual respect.

Efforts are also needed to increase the retention of already trained professionals in developing nations. This is currently a serious problem as many wish to emigrate to countries that offer better salaries or career prospects. Professional development and continuing education can assist by helping personnel remain current and motivated. Typically, these programs are not available.

The use of visiting professionals from industrialized nations is helpful both for developing human resources and for providing continued learning opportunities for those who are providing services. But, as discussed by Kay & Salzman (1994) and others (Cross-Cultural and International Special Interest Group [CCISIG], 2008), this role may be fraught with inherent ethical and professional dilemmas. Should an expatriate practice outside the scope of their usual practice by doing primary health care activities (giving injections, suturing, or educating about family planning or nutrition) for which one has not been trained? How can you respect the concerns of local colleagues by spending time educating them yet not forget the needs and rights of the many under-served PWD? If you upgrade the skills of a local therapist, does that increase the chance for emigration? Are you honest about your motivation or intent in volunteering or working abroad? The permanent use of expatriates is not a solution, and transfer of knowledge and skills to local personnel should be the aim.

In summary, more continuous and comprehensive training, integrated with practical real-life examples and supervised experience, is advised to allow the CRWs to upgrade their level of expertise and problem solving, which subsequently should improve their clients' status. For professional physical therapists (either from a developing nation or those from an industrialized nation who want to work in CBR), the challenge is to transfer our skills to the local professional, CRW, family, or client, and value our multiple roles (educating, advising, providing direct care, and more) for its greater potential impact.

REHABILITATION TECHNOLOGY

Arguably, rehabilitation technology may be the area where the relevance of local culture and economics determines the reality the most. Demystification of rehabilitation technology and an emphasis on improved functional capacity are necessary in CBR. To that end, a number of easy-to-use screening tools and simple technologies have been developed. For example, the ten-question screen (TQ) can be used to identify childhood disability. This very simple instrument, to be used by non-professionals, was developed by a major international collaborative effort (Durkin, Davidson, Hasan, et al., 1994). The TQ asks the respondent if anyone in the household has difficulty with moving, learning, seeing, hearing, etc. It has been adapted to improve its sensitivity and specificity, although there are variations in responses in different countries (Durkin, Davidson, Desai, et al., 1994).

Alternative technologies must also be developed in the arena of adaptive equipment for PWD. It is well recognized that assistive devices can make a huge difference in the lives of the PWD and their caretakers (Glumac, Pennington, Sweeney, & Leavitt, 2009). Low-cost, culturally and economically appropriate adaptive equipment for PWD should be developed locally and with locally available materials whenever possible. This is often referred to as "low tech" adaptive equipment.

The WHO estimates that 1% of the world's population, or about 65 million people, need a wheelchair (WHO, n.d.b). Importing highly technical and expensive equipment is both wasteful and impractical. Imported wheelchairs, orthoses, and prostheses, for example, are extremely expensive, and replacement or repair of parts is often impossible. Yet, sometimes this is the only option, and the benefits to PWD and their families can still be substantial (Glumac, Pennington, Sweeney, & Leavitt, 2009). Even particular models of adaptive aids made for less-developed nations are not universally suitable. Equipment that is appropriate for one country may not be well suited for the terrain and environmental obstacles in another country. Equipment for one person may not take into account the lifestyle of a different person. Personal lifestyle and environmental reality are the most important considerations (Zollars & Ruppelt, 1999).

Crutches can be made from bamboo sticks, leg orthoses from PVC piping and old rubber tires, or a wheelchair from rattan. The development of the Jaipur foot in India (Golin, 1999) and the Jaipur Foot Artificial Limb Center in Bangladesh is a relative success story. In 1971, the war of liberation and huge cyclones led to many amputations. Traditional Western-style prosthetics proved totally inappropriate based on the exorbitant cost and

functional limitations because of the solid ankle cushion heel (SACH) foot and poor durability. Most people in need simply refused to try a prosthesis. The Jaipur foot, in contrast,
allows for people to squat (which is the common sitting position in Bangladesh used for
socializing, eating, and toileting), would survive the local wet climate, and could be made
for a fraction of the price. Nevertheless, the ongoing effort to produce a polyurethane version of the Jaipur foot and to train workers to produce these is a reminder that the process
of development and indigenization is lengthy.

"Paper technology" is another cultural adaptation. This is a specific low-cost, alternative technology for adaptive aids, such as seating devices and table-tops that are socially
acceptable and readily available in any environment. Paper technology can also be used to
fabricate functional household items and works of art to be sold as an income-generating
activity (Finkenflügel, 1999).

Programs must consider further support in this area by offering workshops directed
toward the development, production, and maintenance of appropriate technology. A
recent international workshop on integrated treatment for elephantiasis (secondary to
lymphatic filariasis, the world's second leading cause of permanent disability), leprosy,
and the diabetic foot is an example of how to take into account both the need for appropriate therapeutic footwear and the need to increase the capacity of community workers in
primary health care (Geyer, 2008). Two U.S. physical therapists and pedorthists, under the
auspices of Handicap International, organized a program in Africa. Specifically, the footwear design challenge was to produce footwear with materials that were locally available,
required simple tools and minimal training, were adaptable for a range of therapeutic
interventions and environmental needs, and were low cost (~$3.50) yet durable. The solu-
tion was a sandal constructed of microcellular rubber with straps made from old inner
tubes, with an adjustable buckle closure that was easy to clean and could be worn in wet
and hot conditions. The educational materials, needing to transcend the multicultural
language barriers, focused on clear images and demonstrations and hands-on practice.

Resource manuals are available that describe how to make simple and low-cost rehabilitation equipment that take culture and resource availability into account (Finkenfügal,
1999; Golin, 1999; Helander et al., 1983, 1989; Hotchkiss, 1985; Werner, 1987, 1998; Zollars
& Ruppelt, 1999). There are new guidelines, specifically for use in less resourced settings
that address design, production, supply, and service delivery of manual wheelchairs
(WHO, n.d.b).

SUSTAINABILITY OF CBR

As some of the CBR programs begin to celebrate milestones (such as 10, 20, or 30 years
of service), the issue of future sustainability becomes critical. Sustainability is presumed to
depend upon a perceived need, a readiness to support the need, and support from outside
of the community (Momm & Koenig, 1989; UNESCO, 1994). The PAHO estimates that 30%
of available health resources are wasted (Mesa-Lago, 1992). In particular, there is a lack of
community mid-level managerial personnel. Public policy must include an expectation of
accountability, monitoring of programs, and evaluation of programs (Tarimo & Creese,
1990). Regardless of the organizational structure, attainment of program goals can be affected by administrative problems in areas of hiring, establishing role responsibilities, training
of community-level workers, and determining who is to receive economic benefits and
prestige from the program (Boyce, 1994; Gartner, 1971; Leavitt, 1992; Torrey, Smith, & Wise,
1973; WHO, 1968, 1987; Yee, 1989). It is prudent to be cautious of too extensive, and thus
impractical, initial programming or too rapid expansion. As suggested by Miles (1994), to
facilitate success, it is wise to think easy before difficult, children before adults, and limited
geographic focus as basic axioms. Flexibility and adaptability are certainly key concepts.

Sustainability will likely be enhanced if research and evaluation data are exchanged
among CBR programs and adjustments are made accordingly. The International Center

for the Advancement of Community-Based Rehabilitation (ICACBR), based in Canada, is one example of an organization whose mandate is to contribute to this body of knowledge through research and program evaluation (ICACBR, 2008). It would also be advantageous if there were increased cooperation among all governmental and non-governmental organizations working on disability-related issues. It is logical to argue strongly for increased government involvement initially and a process of decentralization so that the community can increasingly make their own decisions regarding priorities and resource allocation. It would also be ideal to no longer rely solely on charity and uncoordinated voluntary efforts, especially since donor agencies rarely remain involved for the "long haul." In reality, government and NGO funding of "social" programs is often the first to be cut in times of economic austerity. Unfortunately, programs for PWD typically do not have an easy way to become independently sustainable with income-producing programs.

The 3D Projects in Jamaica is an example of a program that flourished during its early years in the 1980s and 1990s but has since had to retreat. Economic decline in Jamaica and the lack of government funding as well as a lack of new international NGO funding sources has led to significant cuts in their early intervention and all other programs. Many of the CRWs have been laid off or had their hours cut, and most of the PWD in the program are no longer visited in their homes (Leavitt, personal observation, 2000-2008). Hurricanes have left the nation with even greater debt and fewer resources. The one institutional rehabilitation program in Jamaica was partially destroyed by a hurricane and a fire and is being rebuilt (see Leavitt, 1992 for a more in depth discussion of the situation in Jamaica. Unfortunately, although published in 1992, little has changed for the better). In 2010, after several years of planning, the 3D Projects may merge with two other similar CBR programs in Jamaica in an attempt to continue with CBR. Surely, the present-day world economic crisis is bound to impact PWD to a greater degree than their able-bodied peers.

Networking with religious and lay leaders, traditional healers, and educational, health, and social service representatives is useful. Generally speaking, successful outcomes from community health programs depend on a match between the culture of the community being served and the health personnel or system providing care. That is, the cultural approaches of the two groups involved in the interaction must be complementary, and the program organization must be attuned to the environmental realities of the community. This is difficult to attain, and many community programs are hampered by disjunctions in cultural beliefs and behaviors.

Thus, national policy and programming should consider supporting individuals whose major responsibility is to ensure that such a match is developed. For example, the applied medical anthropologist may be an important professional to add to the rehabilitation team. This person can develop and test theory, gather data, and propose solutions to problems with a focus on cultural explanations of behavior. Furthermore, the applied anthropologist is often an effective "culture broker"—someone who can help to ensure an ecological, holistic approach by bringing about some communication among various modern and traditional health practitioners or systems and the various people in need of service.

THE EVIDENCE BASE FOR COMMUNITY-BASED REHABILITATION

Determining what cultural and other factors contribute to success in CBR programs could be most important if the general premise regarding public policy relating to disabled persons is to be based on a community model. There is a lack of quantifiable monitoring and evaluative material concerning CBR. Qualitative, descriptive research is also insufficient (WCPT, 2003). To this point, although the literature is increasing, there has not been a systematic review of CBR (Finkenflügel, Wolffers, & Huijsman, 2005; Mitchell, 1999; Wirz & Thomas, 2002). The UN has developed a questionnaire for field testing of some CBR programs (Jonsson, 1994). The questionnaire, known as OMAR (A Guide on Operations, Monitoring and Analysis of Results), includes questions on:

- Relevance (Does the program meet the needs of PWD, the families, and communities and does its purpose remain valid and pertinent?)

- Effectiveness (Did the program meet its objectives in terms of population coverage and benefits for individuals?)

- Efficiency (Were the available resources used most efficiently?)

- Sustainability (Will the program continue once external support is withdrawn?)

- Impact (What effects has the program had on its institutional, technical, economic, and social settings?)

With regard to impact of CBR, the verdict is not clear. Although personal experience has led me to know many individuals who have felt a positive impact through CBR programs, there is conflicting evidence. Benedict Ingstad, a medical anthropologist who was one of the first researchers to evaluate a CBR program, as well as to look at the lives of PWD, is disappointed (see Chapter 5). In *Disability in Local and Global Worlds* (2007), Ingstad writes about the lives of individuals that she has met. A main theme is that PWD that she met in Botswana in 1985 (when evaluating one of the earliest CBR programs) had not been "helped" by the CBR program. Although officially still in place, the respondents reported no contact with the program. Ingstad pointedly states that the role of CBR is to aid PWD in the "bottlenecks" they encounter in their attempts to receive education, receive job training, or support themselves. This has not been accomplished. CRWs were not highly motivated and their nurse supervisors did not support CBR. In the long run, the government did not invest adequately in the program. Furthermore, cultural barriers to rehabilitation in Botswana remain. The Tswana society does not attach meaning to the concept of rehabilitation. Impairments are dealt with, not from the vantage point of the individual with a disability who deserves equal rights and the ability to be empowered, but from the vantage point of what the presence of a PWD means to the family and primary caregiver. It is the family that expects to be given extra resources for taking care of a PWD. There is a mismatch between the ideas behind rehabilitation in CBR and the people of Botswana.

An evaluation of CBR by the WHO Disability and Rehabilitation Programme (DAR) and the Swedish Organizations of Disabled Persons International Aid Association (SHIA) (2002), noted several concerns. Among the most salient are the following:

- CBR programs have not met the needs of very many communities, and even when a community has programming, only some of the people with a disability are served

- CBR continues to regard persons with disabilities as beneficiaries and not as active participants

- Sustainability of CBR has proven a challenge due to lack of government and community resources

Nevertheless, some initiatives were found to be particularly useful—social counseling, training in mobility and daily living skills, facilitating access to loans, and raising community awareness are among the most often cited.

From 2000 to 2002, the WHO, in collaboration with UN Organizations, NGOs, and Disabled People's Organizations, held meetings hosted by the Government of Finland. The report, entitled "International Consultation to Review Community-Based Rehabilitation (CBR)" (WHO, 2003, 2005c), identified four major concerns relevant to strengthening CBR:

1. Community involvement and ownership

2. Multi-sectoral collaboration in CBR

3. The role of Disabled People's Organizations in CBR

4. Scaling up of CBR programs

These points have been addressed already. Having said this, the Report (and a follow up report by the WHO in 2006) (WHO, 2006a), recommends further evidenced-based practice to promote CBR. Lastly, the Report concludes that CBR remains an effective strategy for poverty reduction and calls for increasing human rights for PWD.

Kendall, Buys, and Larner (2000) propose that CBR is ripe with promise, yet recognize that there are also inherent paradoxes to address. For example, the original paradigm shift toward a community model to address a paucity of services for PWD is now more focused on equalization of opportunities and empowerment. However, resources remain incredibly limited and collectivist values of many developing nations are in opposition to independence. In fact, CBR may not harmonize with local beliefs and behaviors. Furthermore, have we adequately developed operational definitions for terms like *empowerment* and *inclusion*? It is suggested that developing working definitions for these constructs will make evaluative research more plausible (Kendall et al.; Wirz & Thomas, 2002).

Additional quantitative and qualitative research will undoubtedly facilitate the development of ideal, culturally-specific models that are more likely to be sustainable and successful (Boyce, 1994). In 2009, the first Asia-Pacific CBR Congress will take place. Some of the issues on the agenda include CBR as a grass-root strategy to promote inclusive development, research, and evidence-based practice in CBR; CBR and implementing the Convention on the Rights of Persons with Disabilities; and more (WHO, 2008c).

COMPARATIVE RESEARCH ON DISABILITY AND REHABILITATION SERVICES

More research about disability and rehabilitation comparing the lives of PWD and the programs that work to effect their everyday lives is needed. The WHO has put great effort into defining a mechanism by which cross-cultural comparisons are possible. This is particularly difficult since the definition of *disability* is not uniform (see Chapter 5). In an effort to help with this task, the WHO developed *The International Classification of Impairments, Disabilities and Handicaps (ICIDH)* in 1980. Revised in 2001, it is now called the *International Classification of Functioning, Disability, and Health (ICF)* (WHO, 2001b).

The ICF is a tool for classifying and comparing disability in a culturally neutral way and further minimizing the use of a bio-medical model of disease. It embodies the idea that everyone, throughout the course of life, can experience a disability rather than disability being a specific set of conditions. The more negative concepts of "impairment," "disability," and "handicap" are replaced by the more neutral terms *body structures/functions, activity* (ability or actual performance), and *participation* (involvement in life situations). The new level, "environmental factors," includes physical, social, and attitudinal variables that constitute a person's life (Ingstad & Whyte, 2007). In summary, disability is defined as "the outcome or result of a complex relationship between an individual's health condition and personal factors and of the external factors that represent the circumstances in which the individual lives" (WHO, 2001b) (see Schumacher, 1999).

PREPARING FOR IMMERSION IN A CROSS-CULTURAL SITUATION: PRACTICAL CONSIDERATION FOR THE EXPATRIATE CONSULTANT

What I consider exotic, charming, enchanting, or captivating, you may consider annoying, distasteful, offensive, or even repugnant. What works for one does not work for another. For some people, the opportunity to work in a cross-cultural setting is the chance of a lifetime. Others might find it a miserable experience. What personal characteristics are likely to foster a successful cross-cultural encounter, especially in a developing country? High on the list are a sense of humor, a sense of adventure, patience, flexibility, tolerance for ambiguity and difference, and cultural sensitivity. Being perceptive, empathic, innovative, organized, and committed to sharing knowledge and skills are also very important. Working in a cross-cultural setting means being able to cope with the unexpected and being prepared for situations never previously encountered. It is doubtful that anyone can be all of these things all of the time, but we can strive toward maintaining some of these attributes as often as possible. Ironically, every professional has some characteristics that are not conducive to a successful encounter. That is, we can be task-oriented, overachievers, and fearful of failure.

Not all physical therapists are suitable for working internationally, especially when the conditions may be enormously different from what one is used to. That being said, a practitioner who does decide to make the journey into another country/culture must aim for cultural competence. First and foremost, it is essential to understand and reflect upon the notion that each of us is immersed in our own culture, with its associated beliefs, attitudes, and behaviors that guide our personal and professional interactions. Furthermore, we need to take a hard look at both our tendency to stereotype as a means to simplify a complex world, and at the inherent biases we hold toward our own way of life and against that of those who are different. We need to acknowledge our tendency to understand life and draw conclusions based on superficial appearances rather than on well-founded knowledge.

In reality, we all tend to be ethnocentric, that is, believing that our own cultural way of life is the norm, the standard by which all others are judged. What we forget is that the next person, from another culture, is also ethnocentric. Thus, the ability to function effectively in another environment is no easy task; cultural competence is easy to espouse, yet very difficult to do. Do not underestimate the obstacles to achieving the goal of cultural competence. A lifetime of existence cannot be so easily molded or manipulated to accept ways that can be very contrary to our own experiences and values (see Chapter 1).

Advance preparation is a critical component to a successful encounter. Factual information about that particular environment is essential (see Assessment of Culture in Chapter 3 for a more thorough discussion). To the untrained observer, it may seem that people "appear" to be similar to each other in another country. Yet, inter- and intra-cultural diversity is often even greater in developing nations, if less obvious. Language and tribal variations are typically both very significant in numbers and in meaning.

Arguably, the most relevant variable is socioeconomic development. The presence of poverty will assuredly influence what kind of rehabilitation is available. Knowledge about geography, language (including verbal and nonverbal communication styles), disease and disability incidence and prevalence, political and health system structure, economic and material resources, history, and cultural value orientations are all helpful, as are population characteristics such as ethnicity, religion, social structure, roles, and beliefs and behaviors associated with illness and disease or disability. Knowledge of customs regarding such things as dress, food, greetings, forms of address, rites of passage, and common courtesies are also key. See Appendix A for some resources published by U.S. governmental and private agencies that provide information about different nations and cultures. Appendix B is a list of resources specific to PT.

Specific to rehabilitation techniques, one must reconsider the standards of practice that are used in one's home environment. For example, in many Asian cultures, people usually squat rather than sit for socializing, eating, and toileting. Thus, if a person has a fractured hip, a goal for the surgical procedure and rehabilitation process would be for a relatively greater range of motion than is typically sought in the West, even at the expense of stability. Also, eating with hands or chopsticks may require different movement patterns and range than is typically used by Westerners, thus necessitating different exercises and activities of emphasis.

In preparing for cross-cultural work, practitioners must also learn the goals and philosophy of the particular project they are working with. What is the background and rationale of the program? Particularly important is whether the program is primarily oriented to service (i.e., the actual implementation of treatment procedures) or to training and educating people who will take over responsibility for the program. Especially relevant to the clinician who is expecting to educate is that methods of teaching and learning differ between cultures. Knowledge transmission in Western cultures, for example, often relies on taking notes and studying written texts, as well as intense discussions with a great deal of interaction between teacher and student. Other cultures rely more on a straight lecture format with few questions and little discussion, and other cultures rely almost entirely on oral training. A written list of exercises, even with diagrams, may not be as effective as demonstrating such exercises. A disjuncture in your goals and the program's goals may lead to disappointment.

Physical therapists need to be mindful of the paradigm shift to become co-participants or partners with PWD and serve as collaborators or consultants rather than managers of rehabilitation activities. They may find it most productive to become more involved with a broader array of activities than heretofore seen as part of one's traditional professional responsibilities. As an example, the professional may become an advocate for the disability rights movement, keeping in mind the ultimate goal is for PWD to become empowered to have the freedom and equal opportunity to make their own choices in life. A focus on changing societal attitudes toward PWD might have a greater impact than an exercise regime. In essence, the "culture of rehabilitation" needs to change and adapt in response to the environment and conditions present in a particular time and place.

CONCLUSION

The last few decades have seen many positive developments with regard to ensuring that PWD live a humane life. In most parts of the world, social processes of urbanization, migration, industrialization, and the expansion of medical knowledge have had a major impact on the care of PWD. PWD are increasingly educated in the regular school system, given vocational training, and receiving physical rehabilitation and appropriate assistive devices to enhance functional outcomes.

The UN Decade of Disabled Persons (1983-1992) represented progress. "Undoubtedly, the major achievement of the Decade was increased public awareness of disability issues among policy makers, planners, politicians, service providers, parents and disabled persons themselves" (Boutros-Ghali, 1992, p. 4). The UN Convention on the Rights of Persons With Disabilities (the Convention), which was passed in 2006, takes to a new level the movement toward a paradigm shift with regard to attitudes and approaches to PWD. The focus is explicitly on social development, human rights, and social justice. It speaks to the application of all categories of rights and how adaptations are required to ensure that PWD can adequately exercise these rights (UN, 2006; WHO, n.d.a). In line with this shift toward linking rights to development, the WHO Action Plan 2006-2111 (WHO, 2006b, 2008b) and the UN Economic and Social Council (2007) call for the mainstreaming of disability issues within the development agenda. Unfortunately, thus far, PWD have remained conspicuously absent, and without their participation, the UN Millennium Development Goals (target date of 2015) will not be reached.

Sound public policy must be both pragmatic and humanitarian. Governments, along with organizations of PWD, rehabilitation professionals, and donor agencies, must continue to form alliances and strive for excellence. The examples in this chapter do not necessarily offer "best practice" rehabilitation models but rather a range of practice realities, including adaptations to meet these realities. The overarching goal for each program should be advocacy—to support and promote changes that would benefit PWD.

As noted in Chapter 1, it is expected that the reader will usefully generalize information learned about one specific geographic location or population group and apply the principles to another context if it is appropriate. We can all learn from the experience of others. I believe we would all agree that we are far from the ideal and have not yet defined best practice models, especially in the developing world.

Ingstad and Whyte (2007) draw the conclusion that all PWD and/or their families, "reach out for programs, visions, and technologies that seem to open broader horizons... [and] that the energizing potential of human-rights declarations, progressive policies, and national statements of intent toward disabled citizens has to be measured in the context of local worlds. For that is where people are acting to make things work, and where the potential may (or may not) be effected and effective as they were intended to be" (Ingstad & Whyte, 2007, pp. 24-25).

Descriptions of the social construction of disability and rehabilitation in communities in both the developed and developing nations remain all too rare. The job of designing and implementing socially and culturally appropriate models of care and the integration of disabled persons into society are far from complete. As appropriate rehabilitation programs incorporating both the more traditional bio-medical model and the emerging more culturally appropriate community and human rights models are advanced (both in the developed and developing world), national and international policymakers must seek to join forces with the local community to foster a positive adaptation process for PWD. Left without rehabilitation, PWD can be a costly drain on society even as they are denied their right to a meaningful life. To those who argue that rehabilitation is too expensive, pragmatists as well as humanitarians can argue that individual nations and the world community cannot afford not to rehabilitate the persons who are disabled.

REFLECTION QUESTIONS

✔ *Are you interested in volunteering or working in a less developed nation?*

✔ *What personality characteristics do you have that would be helpful while working abroad?*

✔ *What would you find particularly frustrating about working abroad?*

✔ *Do you believe rehabilitation is a low priority within the health care systems of the world?*

✔ *Do physical therapists have a professional responsibility to foster a human rights model for people with disability? Why or why not?*

REFERENCES

Ackerknect, E. H. (1971). *Medicine and ethnology: Selected essays.* Switzerland: Hans Huber.

Benton, L. A., Baker, L. L., Bowman, B. R., & Waters, R. L. (1981). *Functional electrical stimulation: A practical clinical guide* (2nd ed.). Downey, CA: Rancho Los Amigos Hospital.

Blum, N., & Fee, E. (2008). Howard A. Rusk (1901-1989): From military medicine to comprehensive rehabilitation. *American Journal of Public Health, 98*(2), 256-257.

Bogdan, R., & Biklen, D. (1977). Handicapism. *Social Policy, 7*(5), 14-19.

Boutros-Ghali, B. (1992). Message of the Secretary General: World programme of action opens way to full participation in society. *Disabled Persons Bulletin, 2,* Publication 64.

Boyce, W. (1994). Research and evaluation in CBR: An integrated model for practice. Asia Regional Symposium on Research and Evaluation in CBR, Bangalore, India, December 5-7, 1994. Kingston, Ontario: Queens University.

Bryant, J. (1970). *Health and the developing world.* Ithaca, NY: Cornell University Press.

Cornielje, H., & Ferrinho, P. (1999). The sociopolitical context of community based rehabilitation developments in South Africa. In R. L. Leavitt (Ed.), *Cross-cultural rehabilitation: An international perspective* (pp. 217-226). London, England: Harcourt Brace and Company.

Cross-Cultural and International Special Interest Group. (2008). Listserv discussions November 2, 2008 through November 8, 2008. Part of the American Physical Therapy Association, Health Policy Section.

Durkin, M. S., Davidson, L. L., Desai, P., Hasan, Z. M., Khan, N., Shrout, P. E., et al. (1994). Validity of the ten questions screened for childhood disability: Results from population based studies from Bangladesh, Jamaica, and Pakistan. *Epidemiology, 5*(3), 283-289.

Durkin, M. S., Davidson, L. L., Hasan, M., Khan, N., Thorburn, M., & Zaman, S. (1994). Screening for childhood disabilities in community settings. In M. J. Thorburn & K. Marfo (Eds.), *Practical approaches to childhood disability in developing countries: Insights from experience and research* (pp. 179-198). Tampa, FL: Global Age Pub.

Elwan, A. (1999). *Poverty and disability: A background paper for the World Development Report.* Washington, DC: World Bank.

Fabrega, H. (1974). *Disease and social behavior: An Interdisciplinary perspective.* Cambridge, MA: MIT Press.

Finkenflügel, H. (1994). *The handicapped community: The relation between primary health care and community based rehabilitation.* Amsterdam, The Netherlands: VU University Press.

Finkenflügel, H. (1999). Paper technology and community based rehabilitation: Cultural adaptation in Zimbabwe. In R. L. Leavitt (Ed.), *Cross-cultural rehabilitation: An international perspective* (pp. 291-300). London, England: Harcourt Brace and Company.

Finkenflügel, H., Wolffers, I., & Huijsman, R. (2005). The evidence base for community-based rehabilitation: A literature review. *International Journal of Rehabilitation Research, 28*(3), 187-201.

Futter, M. J. (2003). Developing a curriculum module to prepare students for community based physiotherapy rehabilitation in South Africa. *Physiotherapy, 89*(1), 13-24.

Gartner, A. (1971). *Paraprofessionals and their performance: A survey of education, health, and social service programs.* New York, NY: Praeger.

Geyer, M. J. (2008). Focus on footwear: An international workshop on integrated treatment for elephantiasis, leprosy, and the diabetic foot. *HPA Resource, 8*(4), 1-6.

Gish, O. (1979). The political economy of primary care and "health by the people": An historical exploration. *Social Science & Medicine, 13C*(4), 203-211.

Glumac, L., Pennington, S., Sweeney, J., & Leavitt, R. (2009). Guatemalan caregivers' perceptions of receiving and using wheelchairs donated for other children. *Pediatric Physical Therapy, 21*, 167-175.

Goerdt, A. (1984). *Physical disability in Barbados: A cultural perspective.* Unpublished PhD dissertation. New York, NY: New York University.

Goffman, E. (1963). *Stigma: Notes on the management of spoiled identity.* Englewood Cliffs, NJ: Prentice Hall.

Golin, L. (1999). Appropriate prosthetics and orthotics in less developed countries. In R. L. Leavitt (Ed.), *Cross-cultural rehabilitation: An international perspective* (pp. 281-290). London, England: Harcourt Brace and Company.

Granger, F. B. (1976). The development of physiotherapy. *Physical Therapy, 56*(1), 13-14.

Groce, N. (1987). Cross cultural research, current strengths, future needs. *Disabilities Studies Quarterly, 7*(3), 1-3.

Groce, N. (1992). *The U.S. role in international disability activities: A history and look towards the future.* New York, NY: Rehabilitation International, and Durham, ND: World Rehabilitation Fund.

Groce, N. E., & Zola, I. K. (1993). Multiculturalism, chronic illness, and disability. *Pediatrics, 91*(5 Pt 2), 1048-1055.

Hanks, J. R., & Hanks, L. M. (1948). The physically handicapped in certain non-occidental societies. *Journal of Social Sciences, 4*, 11-20.

Hazenhyer, I. M. (1946). A history of the American Physiotherapy Association. *Physiotherapy Review, 26*(1) 123-126.

Helander, E. (1993). *Prejudice and dignity: An introduction to CBR.* Washington, DC: UN Development Fund, Publication No. E93-111-B3.

Helander, E. (1999). *Prejudice and dignity: An introduction to community-based rehabilitation* (2nd ed.). New York, NY: United Nations Development Program.

Helander, E. (2000). Guest editorial: 25 Years of community based rehabilitation. *Asia Pacific Disability Rehabilitation Journal, 11*(1), 4-9.

Helander, E., Mendes, P., & Nelson, G. (1983). *Training disabled people in the community: A manual on community-based rehabilitation for developing countries.* Geneva, Switzerland: World Health Organization.

Helander, E., Mendes, P., Nelson, G., & Goerdt, A. (1989). *Training in the community for people with disabilities.* Geneva, Switzerland: World Health Organization.

Hopeful Steps. (2007). Contact CBR. Retrieved November 26, 2008, from http://www.sdnp.org.gy/cbr/contact/contact.htm

Hotchkiss, R. (1985). *Independence through mobility.* Washington, DC: Appropriate Technology International.

Ingstad, B. (1999). Problems with community mobilization and participation in community-based rehabilitation: A case from Botswana. In R. L. Leavitt (Ed.), *Cross-cultural rehabilitation: An international perspective* (pp. 207-216). London, England: Harcourt Brace and Company.

Ingstad, B., & Whyte, S. R. (2007). *Disability in local and global worlds.* Berkeley, CA: University of California Press.

International Center for the Advancement of Community Based Rehabilitation. (2008). Web page. Retrieved September 30, 2009, from http://www.queensu.ca/icacbr/index.html

Jaffer, R., & Jaffer, R. (1994). The WHO-CBR approach: Programme on ideology—some lessons from the CBR experience in Punjab, Pakistan. In M. J. Thorburn & K. Marfo (Eds.), *Practical approaches to childhood disability in developing countries: Insights from experience and research* (pp. 321-340). Tampa, FL: Global Age Pub.

Jelsma, J., & Zhanje, M. (1999). Impact of the Harare parents' groups for children with a disability and their parents: Are caregivers satisfied with the service? In R. L. Leavitt (Ed.), *Cross-cultural rehabilitation: An international perspective* (pp. 329-338). London, England: Harcourt Brace and Company.

Jonsson, T. (1994). OMAR in rehabilitation: A guide on operations, monitoring, and analysis of results. Washington, DC: United Nations Development Program, Interregional Program for Disabled People.

Kaufman, S., & Becker, G. (1986). Stroke: Health care on the periphery. *Social Science & Medicine, 22*(9), 983-989.

Kay, E., & Dunleavy, K. (1996). Community-based rehabilitation: An international model. *Pediatric Physical Therapy, 8*(3), 117-121.

Kay, E., Huong, N. T., & Chau, N. T. M. (1999). Upgrading physical therapy education in Vietnam. In R. L. Leavitt (Ed.), *Cross-cultural rehabilitation: An international perspective* (pp. 269-280). London, England: Harcourt Brace and Company.

Kay, E., & Salzman, A. (1994). Volunteer PTs in developing nations. *PT Magazine, 2*(10), 52-56.

Kendall, E., Buys N., & Larner, J. (2000). Community-based service delivery in rehabilitation: The promise and the paradox. *Disability and Rehabilitation, 22*(10), 435-445.

King, M. (1966). *Medical care in developing countries: A primer on the medicine of poverty and a symposium from Makerere.* New York, NY: Oxford University Press.

Leavitt, R. L. (1992). *Disability and rehabilitation in rural Jamaica: An ethnographic study.* Madison, NJ: Fairleigh Dickenson University Press.

Leavitt, R. L. (Ed.). (1999). *Cross-cultural rehabilitation: An international perspective.* London, England: Harcourt Brace and Company.

Leavitt, R. L. (2008). Personal observations and conversations in Jamaica and India.

Mesa-Lago, C. (1992). *Health care for the poor in Latin America and the Caribbean.* Washington, DC: Pan American Health Organization.

Miles, M. (1994). The 'community base' in rehabilitation planning: key or gimmick? In M. J. Thorburn & K. Marfo (Eds.), *Practical approaches to childhood disability in developing countries: Insights from experience and research* (pp. 287-302). Tampa, FL: Global Age Pub.

Mitchell, R. (1999). The research base of community-based rehabilitation. *Disability and Rehabilitation, 21*(10-11), 459-468.

Momm, K., & Koenig, A. (1989). *Disabled persons bulletin 1.* Geneva, Switzerland: International Labor Office.

Nagler, M. (1993). *Perspectives on disability* (2nd ed.). Palo Alto, CA: Health Markets Research.

National Organization on Disability. (n.d.). Access to independence: Health care access. Retrieved October 29, 2008, from http://www.nod.org/index.cfm?fuseaction=Page.viewPage&pageId=19

O'Toole, B. (1994). Community-based rehabilitation: The Guyana evaluation project. In M. J. Thorburn & K. Marfo (Eds.), *Practical approaches to childhood disability in developing countries: Insights from experience and research* (pp. 341-366). Tampa, FL: Global Age Pub.

Pan American Health Organization. (1993). *Development and strengthening of local health systems in the transformation of national health systems: The rehabilitation services.* Washington, DC: Author.

Pan American Health Organization. (1994a). *Situational analysis of disabilities and rehabilitation in the English speaking Caribbean.* Washington, DC: Author.

Pan American Health Organization. (1994b). Health conditions in the Americas. *Scientific Publication, 524*(Vol. I), Washington, DC: Author

Parnes, P. (2008). Research on disability and development. Toronto, Ontario: International Centre for Disability and Rehabilitation.

Peat, M., & Shahani, M. (1989). *Community based rehabilitation: International perspectives.* Kingston, Ontario: Queen's University.

Periquet, A. (1984). *Community based rehabilitation services: The experiences of Bacolod, Philippines and the Asia/Pacific region.* New York, NY: International Exchange of Experts and Information in Rehabilitation World, Rehabilitation Fund.

Safilios-Rothschild, C. (1970). *The sociology and social psychology of disability and rehabilitation.* New York, NY: Random House.

Sanders, G. (1986). *Lower limb amputations: A guide to rehabilitation.* Philadelphia, PA: F.A. Davis.

Schneider, E., & Segovia, H. (1999). Development of community rehabilitation in Nicaragua: Training people with disabilities to be trainers. In R. L. Leavitt (Ed.), *Cross-cultural rehabilitation: An international perspective* (pp. 191-206). London, England: Harcourt Brace and Company.

Schumacher, K. (1999). International classification of impairments, disabilities and handicaps (ICIDH): A universal framework. In R. L. Leavitt (Ed.), *Cross-cultural rehabilitation: An international perspective* (pp. 113-124). London, England: Harcourt Brace and Company.

Smilkstein, G., Mendis, P., Sanghavi, S., Campbell, J. B., & Kamwendo, K. (1984). The role of physical therapists in primary care in the developing world. *Clinical Management in Physical Therapy, 4,* 24-27.

Stout, S., & O'Toole, B. (1999). Community based rehabilitation with indigenous peoples: A case description from Guyana. In R. L. Leavitt (Ed.), *Cross-cultural rehabilitation: An international perspective* (pp. 181-190). London, England: Harcourt Brace and Company.

Tappen, F. M. (1961). *Massage techniques: A case method approach.* New York, NY: Macmillan.

Tarantola, D. (2005). Global health and national governance. *American Journal of Public Health, 95*(1), 8.

Tarimo, E., & Creese, A. (Eds.). (1990). *Achieving health for all by the year 2000: Midway reports of country experiences.* Geneva, Switzerland: World Health Organization.

Thorburn, M. (1994). *Roles and relationships of CBR services in the community.* Presented at the Asia Regional Symposium on Results and Evaluation in CBR, Bangalore, India. December 5-7, 1994.

Thorburn, M. (1999). Barriers to successful rehabilitation. In R. L. Leavitt (Ed.), *Cross-cultural rehabilitation: An international perspective* (pp. 317-328). London, England: Harcourt Brace and Company.

Thorburn, M. (2008). Comparative policy brief: Status of intellectual disabilities in Jamaica. *Journal of Policy and Practice in Intellectual Disabilities, 5*(2), 125-128.

Thorburn, M., & Marfo, K. (1994). *Practical approaches to childhood disability in developing countries: Insights from experience and research.* Tampa, FL: Global Age Pub.

Torrey, E. F., Smith, D., & Wise, H. (1973). The family health worker revisited: A five year follow-up. *American Journal of Public Health, 63*(1), 71-74.

Turmusani, M., Vreede, A., & Wirz, S. (2002). Some ethical issues in community based rehabilitation initiatives in developing countries. *Disability and Rehabilitation, 24*(10), 558-564.

United Nations. (2007). Economic and Social Council. Retrieved October 2, 2009, from http://www.choike.org/documentos/disab2008.pdf

United Nations. (2006). Convention on the rights of persons with disabilities. Retrieved November 28, 2009, from http://www.un.org/disabilities/default.asp?navid=13&pid=150

United Nations Children's Fund. (1995). The state of the world's children 1995. New York, NY: Oxford University Press.

United Nations Educational, Scientific and Cultural Organization. (1994). *CBR: For and with people with disabilities: A joint position paper.* Publication No. E.81.N.l. New York, NY: International Labor Organization.

United Nations Educational, Scientific and Cultural Organization. (1998). *From special needs education to education for all.* Paris, France: Author.

Werner, D. (1986). *Project Projimo: A village run rehabilitation program for disabled children in Mexico.* Palo Alto, CA: Hesperian Foundation.

Werner, D. (1987). *Disabled village children: A guide for community health workers, rehabilitation workers, and families.* Palo Alto, CA: Hesperian Foundation.

Werner, D. (1998). *Nothing about us without us: Developing innovative technologies for, by and with people with disabilities.* Palo Alto, CA: Health Wrights.

Werner, D. (1983-2008). Newsletter from the Sierra Madre. Palo Alto, CA: Health Wrights.

Westbrook, M. T., Legge, V., & Pennay, M. (1993). Attitudes towards disabilities in multicultural society. *Social Science & Medicine, 36*(5), 615-623.

Wiman, R., Helander, E., & Westland, J. (2002). Meeting the needs of people with disabilities—New approaches in the health sector. Washington, DC: World Bank.

Wirz, S., & Thomas, M. (2002). Evaluation of community-based rehabilitation programmes: A search for appropriate indicators. *International Journal of Rehabilitation Research, 25*(3), 163-171.

World Confederation for Physical Therapy. (2003). *WCPT Briefing Paper: Primary health care and community based rehabilitation: Implications for physical therapy based on a survey of WCPT's member organizations and a literature review.* London, England: Author.

World Health Organization. (1968). Training manual of medical assistants and similar personnel. *Technical Report Series,* No. 385. Geneva, Switzerland: Author.

World Health Organization. (1981). Disability prevention and rehabilitation. *Technical Report Series,* No. 668. Geneva, Switzerland: Author.

World Health Organization. (1984). *World health: Rehabilitation for all.* Geneva, Switzerland: Author.

World Health Organization. (1987). *The community health worker: Working guide, guidelines for training, guidelines for adaptation.* Geneva, Switzerland: Author.

World Health Organization. (2001a). *Future trends and challenges in rehabilitation.* Geneva, Switzerland: Author.

World Health Organization. (2001b). *International classification of Functioning, Disability and Health (ICF).* Geneva, Switzerland: Author.

World Health Organization. (2003). *International consultation to review community-based rehabilitation (CBR).* Geneva, Switzerland: Author.

World Health Organization. (2005a). World report on disability and rehabilitation. Retrieved October 3, 2007, from http://www.who.int/disabilities/publications/dar_world_report_concept_note.pdf

World Health Organization. (2005b). Fifty-eighth World Health Assembly. Retrieved October 2, 2009, from http://www.who.int/mediacentre/events/2005/wha58/en/index.html

World Health Organization. (2005c). *2nd Meeting Report on the development of guidelines for Community Based Rehabilitation (CBR)*. Geneva, Switzerland.

World Health Organization. (2006a). Disability and rehabilitation: WHO action plan 2006-2111. Retrieved October 3, 2007, from http://www.who.int/disabilities/publications/dar_action_plan_2006to2011.pdf

World Health Organization. (2006b). Report of the 4th meeting on development of CBR guidelines. December 11-15, 2006, Geneva, Switzerland. Retrieved October 3, 2007, from http://www.who.int/disabilities/030507_CBR_guideline_3rd_meeting_report.pdf

World Health Organization. (2008a). World health report 2008—Primary health care (now more than ever). Retrieved November 28, 2008, from http://www.who.int/whr/2008/en/index.html

World Health Organization. (2008b). Disability and rehabilitation. Retrieved November 1, 2008, from http://www.who.int/disabilities/en

World Health Organization. (n.d.a). Concept note: World report on disability and rehabilitation. Retrieved October 3, 2007, from http://www.who.int/disabilities/publications/dar_world_report_concept_note.pdf

World Health Organization. (n.d.b). New guidelines released on wheelchairs to support users in developing countries. Retrieved November 26, 2008, from http://www.who.int/disabilities/publications/technology/wheelchairguidelines/en

World Health Organization, Swedish Organizations of Disabled Persons International Aid Association. (2002). *Community based rehabilitation as we have experienced it: Voices of persons with disabilities*. Retrieved November 19, 2008, from http://whqlibdoc.who.int/publications/9241590432.pdf

World Health Organization, UNICEF. (1978). *Report of the international conference on PHC (Alma-Ata, U.S.SR)*. Geneva, Switzerland: Author.

Wright, B. A. (1983). *Physical disability: A psychosocial approach* (2nd ed.). New York, NY: HarperCollins.

Yee, H. (1989). *Training of rehabilitation persons in Micronesia*. Presented at the Annual American Physical Therapy Association Meeting, Nashville, TN.

Young, J. C., & Garro, L. Y. (1982). Variations in the choice of treatment in two Mexican communities. *Social Science & Medicine, 16*(16), 1453-1465.

Zaman, S., & Munir, S. (1994). Meeting the challenge of implementing services for handicapped children in Bangladesh. In M. J. Thorburn & K. Marfo (Eds.), *Practical approaches to childhood disability in developing countries: Insights from experience and research* (pp. 161-175). Tampa, FL: Global Age Pub.

Zola, I. K. (1982). *Missing pieces: A chronicle of living with a disability*. Philadelphia, PA: Temple University Press.

Zollars, J. A., & Ruppelt, P. (1999). Appropriate assistive technology. In R. L. Leavitt (Ed.), *Cross-cultural rehabilitation: An international perspective* (pp. 125-136). London, England: Harcourt Brace and Company.

The Practice of Cultural Competence in the 21st Century

Ronnie Leavitt, PhD, MPH, PT

The new millennium is well underway, and the recognition of the necessity of cultural competence is expected to grow. Cultural competence depends upon continuing self-assessment regarding the importance of culture, acceptance and respect for difference, vigilance toward the dynamics of differences, ongoing expansion of cultural knowledge and resources, and adaptation of services to meet the needs of a particular individual or group (Cross, Bazron, Dennis, & Isaacs, 1989). Historically, the available models for the provision of care have generally relied on the values and belief systems of the "majority" (i.e., the white, middle-class person). These models have been culturally insensitive by denying the realities of alternative systems of thinking and doing. Today, however, there are several factors in play that must alter the previous paradigm. First, the "majority" is becoming the "minority." Second, there is now a greater awareness of the limitations of biomedicine, a system based solely on a biological understanding of the human being. There is now a greater understanding of the need to pay attention to the material and non-material socio-cultural factors when providing care. In the pluralistic medical systems that exist throughout the world, there is the recognition of the presence and utility of a range of health care beliefs and behaviors, as well as of practitioners of care. Related to this are the increasing requirements by regulatory bodies to address this matter, in part, through cultural competence. Third, health disparities among people of different racial and ethnic groups are of grave concern to the U.S. health care system, as is the impact from such disparities on cost to the system and quality of human life. Interest is rising in the need to provide health care in a more effective and efficient way, to maximize limited resources, and to meet an ever-expanding array of health concerns, including those having to do with disability and rehabilitation.

R. L. Leavitt (Ed.).
Cultural Competence: A Lifelong Journey
to Cultural Proficiency (pp. 227-244).
© 2010 SLACK Incorporated

This chapter will suggest ways to foster the development of a culturally competent physical therapist through changes in the educational curricula and professional practice patterns, as well as specific strategies that are practical to carry out as an individual or organization. Through these efforts, the lifelong journey to cultural proficiency is propelled forward.

FOSTERING THE DEVELOPMENT OF A CULTURALLY PROFICIENT PHYSICAL THERAPIST

PHYSICAL THERAPIST EDUCATION

To achieve cultural competence and show a commitment to a new vision of health care, professionals, either in training or in practice, must be exposed to the process of recognizing one's own cultural identity and worldview and learning about others' cultural value system. The assumption is that competency in recognizing bias, prejudice, and discrimination and our discomfort when faced with difference, using cultural resources, and overcoming cultural barriers can be learned. An understanding of socio-cultural variables in the health care setting and an individual client's worldview is expected to lead to an improved clinical encounter with better functional outcomes for the patient and a more rewarding personal experience for the physical therapist. As Ibrahim (1995) proposes: "Each individual in a professional-consumer dyad [should] be viewed as a unique 'cultural entity' with an emphasis on the individual's 'subjective reality' or worldview… [This] can lead to professional-consumer cultural matching" (pp. 194-195). Nonetheless, "The helping professions are still seeking viable theories and models for training that would prepare service providers to provide valid, effective, reliable, and ethical professional services in a culturally diverse society" (Ibrahim, p. 190).

Historically, few practicing medical or rehabilitation professionals have been suitably educated on the issues associated with the delivery of cross-cultural health care. Many have long argued that there is no time in the curriculum to add material that is not bio-medically (clinically) oriented. Often, education has ignored the influence of socioeconomic status, religion, race, or ethnicity, as well as the presence of differing explanatory models or differing verbal and non-verbal communication or learning styles. Strategies to overcome potential barriers resulting from misunderstandings have been sorely lacking, and few schools or training programs provide adequate instruction about the relationship of culture to health. Yet, there is increasing literature supporting a social humanistic perspective to physical therapy education as opposed to a bio-medical perspective (Lundström, 2008).

To foster change in this regard, professional groups have begun to recommend specific areas of content for teaching health professionals. One of the first was the "Recommended Core Curriculum Guidelines on Culturally Sensitive and Competent Health Care" for residents in training (Like, Steiner, & Rubel, 1996). Specific recommendations for required attitudes, knowledge, and skills were listed. A few examples of the "higher level" recommendations that might lead to cultural proficiency are noted below (Like et al.):

- *Attitudes*: Understanding the limitations of cultural analysis and the role played by a range of forces (historical, political, economic, technologic, and environmental) in shaping the health care delivery system as it is today; A moral and ethical obligation to challenge the forms of bias, prejudice, and discrimination as they occur within the health care system and society

- *Knowledge*: An understanding of cultural perspectives on medicine and public health (e.g., Kleinman's typology of health sectors; sociocultural determinants of health and wellness); Cultural assumptions and their influence on the U.S. health care system (e.g., privilege/disadvantage; power/powerlessness/critical consciousness)

- *Skills*: Using a negotiated approach to clinical care (eg. LEARN model; Explanatory Model); Identifying how one's clinical values and assumptions affect clinical decision making (Like et al., 1996)

Incorporating cultural competence as a subject matter into physical therapy education is no longer an option to be debated by individual educational programs. However, "how to" and "to what degree" are still questions to be tackled. The American Physical Therapy Association (APTA) Committee on Cultural Competence has developed a "Blueprint for Teaching Cultural Competence in Physical Therapy Education" (APTA, 2008a). As specified in Chapter 1, the need for cultural competence is embedded within several APTA documents including the "Normative Model of Physical Therapist Professional Education and for Physical Therapist Assistant Education" and the evaluative criteria for accreditation of educational programs (i.e., Commission on Accreditation of Physical Therapy Education [CAPTE] documents) (APTA, 2008b). The APTA recognizes cultural competence as a component of "best practice" in providing physical therapy care.

The Blueprint is based on the conceptual frameworks of Cross et al. (1989) and Campinha-Bacote (2007) and the idea that a holistic model of cultural competence is a developmental process to be learned throughout one's career from a variety of learning experiences (see Chapters 1 and 3). This model requires the student to:

- Examine self through reflective practice
- Learn about the diversity dimensions that influence health outcomes and affect the human experience both positively and negatively
- Recognize the need for a patient-centered approach to delivery of culturally competent physical therapy services
- Value effective communication between the patient and the therapist as a fundamental for delivery of culturally competent care
- Apply core knowledge about culture, belief systems, and traditions to enhance the patient-therapist interaction

Furthermore, cultural competence education should provide knowledge, attitudes, and skills that can enhance best practice models of care to improve health care delivery and reduce health disparities.

Teaching methodology will differ in different programs and no one model has been shown to be most effective (Lipson & Desantis, 2007). Possibly the first question to undertake is how to modify the medical model of education to become more holistic/socio-cultural in nature. This is a transformative approach, whereby the policy, mission, and curricula is altered to embrace multiculturalism. Generally, it is best if culture can be viewed as a broad construct, to be integrated throughout the curriculum with content included in a progressive manner (with strands being added to over time) using a range of training strategies. That is, content addressing cultural competence can be integrated into clinical related didactic and practicum courses as well as in the professional courses (e.g., management, research, education, and others). Romanello (2007) reported on a physical therapist education program that integrated cultural competence into its curriculum in four ways:

1. By developing a strategic plan to encourage faculty to become committed to diversity
2. By immersing faculty and students in diverse environments (possibly through in-country or international service learning experiences in addition to clinical practica)
3. By using artifacts, language, and teaching methods to raise diversity to a conscious level
4. By incorporating reflection and discussion that encourages people to discover their own cultural values and beliefs, as well as those of others

---

A REMINDER: THE NATURE OF STEREOTYPING

It is our duty to recognize that we all have stereotypes and that we must constantly evaluate them and the effect they are having on our personal and professional lives. Stereotyping is a significant barrier to achieving cultural competence.

Stereotyping has been learned from early childhood through messages that we receive from society at large (media, schools, religious institutions, and more) and through our family. Some of these are overt and purposeful, but many are subtle, subconscious, and passed on without mal-intent.

Learned stereotypes become "mental tapes" that affect what we think and how we act. They become automatic and internalized. Stereotyping is a shortcut version of perception not based on reality. We place someone in a particular mental file not based on information gained from personal experience, but from our conscious or unconscious beliefs about a general group to which the person belongs.

Students need to be held accountable to this content as they would clinical elements of care. Wong and Blissett (2007) have proposed reflective writing as one means of assessment. Appreciable changes in physical therapy educational content and experiences should lead to changes in best clinical practice models.

The Tool for Assessing Cultural Competence Training (TACCT), developed by Lie, Boker, and Cleveland (2006) for the Association of American Medical Colleges (AAMC) is one suggested instrument by which to measure the success of cultural competency training. This instrument addresses knowledge (K), skills (S), and attitudes (A) within five domains (AAMC, n.d.):

1. Cultural competence rationale, context, and definition (K= identify patterns of national data on disparities; S= use assessment tools; A= value importance of diversity in health care)

2. Key aspects of cultural competence (K= describe challenges in cross-cultural community; S= elicit information in family-centered context; A= nonjudgmental listening to health beliefs)

3. Impact of stereotyping on medical decision making (K= describe community partnering strategies; S= engage in reflection about own beliefs; A= value the need to address personal bias)

4. Health disparities and factors influencing health (K= discuss barriers to eliminating heath disparities; S= propose a community-based health intervention; A= recognize disparities amenable to intervention)

5. Cross-cultural clinical skills (K= list ways to enhance patient adherence; S= use negotiating and problem-solving skills; A= respect patient's cultural beliefs) (AAMC, n.d.)

Non-curricular factors associated with the educational program environment (i.e., degree of diversity among the student body, faculty, and staff), geographic environment, and scholarly efforts are also important in fostering cultural competence. With regard to the need to increase ethnic and racial diversity (as well as other kinds of diversity) of the student body, the APTA has identified increasing the diversity within the profession as one of six actions necessary to fulfill its mission statement. Johanson (2007) studied what factors students considered when choosing a PT educational program. With regard to people of color, the most important considerations were positive interaction with students, financial aid, and number of prerequisites.

In-depth interviews of 15 nursing students of color identified eight themes regarding their experiences in a predominantly White nursing program. The themes were loneliness and isolation, differentness, absence of acknowledgment of individuality from teachers, peers' lack of understanding and knowledge about cultural differences, lack of support

In an effort to increase self-reflection, there are any number of simple exercises or more formal train-ing packages. Here are two suggestions that help individuals recognize their own culture, are very simple, can be adapted to any time frame, and cost nothing:

- **The Name Game**: Instruct participants to speak about their name (first or last). This will intro-duce concepts of self-identity, pride in cultural background and ethnic heritage, and gender issues. It can be used effectively with people who already know each other or as an ice breaker when people are first meeting each other.

- **The Artifact Game**: Instruct people to bring in something from home that will help other people understand who they are. This will allow a person to self reflect on what is important to his or her identity and allow others to ask questions that will increase participants' under-standing of each other.

from teachers, coping with insensitivity and discrimination, determination to build a bet-ter future, and overcoming obstacles (Gardner, 2005). Although Johanson (2007) did not specifically define the concept of fostering positive relationships within the department, it is logical that this would go a long way toward lessening the specific concerns cited by Gardner.

Saha, Guiton, Wimmers, and Wilkerson (2008) published the results of a survey of over 20,000 medical students from 118 U.S. medical schools and found that White students who attend racially diverse medical schools felt better prepared to care for racial and eth-nic minority patients than students at less diverse schools. The outcome measures used were self-rated preparedness to care for people from another background, attitudes about equity and access to care, and intent to practice in an underserved area. The study also suggested that positive interactions among students needs to be encouraged in order to achieve the most benefit.

TOWARDS A PUBLIC HEALTH PERSPECTIVE IN REHABILITATION: HEALTH PROMOTION AND DISEASE PREVENTION

Health was previously defined as simply the absence of disease. Now the definition of health includes physical, social, and mental well-being. The health system is no longer merely concerned with adding years to life, but rather advancing the quality of life for people and the reduction of health disparities within society. Should not the physical therapist play a role in these goals? Isn't it likely that being a culturally competent practi-tioner can assist in making these goals possible?

Rehabilitation professionals are conventionally reactive. They address an impairment, disability, or handicap at the individual level and focus on specific needs of a patient. However, there is a new paradigm developing within the health care field that is more pro-active and oriented to both public health and human rights. Public health is the sci-ence and art of preventing disease, prolonging life, and promoting mental, social, and physical health through organized community efforts. The emphasis, by definition, is on the health interests of the community or collective efforts and responsibilities and not on the individual. In a public health paradigm, health care workers, including physical thera-pists, need to consider the social and cultural determinants of health and ill-health and healing processes. Yet, there remains doubt about what exactly these determinants are (most of the research focuses on socioeconomic status as the principle variable). The mod-ern human rights movement focuses more on societal conditions and the promotion and protection of human rights and dignity. This approach considers the whole human being who has been vulnerable to a range of pathogens and unhealthy conditions as a result of how the person is treated by society—the need for inclusiveness and tolerance is recognized. Accordingly, this new paradigm will logically pay more attention to people with disabilities, a group of individuals with whom physical therapists work (Mann, 2006).

Physical therapists know that reducing and eliminating health disparities is a substantial problem in the U.S. The determinants of health are myriad and it is often difficult to tease out which specific variables are most important for a given outcome. A comprehensive public health approach to target these determinants by focusing on health promotion and disease prevention makes sense. An investment of $10 per person could save the U.S. more than $16 billion annually within five years, with a $5.50 return of every dollar spent (Trust for America's Health, 2009). Although an in-depth discussion of health promotion and disease prevention is outside the scope of this chapter, the *Guide to Physical Therapist Practice* (APTA, 2001) states, "Physical therapists are involved in prevention; in promoting health, wellness, and fitness; and in performing screening activities." Health promotion and disease prevention (primary, secondary, and tertiary) programs should be culture-specific, include input from the people involved, and address a person's explanatory model. One size does not fit all.

After an adequate assessment of individuals and the community (e.g., statistics on individual health status; community needs; available resources; the ability to collaborate with clergy, community leaders, and like-minded agencies) has been completed and goals have been established, a program targeted to the specific population can be developed. Certain considerations are likely to be apparent: people may not speak English fluently and thus hiring personnel who are from the community and who are bicultural is ideal, the group may have a relatively large number of uninsured people (except for Medicare), and there may be identifiable normative cultural value systems (e.g., importance of family, respect for elders, desire for *personalismo*). An additional key program goal will ideally include teaching people, especially those who have not completely acculturated, to advocate for their health care and patient rights.

Some public health activities seem well-suited to physical therapy: pre- and postnatal exercise programs, therapeutic and recreational exercise for children with special needs or the frail elderly, educating the public about preventive measures based on ergonomic principles, fall prevention, and more. For example:

- Immigrants are a particularly vulnerable population. Immigrant children of all backgrounds appear to get even less vigorous exercise than their U.S.-born counterparts. Suggestions as to why this is so focus on socioeconomic status and neighborhood safety. How can physical therapists be involved in increasing exercise for children/organizing community sports teams?

- All Hispanic subgroups are less active than non-Hispanic White people, yet there is significant heterogeneity among Hispanic sub-groups. For men, socio-demographic factors accounted for the disparity in part, but among women, the disparities persisted despite multivariate adjustments (Neighbors, Marquez, & Marcus, 2008). What interventions can physical therapists help to develop and carry out?

- When a patient is seen by a physical therapist, does the therapist ask questions about lifestyle, nutrition, general physical activity, and others? Can the physical therapist become involved in general health education with their clients?

As suggested by Cornielje (1999), critical to an expansion of the public health role of physical therapists is:

- A more proactive approach that focuses on education, promotion of healthy lifestyles, and prevention of disability

- A shift toward a social approach to rehabilitation whereby the ultimate goal is the equalization of opportunity and the integration of PWD into society

- A change from being a manager of our patients to a resource
- Stronger political representation of rehabilitation workers in the disability rights movements and community-based care

THE RESEARCH IMPERATIVE: THE ROLE OF CULTURE IN TESTS AND MEASURES, AND RESEARCH QUESTIONS

To be culturally proficient, physical therapists must do cross-cultural research. Thus far, the most typical research participant is a White male. The under-representation of women and people of different ethnic backgrounds is significant because it inhibits knowledge about differences in clinical responses and how to best decrease health disparities. Lack of minority representation in clinical research studies has been attributed to history, education, culture, language, income and wealth, geography, racial identity, prejudice, paternalism, and other social deterrents. Public Law 103-43 (Giger et al., 2007) was passed in an effort to ensure outreach programs to recruit and retain women and members of "minority" groups as subjects in clinical research. This inclusion remains an explicit criterion in the review of applications for National Institutes of Health (NIH) funding. Furthermore, research should be conducted with culturally appropriate interventions related to specific groups (Giger et al.).

Qualitative and quantitative research can aid in the development of cultural competence by increasing our understanding of particular populations. For example, what is the meaning of disability for a particular patient and for their family? Does a patient partake in other means of treating the disability besides coming to physical therapy? If so, what is the efficacy of such treatment? (The National Institutes of Health, National Center for Complementary and Alternative Medicine has identified the efficacy of complementary and alternative medicine [CAM] as a priority). How does the explanatory model of the patient differ from that of the therapist? Research to develop culturally valid standardized screening instruments (and best practice interview techniques), culture-specific functional outcome measures, and patient satisfaction scales are all important goals.

One important line of inquiry would be to identify very specific attributes required by health professionals to be culturally competent with a specific cultural group. For example, Wittig (2004) surveyed nursing students, some of whom were expected to work in the Indian Health Service, and identified four knowledge themes (general cultural factors, spiritual and religious beliefs, health and risk factors including dietary habits, and self-knowledge and reflection), two skill themes (basic nursing skills, effective communication skills), and two attitude/value themes (open-minded, nonjudgmental, and caring; and respect for diversity) that were critical.

Another domain to research relates to physical therapy tests and measures. Scales to assess patient status and intervention efficacy have generally been standardized for the Euro-American culture and lifestyle, yet in the U.S., people of non-Euro-American heritage are at greater risk for disability and have greater secondary complications and mortality rates associated with disability. Merely translating an assessment tool into another language is insufficient. For example, an analysis of the Denver Developmental Screening Test (DDST), a commonly used pediatric instrument, has indicated that some developmental skills emerge at significantly different ages for Alaska Native children compared with a group of white, middle-class children in the U.S. (Kerfeld, Guthrie, & Steward, 1997).

Similarly, Gannotti, Handwerker, Groce, and Crux (2001) found differences in the scores on the Pediatric Evaluation Disability Inventory (PEDI) when comparing the scores obtained from a population of children living in Puerto Rico with the norms developed in the U.S. Gannotti et al. noted several social customs that affected the age at which developmental skills were expected to occur. For example, young children in Puerto Rico, in contrast to White children in the U.S., typically use a bottle at night for up to 6 or 7 years, might not use a fork for fear of injury, might wear diapers for public outings to avoid the use of public restrooms, and might not learn to put on socks or tie their shoes because they wear sandals secured with Velcro all year. Puerto Rican parental expectations for their children with disabilities are influenced by the Puerto Rican values of interdependence, *añoñar* (pampering or nurturing behaviors), and *sobre protectiva* (overprotectiveness).

Nixon-Cave (2001), in a qualitative study, examined the influence of cultural/ethnic beliefs and values and the environment on the motor development of young children ages 12 to 18 months in three different ethnic groups. The study found similarities and differences in childrearing practices across Anglo-European, Hispanic/Latino, and African American families that influence the development of motor skills. The results indicate that the parent's cultural and ethnic background, parental knowledge, and handling and interaction with the infant have a relationship to the rate of motor development. Hispanic/Latino and African American parents who tend to use more physical handling (including sibling and extended family handling), along with specific play activities, have children whose gross motor development was accelerated. They were also more likely to use grandparents and elders in the community as a source of knowledge concerning childrearing practices. Using the Peabody Developmental Motor Scales (PDMS), the African American children had a motor developmental age of 1 to 4 months above chronological age and Hispanic/Latino children had a motor developmental age of 1 to 2 months above chronological age.

Physical therapists must ask: Are the DDST, PEDI, or PDMS appropriate tests to use to evaluate children's development if the expected developmental age is different for the cultural group in which the child lives? Alternatively, after exploring the beliefs about disability in the family, is a change in the developmental milestone of a child with a disability more or less important than a change in the effect that child will have on the life of the family?

For adults, Duncan (2002) has validated a new Stroke Impact Scale for 14 culturally and linguistically diverse European groups. However, it has not been validated on people from South and Central America, Asia, or the Caribbean, where most immigrants to the U.S. are from. Typically used functional tests do not take into account activities such as eating with chopsticks, eating with hands, sitting on the floor, or moving in and out of the squat position. These activities may be everyday requirements for people from Asia or Africa. Determining culture-specific norms for functional activities also can help the clinician avoid using ethnocentric standards when assessing areas such as cognition, language skills, learning style, gross motor skills, and fine motor skills (Lynch & Hanson, 1998).

Furthermore, best practice intervention methods might vary according to cultural context. In Coyne (2001), physical therapist Lynda Woodruff cited several examples of how physical therapists might modify examination procedures and interventions when treating people with darker skin color:

- It is more difficult to see redness on dark skin; therefore, the effects of infection are more difficult to assess.

- The presence of keloid tissue scarring after a burn, which occurs in some African American and Arab American patients, and the use of cocoa butter as a treatment of choice for burns may decrease the durability of pressure bandages.

- A child with sickle cell anemia may benefit from exercise in a pool because the buoyancy of water can support the weight of the limbs and help reduce the pain caused by movement.

Cross-cultural research is also necessary because the APTA has charged physical therapists with the responsibility of contributing to the body of knowledge that will help to eliminate health disparities in their own practices and more widely. Guided by RC 41-03, the APTA has developed strategies and guidelines for identifying and addressing racial and ethnic disparities in utilization, outcome, and access to physical therapy services (APTA, 2003). By reflecting on the current literature, there is widespread support for the presence of health disparities in medical screening, intervention, access, and outcomes in patients who have actively participated in rehabilitation programs, as well as with patients who have diagnoses that pre-dispose them to interaction with physical therapists. Physical therapists must now consider their own roles in contributing to the presence (or absence) of health disparities, especially in patient populations where disparities in community reintegration have been identified and in the area of interventions where limited evidence is currently available. A key step might be as simple as committing to measuring outcomes or taking note of racial or ethnic demographics. See Chapter 6 for examples of present research findings regarding disparities within physical therapy practice.

In addition to the questions posed above, the physical therapist can be involved in research to discover the relative value of different cultural competence methods and programs. What does cultural competence actually accomplish? As noted in Chapter 3, definitive answers have been elusive. The U.S. Department of Health and Human Services (HHS), Office of Minority Health, Agency for Healthcare Research and Quality (AHRQ) (Fortier & Bishop, 2004), has set a research agenda that focuses on questions relating to:

- *Access and outcomes*: Which interventions increase access for people and/or improve health-related outcomes?

- *Quality and decrease in errors*: Which interventions increase the likelihood of appropriate care and/or reduce the incidence of medical errors?

- *Cost*: Which interventions are cost effective?

- *Comparative analyses*: Which interventions work best under which circumstances?

In summary, cross-cultural research must link theoretical models to practice including outcome measures. It will impact cultural competence and help lead to cultural proficiency—that is, when cross-cultural research is held in high regard, is disseminated, and new approaches are developed in response to need.

PHYSICAL THERAPISTS AS CULTURE BROKERS

Physical therapists may be in the unique position of serving as culture brokers between the health care system and the patient and their family because of the prolonged nature of rehabilitation services. Being a culture broker entails bridging the gap between two people with two different worldviews. In essence, it is a means to mediate conflict for the greater good of the patient. By being well-versed in the theory and practice of cultural competence, physical therapists can educate other health professionals about various cultural styles (such as different verbal and nonverbal ways to communicate or different preferred ways of learning). A physical therapist may help other rehabilitation professionals understand medical pluralism (the existence and use of many different health care alternatives within societies) and therefore the possibility that the patients may be, to varying degrees, intertwining "modern" or "Western" medicine with "indigenous" or "folk" medicine (Fabrega, 1974; Young & Garro, 1982).

To be a culture broker, the physical therapist should learn as much as possible about the relevant traditional practices and practitioners in the community. A physical therapist doing home visits may discover that Hispanic women commonly give their infants Manzanilla tea to control colic. The therapist can then share this observation with the nurses responsible for WIC (Women, Infant, and Children) programs so that they can adapt appropriate guidelines for feeding practices. Therapists might ask their patient or client to bring them to a traditional healing ritual. A physical therapist working in an

Hispanic/Latino neighborhood or with Hispanic/Latino patients might become familiar with the local *botonica* (herbal and religious shop). Physical therapists should be concerned about patient welfare if the traditional healer prescribes an unhealthy, dangerous remedy (although not typical, it is possible). Clinicians may want to think in terms of multiple treatment options, or mutual adaptation—each serving its own purpose. Resources on the beliefs and behaviors of a particular cultural group can be found in Appendix C.

In summary, the best scenario for avoiding or reducing conflict and encouraging collaborative relationships among health care providers and patients would involve the physical therapist serving as a "culture broker," or a link that connects the patient, the traditional healers, and the mainstream health care system.

PREPARING FOR IMMERSION IN A MULTICULTURAL ENVIRONMENT

Becoming culturally competent is the key ingredient to help physical therapists practice in a cross-cultural environment. Gaining cultural skills and knowledge about a person's and a cultural group's way of life and worldview is bound to encourage adaptations of practice. Yet, clinicians are still likely to experience "culture shock."

CULTURE SHOCK

When working cross-culturally—whether in their own nation or in another country—physical therapists are likely to experience *culture shock*. The term describes the more pronounced reactions to the psychological disorientation most people experience when immersed in a culture markedly different from their own. Some degree of culture shock is almost inevitable, and more often than not, it does not stem from any single event or series of events that you may easily confront. Rather, cumulative pressures develop from having your values constantly questioned. Your belief in your own culture and your ethnocentrism is threatened. You are cut off from familiar cultural cues and known patterns (Kohls, 2001).

Culture shock is a cyclical phenomenon involving four basic phases of adjustment. When you arrive in a new environment, you are likely to experience a sense of euphoria for a period of several weeks as you see and absorb new experiences. Later you will probably undergo a period of more pronounced, more unpleasant symptoms as you enter the second stage of culture shock. Differences that once seemed exciting or exotic become overwhelming and a source of anger. Differences associated with the non-material, less-obvious value systems can especially affect you as it becomes clear that you and your client see the world from different vantage points. As previously noted (see Chapters 4 and 9), perhaps the most difficult cultural differences to overcome psychologically, especially for those practicing according to the Western bio-medical model, relate to pace of life and notion of time. Physical therapists are action-oriented and often less forgiving about such things as missed appointments, being late, "red tape," bureaucratic delays, and a sense that time is an unimportant concept. Combine this with the stressors of having to be "productive" at all times, or, if abroad, living and working under different physical conditions and an ambiguous situation, and culture shock becomes likely. Symptoms of this stage may include homesickness for something more familiar, withdrawal, irritability, stereotyping of and hostility toward the patients/hosts, a lessened ability to work effectively, and physical ailments.

With time, there is a gradual adjustment and a level of appreciation for, and comfort with, the alternative cultural viewpoints. With a general understanding of cultural value systems, for example, a tendency toward collectivism (versus individualism) or past orientation (versus present or future orientation), this third stage leads to a better understanding of the logical reasons behind some of the behaviors that are most frustrating. If one remains in an environment for an extended period of time, you may adapt and become more accepting and appreciative of the multicultural environment or even become bicultural. However, do not underestimate how difficult it is to fully adapt to another culture.

If you are working abroad, once back in a more familiar environment, you may experience a reverse culture shock. One is likely to undergo initial elation over being home again, but then, more quickly than you did while living in the other culture, you may experience depression and frustration and find difficulty adjusting. Back home, you expect things to be the same as before, but you are often changed by the cross-cultural experience. Many, for example, find "Western" lifestyles to be wasteful and lavish. Underlying value systems, such as the expectation to be action-oriented and time bound, no longer seem that important. Also, you may want to share your experiences with others, yet colleagues and friends are not all that interested. Giving talks and presentations to interested groups can be a way of channeling your enthusiasm to those who share your interests. Again, being aware of this phenomenon, and seeking out others who have gone through a similar situation, is likely to be helpful.

In a sense, culture shock is an occupational hazard of cross-cultural immersion—either in the U.S. or elsewhere. There are no easy remedies, but some things can help lessen its impact. Admitting to your ethnocentrism and understanding your own culture are the first steps. Learn more about yourself and your own culture through the eyes of your hosts. Also, continue to learn about the particular culture in which you are working. Ask questions and be astute in your observations. Have realistic expectations of yourself and others and remember that problems and challenges are inevitable. The more respect that you show for the people and culture, the more respect you are likely to command and the more effective a consultant/clinician you are. Additionally, be realistic about how much you can accomplish during a particular time period. It can be disheartening to leave a site with the realization that you have only made a dent and that many needs are left yet unmet. Similarly, within the U.S., it can be equally disheartening to recognize that physical therapy may be just one tiny element of what is needed for your patient to have a better quality of life. However, the gratitude you will receive from PWD and colleagues in a cross-cultural immersion is likely to be one of the richest rewards of your life. You may actually gain more than you have given.

BECOMING CULTURALLY COMPETENT: PRACTICAL STRATEGIES TO FACILITATE CULTURAL PROFICIENCY

In order to ensure that the American health care system better responds to the needs of an increasingly diverse patient population, a growing number of health care organizations and agencies are addressing the issue of cultural competence. Cultural competence alone will surely not solve all of the problems we face with regard to patient outcome (including health disparities and inequities) and job satisfaction, but it is a good start. Furthermore, the physical therapist might actively attempt to formalize larger scale, political change through legislative or political action by engaging in the process of advocating for and developing disability rights groups or support systems for people facing multiple barriers to optimal physical therapy services. This suggests the need for practitioners to redefine their role more broadly than they have in the past.

The information in this book provides the PT with knowledge to enhance cultural competence; hopefully, the process is bounded by openness, curiosity, and respect. There are a wide variety of specific assessment tools, multicultural training methods and exercises, and checklists that can assist in the preparation of a culturally proficient physical therapist. The following is a conglomeration of questions to ask yourself that can lead to practical strategies to encourage cultural competence in a climate in which multiculturalism is the norm. Multiculturalism encompasses cultures that differ in age, color, ethnicity, sex, national origin, political ideology, race, religion, and sexual orientation and includes the presence and participation of those with disabilities and those from differing socio-economic backgrounds.

Oftentimes, organizations and individuals use distancing strategies (i.e., excuses) to avoid taking steps necessary for change. For example, with regard to hiring practices, excuses typically heard are that there are few people of color in the community to fill positions, or it is a hassle and expense to look outside of the usual hiring network, or color-blind hiring is what is ethical. These distancing behaviors will not encourage change. Don't be afraid to have open discussions so that people can air their concerns, learn from each other, and thus be more open to change. As an organization or practice becomes multicultural, cultural competence is imperative. For an individual to function in a multicultural environment, cultural competence is an imperative. Examples of questions to ask yourself follow.

ORGANIZATIONAL POLICY CONSIDERATIONS

- Does the mission statement of the organization have a commitment to cultural competence?

- Do the budget and the strategic plans (with regard to practice, education, research, policy, and advocacy) of the organization demonstrate a commitment to culturally competent practice?

- Does the organizational leadership set a good example with regard to their approach to a diverse range of client cultural ways of life?

- Does the organization know the community demographic data, needs, health care practices, and barriers to care?

- Is the organization committed to cultural competence training for health care personnel?

- Has the organization become aware of, and abided by, the state, federal, and professional organization standards requiring cultural competence?*

- Does the organization work to build culturally appropriate resource networks?

HUMAN AND PERSONNEL CONSIDERATIONS

- What is the ethnic background of the staff and the board of directors? Is there a commitment to a diverse workforce? Is there an effort to hire people who speak the same languages as the patients or staff that is bicultural?

- If you drew an organizational chart, what would it look like? Who is in a position of power? Who is at the bottom of the hierarchy?

---

*For example, to ensure that the health care system better responds to the needs of an increasingly diverse patient population, the HHS Office of Minority Health has developed National Standards for Culturally and Linguistically Appropriate Services in Health Care (2001). The 14 standards are organized by themes: culturally competent care (Standards 1 to 3), language access services (4 to 7), and organizational supports for cultural competence (8 to 14). Although these standards are intended to be inclusive of all cultures, they are particularly designed to assist in the elimination of racial and ethnic health disparities in the U.S. by making the health care environment more inviting to those groups who historically have experienced unequal access to health services. Specific ways to put culturally and linguistically appropriate services into action are found in the document. For example, Standard 2 states that diversity is a necessary but not sufficient condition to achieve a culturally competent organization. The notion of a diverse staff includes all personnel from maintenance to administrative to medical professionals. The use of proactive incentives, mentoring programs, staff education, and training are all given forethought to avoid the need for resolution of conflict.

- Who is the "face to the wider world" for the organization? Who represents the organization?

- Are the employee benefits meeting the needs of individuals with unique circumstances?

- Is there a commitment to ongoing discussion and training on issues of cultural competence at the staff/board level?

- Has the organization established collegial and collaborative relationships with other relevant community groups to improve the health status of patients?

- Are there clear recruitment and retention/affirmative action goals for the organization? Does everyone in the organization understand the meaning of affirmative action and know these goals?

- Do the White people in the organization value working in a diverse setting? How is this evident?

- Is there a safe forum for people to learn how they may have unknowingly excluded or slighted their colleagues?

- Has anyone ever been rewarded in any way for their efforts to become culturally competent? Has anyone in the organization ever been penalized in any way for their inappropriate behavior?

- Is there a specific survey to assess patient and staff satisfaction with the facility and personnel?

ENVIRONMENTAL CONSIDERATIONS

- What images decorate the space?

- What magazines are placed in public meeting spaces and/or in the waiting area? Are publications in more than one language? Do pictures in the literature look like the people who frequent the facility?

- Are bicultural or bilingual interpreters available to clients with limited English proficiency? Are the signs around the workplace in more than one language?

- What types of foods are served at group gatherings?

- Does the organization follow the Christian calendar? Do people of a different religious faith have the option to observe their holidays?

- Who considers the "fun" days (group picnics, parties, dinners, etc.) fun?

- Is the workplace fully wheelchair accessible?

- Is public transportation available to come to the practice?

- Are the workplace hours of operation conducive to meeting the needs of the clients?

MOVING FROM CONCERN TO ACTION: PERSONAL INVENTORY

- Have I consciously thought about my own cultural identity and come to realize how much it is a part of who I am? For example, does my name have a relationship to my ancestors' ethnic identity? What belongings in my home are meaningful to me and why? Do my preferences regarding food, music, clothes, and so forth give an indication of who I am? Do I have health beliefs and behaviors that have been passed down to me from my ancestors?

- Have I spent some time reflecting on my own childhood and upbringing and analyzing where, how, and when I was receiving cultural, ethnocentric, and racist messages?

- Have I spent some time recently looking at my own attitudes and behaviors as an adult to determine how I am contributing to or combating ethnocentrism? Do I recognize that I may be prejudiced and may stereotype even if it is unconscious?

- Have I intentionally and aggressively sought to educate myself on other cultural ways of life and on issues of bias and racism by talking with others, viewing films and videos, finding reading material, attending lectures, or joining a study group?

- Have I evaluated my use of language, light and dark imagery, and other terms or phrases that might be degrading or hurtful to others? Do I make comments or jokes about cultural groups?

- Have I grown in my awareness of subliminal messages in television programs, advertising, and news coverage?

- Have I supported political candidates or contributed financially to an agency, fund, or program that actively confronts the problems of inequality and discrimination or enhances my patients' likelihood of receiving more culturally competent health care?

- Have I worked directly or indirectly to dispel misconceptions, stereotypes, prejudices, and other adverse feelings that members of one group have against members of another group? For example, have I openly disagreed with an insensitive comment, joke, reference, or action among those around me?

- Have I taken the initiative in dispelling prejudices, stereotypes, and misunderstandings among staff and discouraging or preventing patterns of informal discrimination, segregation, or exclusion of individuals?

- Do I listen with an open mind to members of other groups, even if their communications are initially disturbing or divergent from my own thinking? Do I welcome constructive feedback from others about how I relate to people from different cultures?

MOVING FROM CONCERN TO ACTION: PROFESSIONAL INVENTORY

- Have I asked my patients appropriate questions about their culture and way of life and let them know I have a lot to learn?

- Have I made the necessary adaptations to ensure that my client and I are able to communicate effectively?

- Have I recognized that my clients may be from a different socio-economic class than I am? Have I considered a sliding scale for fees? Do I assume my client has the same comforts and capabilities for a home program as I might? Do I recognize the need to minimize potential barriers to service for my clients?

- Have I considered doing research that includes people of diverse backgrounds to enable the profession of physical therapy to become more culturally proficient? For example, have I considered the need for assessment tools that address culture-specific functional tasks such as squatting or eating with chopsticks?

- Have I made overtures toward traditional healers to collaborate and increase my understanding of their ideas and ways?

- Does my clinic conduct inspire patients to respect one another and be open and honest in their communications with others and with me?

- Have I adapted my physical therapy examination and intervention to reflect my patient's culture and desires?

- Have I worked toward aiding my patients to navigate the health care system as needed?

CONCLUSION

In this millennium, national population patterns will continue to shift, and physical therapists will increasingly be required to practice in less familiar multicultural settings. The challenges to delivering effective and humanistic care will become even greater than they are today.

An understanding of the socio-cultural variables in the health care setting and of an individual patient or client's worldview is believed to lead to an improved clinical encounter. Clinicians increasingly understand that the client will likely discard a culturally inappropriate intervention and the physical therapy service would be rendered ineffective. A health care interaction that incorporates negotiation and preservation of cultural health-related beliefs and practices will likely increase treatment adherence and self-efficacy for both parties (Kavanagh, Absalom, Beil, & Schliessmann, 1999). Physical therapists need to strive for cross-cultural efficacy (Núñez, 2000), the ability of a caregiver to be effective in interactions that involve individuals of different cultures by ensuring that neither the caregivers' nor patients' culture is the preferred or the more accurate view.

The culture of the individual client, physical therapist, physical therapy institution, and the broader society each contribute to our daily lives. When cultures clash consciously or unconsciously, overtly or subtly, health care is likely to be impacted, most often negatively. When physical therapy providers and institutions are able to identify or anticipate the potential clashes and seek ways to overcome potential cultural barriers, the profession moves toward more culturally congruent care with all of the respective benefits, including the lessening of health disparities. Removal of barriers, whether in the form of access to a practitioner who is more similar to the patient, correction of stereotype and bias, or physical ability to access physical therapy, will improve interactions with patients. With these efforts, better physical therapy can be provided to the greatest number of individuals, regardless of cultural background or status. Tervalon and Murray-García (1998) refer to the process as cultural humility, or a lifelong commitment to self-evaluation and self-critique, which requires readdressing the power imbalances (i.e., barriers) in the client-health care professional relationship and developing mutual beneficial partnerships with communities on behalf of individuals and defined populations.

Constructive movement toward the future requires a vision. The vision can be obtained by pooling our ideas and resources and seeking a commitment from all of those involved in the rehabilitation process. For physical therapists, there is a special moral and political imperative to assist persons with disabilities to maximize their human potential by fulfilling their life's goals. Included in this obligation is the idea that all consumers of care, no matter what their specific identity, deserve respect and the very best that a professional has to offer. To have the most impact on diminishing the disability status of a client, the physical therapist must understand how disability is socially constructed for that particular individual and the socio-cultural context in which that person lives. The physical therapist needs to learn how to learn culture rapidly and effectively. We need to master the knowledge and skills necessary to feel comfortable and communicate effectively with people of similar and dissimilar backgrounds in any situation involving a group of people of diverse ethnocentric backgrounds. This knowledge and skill then needs to be translated into effective holistic caring for the individual and/or family unit within a meaningful cultural context. This requires the physical therapist to be culturally competent and, more ideally, culturally proficient. The path of intercultural learning to cultural proficiency is a conscious, lifelong effort. There will be errors in judgment and practice, probably for as long as we live, but cultural competence can be learned and nurtured. Physical therapists, in acknowledging the uniqueness of the individuals with whom we work, then face the challenge of embracing (and enjoying) diversity and differences, reshaping practice protocols, redefining research priorities, and developing the most appropriate service models and public policy to benefit people with disability. Quality of life outcome measures for our clients and our personal professional satisfaction should be enhanced.

REFERENCES

American Physical Therapy Association. (2001). *Interactive guide to physical therapist practice with catalog of tests and measures: Version 1.0.* Alexandria, VA: Author.

American Physical Therapy Association. (2003). Health disparities: Information and funding sources. Retrieved December 16, 2008, from http://www.apta.org/AM/Template.cfm?Section=Home&CONTEN TID=62954&TEMPLATE=/CM/ContentDisplay.cfm

American Physical Therapy Association. (2008a). Blueprint for teaching cultural competence in physical therapy education. Retrieved December 16, 2008, from http://www.apta.org/AM/Template. cfm?Section=Minority_Affairs1&Template=/CM/ContentDisplay.cfm&ContentID=49345

American Physical Therapy Association. (2008b). Web site. Retrieved December 16, 2008, from http://www.apta.org

Association of American Medical Colleges. (n.d.). Tool for Assessing Cultural Competence Training. Retrieved December 10, 2009, from http://www.aamc.org/meded/tacct/start.htm

Campinha-Bacote, J. (2007). *The process of cultural competence in the delivery of healthcare services: The journey continues* (5th ed.). Cincinnati, OH: Transcultural C.A.R.E Associates.

Cornielje, H. (1999). Towards a public health perspective on rehabilitation. In R. L. Leavitt (Ed.), *Cross-cultural rehabilitation: An international perspective* (pp. 365-373). London, England: Harcourt Brace and Company.

Coyne, C. (2001). Cultural competency: Reaching out to all populations. *PT Magazine, 9*(10), 44-50.

Cross, T. L., Bazron, B. J., Dennis, K. W., & Isaacs, M. R. (1989). *Towards a culturally competent system of care: A monograph on effective services for minority children who are severely emotionally disturbed.* Washington, DC: CASSP Technical Assistance Center, Georgetown University Child Development Center.

Duncan, P. (2002). *The Stroke Impact Scale.* Boston, MA: Paper presented at American Physical Therapy Association Combined Sections Meeting.

Fabrega, H. (1974). *Disease and social behavior: An interdisciplinary perspective.* Cambridge, MA: MIT Press.

Fortier, J. P., Bishop, D. (2004). *Setting the agenda for research on cultural competence in health care: Final report.* Edited by C. Brach. Rockville, MD: U.S. Department of Health and Human Services, Office of Minority Health, and Agency for Healthcare Research and Quality.

Gannotti, M. E., Handwerker, W. P., Groce, N. E., & Crux, C. (2001). Sociocultural influences on disability status in Puerto Rican children. *Physical Therapy, 81*(9), 1512-1523.

Gardner, J. (2005). Barriers influencing the success of racial and ethnic minority students in nursing programs. *Journal of Transcultural Nursing, 16*(2), 155-162.

Giger, J., Davidhizar, R. E., Purnell, L., Harden, J. T., Phillips, J., & Strickland, O. (2007). American academy of nursing expert panel report: Developing cultural competence to eliminate health disparities in ethnic minorities and other vulnerable populations. *Journal of Transcultural Nursing, 18*(2), 95-102.

Ibrahim, F. (1995). Multicultural influences on rehabilitation training and services: The shift to valuing non-dominant cultures. In O. C. Karan & S. Greenspan (Eds.), *Community rehabilitation services for people with disabilities* (pp. 187-205). Boston, MA: Butterworth-Heinemann.

Johanson, M. A. (2007). Factors influencing students' selection of physical therapist programs: Differences between men and women and racial/ethnic groups. *Journal of Physical Therapy Education, 21*(1), 22-32.

Kavanagh, K., Absalom, K., Beil, W., Jr., & Schliessmann, L. (1999). Connecting and becoming culturally competent: A Lakota example. *Advances in Nursing Science, 21*(3), 9-31.

Kerfield, C. I., Guthrie, M. R., & Steward, K. B. (1997). Evaluation of the Denver II as applied to Alaska Native children. *Pediatric Physical Therapy, 9*(1), 23-31.

Kohls, L. R. (2001). *Survival kit for overseas living: For Americans planning to live and work abroad* (4th ed.). Boston, MA: Nicholas Brealey Publishing.

Lie, D., Boker, J., & Cleveland, E. (2006). Using the tool for assessing cultural competence training (TACCT) to measure faculty and medical student perceptions of cultural competence instruction in the first three years of the curriculum. *Academic Medicine, 81*(6), 557-564.

Like, R. C., Steiner, R. P., & Rubel, A. J. (1996). STFM Core Curriculum Guidelines. Recommended core curriculum guidelines on culturally sensitive and competent health care. *Family Medicine, 28*(4), 291-297.

Lipson, J. G., & Desantis, L. A. (2007). Current approaches to integrating elements of cultural competence in nursing education. *Journal of Transcultural Nursing, 18*(1 Suppl), 10S-20S.

Lundström, L. G. (2008). Further arguments in support of a social humanistic perspective in physiotherapy versus the biomedical model. *Physiotherapy Theory and Practice, 24*(6), 393-396.

Lynch, E. W., & Hanson, M. J. (1998). *Developing cross-cultural competence: A guide for working with children and their families.* Baltimore, MD: Brookes Publishing Company.

Mann, J. (2006). Health and human rights: If not now, when? *American Journal of Public Health, 96*(11), 1940-1943.

Neighbors, C. J., Marquez, D. X., & Marcus, B. H. (2008). Leisure-time physical activity disparities among Hispanic subgroups in the United States. *American Journal of Public Health, 98*(8), 1460-1464.

Nixon-Cave, K. (2001). *Influence of cultural/ethnic beliefs and behaviors and family environment on the motor development of infants 12-18 months of age in three ethnic groups: African-American, Hispanic/Latino and Anglo-European.* Unpublished dissertation. Philadelphia, PA: Temple University.

Núñez, A. E. (2000). Transforming cultural competence into cross-cultural efficacy in women's health education. *Academic Medicine, 75*(11), 1071-1080.

Romanello, M. L. (2007). Integration of cultural competence in physical therapist education. *Journal of Physical Therapy Education, 21*(1), 33-39.

Saha, S., Guiton, G., Wimmers, P. F., & Wilkerson, L. (2008). Student body racial and ethnic composition and diversity-related outcomes in U.S. medical schools. *Journal of the American Medical Association, 300*(10), 1135-1145.

Tervalon, M. & Murray-García, J. (1998). Cultural humility versus cultural competence: A critical distinction in defining physician training outcomes in multicultural education. *Journal of Health Care for the Poor and Underserved, 9*(2), 117-125.

Trust for America's Health. (2009). *Prevention for a healthier America: Investments in disease prevention yield significant savings, stronger communities.* Washington, DC: Author. Retrieved October 5, 2009, from http://healthyamericans.org/reports/prevention08/Prevention08.pdf

U.S. Department of Health and Human Services, Office of Minority Health. (2001). *National standards on culturally and linguistically appropriate services in health care—Final report.* Washington, DC: Author.

Wittig, D. R. (2004). Knowledge, skills, and attitudes of nursing students regarding culturally congruent care of Native Americans. *Journal of Transcultural Nursing, 15*(1), 54-61.

Wong, C. K., & Blissett, S. (2007). Assessing performance in the area of cultural competence: An analysis of reflective writing. *Journal of Physical Therapy Education, 21*(2), 40-47.

Young, J. C., & Garro, L. Y. (1982). Variation in the choice of treatment in two Mexican communities. *Social Science & Medicine, 16*(16), 1453-1465.

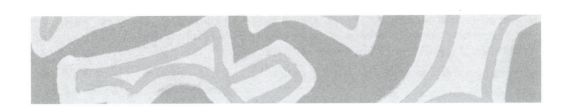

Appendix A

RESOURCES FOR ADDITIONAL INFORMATION
ON CULTURES OUTSIDE OF THE UNITED STATES

This list focuses primarily on resources produced in the U.S. Other nations have similar resources.

1. **Background notes**. Published by the U.S. State Department; 170 countries are covered. Between 6 and 10 pages long, they cover geography, people, history, government, political conditions, economy, and foreign relations, often with suggested reading. Available from the Superintendent of Documents, Government Printing Office, Washington, DC 20402-9325. For information, call +1 (202) 647-6575.

2. **Bibliographic surveys**. These are annotated bibliographies. Ten volumes are available from the Superintendent of Documents, U.S. Government Printing Office, Washington, DC 20402-9325.

3. **Business customs and protocol**. This series is produced primarily for business people by the Stanford Research Institute. The series concentrates on how to get started, how to get things done, and how to facilitate mutual understanding. Available from Stanford Research Institute International, 333 Ravenswood Avenue, Menlo Park, CA 94025.

4. **Country studies** (formerly called Area Handbooks). These valuable resources are updated regularly. They are prepared by the Foreign Area Studies Group at American University. These include 108 different countries covered to varying degrees of thoroughness. Also available from the Superintendent of Documents, U.S. Government Printing Office, Washington, DC 20402-9325. For information, call +1 (202) 647-6575.

5. **Country updates**. These summarize important information that the foreign resident might need. Available from Intercultural Press, Inc, PO Box 768, Yarmouth, ME 04096.

6. **Culturegrams.** These are published by Brigham Young University and cover 96 countries. The reports are brief, but cover customs and courtesies, the people, lifestyles, and a small map. They contain information about local customs, and there is an emphasis on practical tips on how to get along. Available from David M. Kennedy Center for International Studies, Publication Services, 280 HRCB, Provo, UT 84602, or call +1 (801) 378-6528.

7. *Encyclopedia of the Third World*. There are three volumes in the series, which can be consulted in the reference section of most libraries. Published by Facts on File, 460 Park Avenue South, New York, NY 10016.

8. **Human relations area file**. A tremendously valuable resource, but probably one that contains more information than the average person needs. It provides access to voluminous entries of an anthropological nature for many cultures and subcultures around the world. If you want to be thoroughly prepared, it is a gold mine of information. Many major university libraries house copies of the HRAF on microfiche. Information can be obtained from Human Relations Area File, 755 Prospect Street, New Haven, CT 06511.

9. **Professional organization special interest groups**. For example, the Cross-Cultural and International Special Interest Group (CCISIG) of the American Physical Therapy Association has additional resources and the names of individuals who have worked internationally.

10. **Other sources of information**:

   - Chamber of Commerce

   - Church and missionary societies

   - The embassy of the host country. Many also have Offices or Ministers of Tourism, which are frequently located in New York City, or the capital of your own country.

   - Universities and colleges in your area. The departments of anthropology and public health are likely to be the most useful.

   - Foreign exchange students

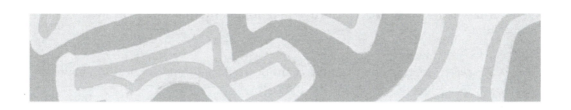

Appendix B

RESOURCES FOR PHYSICAL THERAPISTS
INTERESTED IN GLOBAL HEALTH

1. **Cross Cultural and International Special Interest Group (CCISIG)**
   - Join the CCISIG listserv to receive timely notices via email about volunteer and paid positions in other countries, global health conferences, international service-learning opportunities, international clinical education opportunities, and global health resources.
   - Download the CCISIG Resource Guide for International Service-Learning in Physical Therapy Education (free to all CCISIG members)

2. **World Confederation for Physical Therapy**: www.wcpt.org
   - View messages from PTs around the world on the various forums, including the Forum for International Work & Study. Also, it is free to post your own messages or questions at www.wcpt.org/smfforum/index.php
   - If you are interested in working in the UK or Canada, see links at www.wcpt.org/node/29608
   - If you are interested in working in other countries, find the link to their PT organizations at www.wcpt.org

3. **Health Volunteers Overseas (HVO)**: www.hvousa.org
   - HVO is a private nonprofit organization dedicated to improving the availability and quality of health care in developing countries through the training and education of local health care providers. HVO includes Physical Therapy Overseas, a division run for physical therapists by physical therapists.

4. **World Health Organization (WHO) Disability and Rehabilitation (DAR) Team**
   - DAR's mission is to enhance the quality of life for people with disabilities through national, regional, and global efforts: www.who.int/disabilities/en
   - Contact pedersenr@who.int to sign up for WHO Disability and Rehabilitation Newsletter, which is distributed by email three times per year.

5. **International Centre for Disability and Rehabilitation (ICDR)**: www.icdr.uto-ronto.ca

   - ICDR focus includes:
     - o *Teaching*: Offering opportunities to influence the education of health care providers and students in Canada and internationally
     - o *Research and evaluation*: Contributing to new knowledge on rehabilitation issues in various cultural and ethnic settings
     - o *Service delivery*: Developing programs that provide appropriate services in countries with developing and transitional economies
   - See www.icdr.utoronto.ca/Files/PDF/8181722c29918ee.pdf for the 2008 report, "Research on Disability and Development"

6. **Global Health Educators Consortium (GHEC)**

   - GHEC is a consortium of faculty and health care educators dedicated to global health education in North American health professions schools and residency programs (information quoted from http://globalhealthedu.org/pages/default.aspx)
   - See *Resources for Developing Global Health Curricula: A Guidebook for U.S. Medical Schools*
   - See "Modules for Disability and Rehabilitation in Developing Countries" and other global health teaching modules

7. **Center for International Rehabilitation Research Information and Exchange (CIRRIE)**: http://cirrie.buffalo.edu

   - CIRRIE facilitates the sharing of information and expertise in rehabilitation research between the U.S. and other countries through a wide range of programs. CIRRIE offers resources and links to resources, such as:
     - o Disability in the Middle East
     - o Disability and Social Responses in Some Southern African Nations
     - o Disability and Social Responses in Afghanistan and Pakistan
     - o http://cirrie.buffalo.edu/bibliography/index.html

8. **United Nations**

   - Convention on the Rights of Persons with Disabilities: www.un.org/disabilities

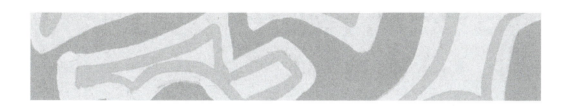

Appendix C
Resources for Establishing a Culturally Competent Practice

The following is a list of resources that can assist you to become culturally proficient. It is by no means all inclusive, but rather an effort to entice you to explore the available information more fully.

America's Health Insurance Plans. (2005). *Tools to address disparities in health: Data as building blocks for change.* Retrieved December 10, 2009, from http://www.ahip.org/content/default.aspx?docid=10761

American Medical Association. (2007). Educating physicians controversies challenges health: Health care disparities among racial/ethnic minority patients. Retrieved October 5, 2009, from http://www.ama-assn.org/ama/pub/physician-resources/public-health/general-resources-health-care-professionals/educating-physicians-controversies-challenges-health/health-care-disparities-among-racialethnic-minority.shtml

American Physical Therapy Association. International Affairs. Retrieved October 5, 2009, from http://www.apta.org/AM/Template.cfm?Section=International_Affairs1&Template=/TaggedPage/TaggedPageDisplay.cfm&TPLID=64&ContentID=13004

American Physical Therapy Association. Minority Affairs. Retrieved October 5, 2009, from http://www.apta.org/AM/Template.cfm?Section=Minority_Affairs1&Template=/TaggedPage/TaggedPageDisplay.cfm&TPLID=417&ContentID=63007

Anand, R. (2006). *Cultural competence in health care: A guide for trainers* (4th ed.). Washington, DC: National Multicultural Institute.

Anti-Defamation League. (2009). A world of difference institute: A classroom of difference. Retrieved October 5, 2009, from http://www.adl.org/education/edu_awod/awod_classroom.asp

Bonder, B., Martin, L., & Miracle, A. W. (2001). *Culture in clinical care.* Thorofare, NJ: SLACK Incorporated.

Boston Healing Landscape Project. (2007). Cultural competency in US health care. Retrieved October 5, 2009, from http://www.bu.edu/bhlp/pages/resources/cultural_competency/overview.html

Brooks, S. (2003). Religious issues. In M. Thompson & J. Okubo (Eds.), *Cultural diversity of older Americans.* Washington, DC: American Physical Therapy Assosication, Section on Geriatrics.

Center for Cross Cultural Health. (n.d.). Web site. Retrieved October 5, 2009, from http://www.crosshealth.com

Center for the Health Professions. (n.d.). Web site. Retrieved October 5, 2009, from http://old.futurehealth.ucsf.edu/?tabid=290

Center for International Rehabilitation Research Information and Exchange (CIRRIE). Web site. Retrieved October 5, 2009, from http://cirrie.buffalo.edu

Champlain Valley Area Health Education Center. (2007). *Cultural competency for health care providers.* Retrieved October 5, 2009, from http://www.cvahec.org/documents/CulturalComptencyforHeatlhCareProviders2007_11.8.07.pdf

Cross-Cultural and International Special Interest Group (CCISIG).

Dickerson-Jones, T. (1993). *Fifty activities for managing cultural diversity.* Amherst, MA: Human Resource Development Press.

DiversityRx. (2003). Models and practices. Retrieved October 5, 2009, from http://www.diversityrx.org/HTML/MODELS.htm

Doctors in Touch. (n.d.). Web site. Retrieved October 5, 2009, from http://www.doctorsintouch.com/courses_for_CME_credit.htm

Galanti, G. A. (1997). *Caring for patients from different cultures: Case studies from American hospitals* (2nd ed.). Philadelphia, PA: University of Pennsylvania Press.

Goode, T. (1989). *Promoting cultural and linguistic competence self-assessment checklist for personnel providing services and supports in early intervention and childhood settings.* Washington, DC: Georgetown University Child Development Center, UAP.

Grainger-Monsen, M., & Haslett, J. (2003). *Worlds apart: A four-part series on cross-cultural healthcare.* United States: Fanlight Productions.

Health Resources and Services Administration. (2009). Cultural competence resources for health care providers. Retrieved October 5, 2009, from http://www.hrsa.gov/cultural-competence

Huff, R. M., Kline, M. V. (1999). *Promoting health in multicultural populations: A handbook for practitioners.* Thousand Oaks, CA: Sage Publications.

Johns Hopkins School of Public Health Bloomburg. (n.d.). Hopkins Center for Health Disparities Solutions. Retrieved October 5, 2009, from http://www.jhsph.edu/healthdisparities/index.html

Lambert, J. (1994). *Fifty activities for diversity training* (3rd ed.). Amherst, MA: Human Resource Development Press.

Lattanzi, J. B. (2003). Overview of cultural competency: Considerations for older adults. In M. Thompson & J. Okubo (Eds.), *Cultural diversity of older Americans.* Washington, DC: American Physical Therapy Assosication, Section on Geriatrics.

Lattanzi, J. B., & Purnell, L. D. (2005). *Developing cultural competence in physical therapy practice.* Philadelphia, PA: F.A. Davis.

Leavitt, R. L. (2002). Developing cultural competence in a multicultural world: Part I. *PT Magazine, 10*(12), 36-48.

Leavitt, R. L. (2003). Developing cultural competence in a multicultural world: Part II. *PT Magazine, 11*(1), 56-70.

Lynch, E. W., & Hanson, M. J. (Eds.). (1998). *Developing cross-cultural competence: A guide for working with young children and their families* (2nd ed.). Baltimore, MD: Brookes Publishing Company.

Management Sciences for Health. (n.d.). The providers guide to quality and culture. Retrieved October 5, 2009, from http://erc.msh.org/mainpage.cfm?file=1.0.htm&module =provider&language=English

Medline Plus. (2008). Population groups. Retrieved December 10, 2009, from http://www.nlm.nih.gov/medlineplus/populationgroups.html

Müller-Ebeling, C., Rätsch, C., & Storl, W. (2003). *Witchcraft medicine: Healing arts, shamanic practices, and forbidden plants.* Rochester, VT: Inner Traditions.

Mutha, S., Allen, C., & Welch, M. (2002). *Toward culturally competent care: A toolbox for teaching communication strategies.* San Francisco, CA: Regents of the University of California.

Nakamura, R. M. (1998). *Health in America: A multicultural perspective.* San Francisco, CA: Benjamin-Cummings Publishing Company.

National Center for Cultural Competence. (n.d.). Cultural competence health practitioner assessment (CCHPA). Retrieved October 5, 2009, from http://www11.georgetown. edu/research/gucchd/nccc/features/CCHPA.html

National Network of Libraries of Medicine. (n.d.). Minority health. Retrieved December 10, 2009, from http://nnlm.gov/mcr/resources/community/minority.html

Patient and Family Education Services. (n.d.). Cultural clues. Retrieved October 5, 2009, from http://depts.washington.edu/pfes/CultureClues.htm

Purnell, L. D. (2003). Cultural competence for the physical therapists: Working with clients with alternative lifestyles. In M. Thompson & J. Okubo (Eds.), *Cultural diversity of older Americans.* Washington, DC: American Physical Therapy Assosication, Section on Geriatrics.

Putsch, B., SenGupta, I., Sampson, A., & Tervalon, M. (2003). *Reflections on the CLAS Standards: Best practices, innovations and horizons.* Retrieved October 5, 2009, from http://www.omhrc.gov/assets/pdf/checked/reflections.pdf

Royeen, M., & Crabtree, J. L. (2005). *Culture in rehabilitation: From competency to proficiency.* Upper Saddle River, NJ: Prentice Hall.

Satcher, D., & Pamies, R. (2005). *Multicultural medicine and health disparities.* New York, NY: McGraw-Hill.

Spector, R. E. (2000). *Cultural diversity in health and illness* (5th ed.). Upper Saddle River, NJ: Prentice Hall.

Teaching Tolerance. Biannual publication of the Southern Poverty Law Center. Montgomery, AL.

Thompson, M., & Okubo, J. (Eds.). (2003). *Cultural diversity of older Americans.* Washington, DC: American Physical Therapy Assosication, Section on Geriatrics.

Transcultural Nursing Society. (2009). Web site. Retrieved October 5, 2009, from http://www.tcns.org

U.S. Department of Health and Human Services, Office of Minority Health. (2007). National standards for culturally and linguistically appropriate services (CLAS) in health care. Retrieved October 5, 2009, from http://minorityhealth.hhs.gov/templates/browse. aspx?lvl=2&lvlid=15

U.S. Department of Health and Human Services, Office of Minority Health. (2008). Cultural competency. Retrieved October 5, 2009, from http://minorityhealth.hhs.gov/templates/browse.aspx?lvl=1&lvlID=3

Wilson-Stronks, A., & Galvez, E. (2009). Hospitals, language, and culture: A snapshot of the nation. Retrieved October 5, 2009, from http://www.jointcommission.org/PatientSafety/HLC/about_hlc.htm

Wilson-Stronks, A., Lee, K., Cordero C., Kopp, A, & Galvez, E. (2008). *One size does not fit all: Meeting the health care needs of diverse populations*. Oakbrook Terrace, IL: The Joint Commission.

SPECIFIC CULTURES, HEALTH BELIEFS, AND BEHAVIORS RESOURCES

Emergency and Community Health Outreach Broadcast: Mass Dispensing of Medicine, August 2006:

- Khmer link: http://www.echominnesota.org/index.cfm/p/tvArchive/l/km/tvID/23
- Somali link: http://www.echominnesota.org/index.cfm/p/tvArchive/l/so/tvID/23
- Vietnamese link: http://www.echominnesota.org/index.cfm/p/tvArchive/l/vi/tvID/23
- Spanish link: http://www.echominnesota.org/index.cfm/p/tvArchive/l/es/tvID/23
- Hmong link: http://www.echominnesota.org/index.cfm/p/tvArchive/l/hmn/tvID/23
- Lao link: http://www.echominnesota.org/index.cfm/p/tvArchive/l/lo/tvID/23

Gehrke-White, D. (2006). *The face behind the veil: The extraordinary lives of Muslim women in America*. New York, NY: Citadel Press.

Jewish Healing Foundation. (2007). Integrating religion and spirituality into the body and soul. Retrieved October 5, 2009, from http://www.jewishhealing.com

Kriebel, D. W. (n.d.). Powwowing: A persistent American esoteric tradition. Retrieved October 5, 2009, http://www.esoteric.msu.edu/VolumeIV/Powwow.htm

Leavitt, R. L. (1992). *Disability and rehabilitation in rural Jamaica: An ethnographic study*. Rutherford, NJ: Fairleigh Dickinson University Press.

Ling, W. (2003). An overview of east Asian cultures for physical therapists. In M. Thompson & J. Okubo (Eds.), *Cultural diversity of older Americans*. Washington, DC: American Physical Therapy Assosication, Section on Geriatrics.

National Network of Libraries of Medicine. (n.d.). Minority health. Retrieved October 5, 2009, from http://nnlm.gov/mcr/resources/community/minority.html

African American and Black culture and health:

- Van Gelder, S. (1993). Remembering our purpose: The teachings of indigenous cultures may help us go beyond modernity. In Context, 34. Retrieved October 5, 2009, from http://www.context.org/ICLIB/IC34/Some.htm
- Writings on the Wall. (2008). Articles, essays and interviews on African diaspora religion and culture. Retrieved October 5, 2009, from http://www.mamiwata.com/articles1.html

Avila, E., & Parker, J. (2000). *Woman who glows in the dark: A curandera reveals traditional Aztec secrets of physical and spiritual health*. New York, NY: Tarcher.

Braithwaite, R. L., & Taylor, S. E. (Eds.). (2001). *Health issues in the Black community* (2nd ed.). San Francisco, CA: Jossey-Bass.

Gary-Williams, G. (2003). African Americans: Young-old and older—65 years and beyond. In M. Thompson & J. Okubo (Eds.), *Cultural diversity of older Americans.* Washington, DC: American Physical Therapy Assosication, Section on Geriatrics.

Somé, M. P. (1995). *Of water and the spirit: Ritual, magic and initiation in the life of an African shaman.* New York, NY: Penguin Books.

Somé, M. P. (1999). *The healing wisdom of Africa: Finding life purpose through nature, ritual, and community.* New York, NY: Tarcher.

Hmong culture:

- WWW Hmong Homepage. (n.d.). Web site. Retrieved October 5, 2009, from http://www.hmongnet.org
- Gary Yia Lee. (n.d.). Web site. Retrieved October 5, 2009, from http://www.garyyialee.com

Fadiman, A. (1997). *The spirit catches you and you fall down: A Hmong Child, her american doctors, and the collision of two cultures.* New York, NY: Farrar, Straus, and Giroux.

Hmong Health. (n.d.). Web site. Retrieved October 5, 2009, from http://www.hmong-health.org/

Latin American and Hispanic culture:

- Soundprint. (n.d.). Curanderismo: Folk healing in the southwest. Retrieved October 5, 2009, from http://soundprint.org/radio/display_show/ID/288/name/Curanderismo:+Folk+Healing+in+the+Southwest

Aguirre-Molina, M., Molina, C. W., Zambrana, R. E. (Eds.). (2001). *Health issues in the Latino community.* San Francisco, CA: Jossey-Bass.

American Medical Association. (2007). Strategies to improve communication with Latino/Hispanic patients. Retrieved October 5, 2009, from http://www.ama-cmeonline.com/lep_com_strategies

Leavitt, R. L. (2003). Developing cultural competence: Working with older adults of Hispanic origin. In M. Thompson & J. Okubo (Eds.), *Cultural diversity of older Americans.* Washington, DC: American Physical Therapy Assosication, Section on Geriatrics.

National Council of La Raza. (n.d.). Web site. Retrieved October 5, 2009, from http://www.nclr.org

Native American culture and health:

- Center for Health and Healing. (n.d.). Native American history and philosophy. Retrieved October 5, 2009, from http://www.healthandhealingny.org/tradition_healing/native-history.html
- Native American Culture. (2008). Health. Retrieved October 5, 2009, from http://www.ewebtribe.com/NACulture/health.htm
- Native Languages of the Americas. (n.d.). Native American cultures. Retrieved October 5, 2009, from http://www.native-languages.org/home.htm
- WWW Virtual Library. (n.d.). American Indians. Retrieved October 5, 2009, from http://www.hanksville.org/NAresources/indices/NAknowledge.html

Cochran, T. M. (2003). Rehabilitation and Native American elders. In M. Thompson & J. Okubo (Eds.), *Cultural diversity of older Americans.* Washington, DC: American Physical Therapy Assosication, Section on Geriatrics.

Mehl-Madrona, L. (1998). *Coyote medicine: Lessons from Native American healing.* New York, NY: Touchstone Publishing.

LANGUAGE/INTERPRETATION SERVICES

Ethnomed. (n.d.). Web site. Retrieved October 5, 2009, from http://ethnomed.org

Healthy Roads Media. (n.d.). Web site. Retrieved October 5, 2009, from http://healthy-roadsmedia.org

International Medical Interpreters Association. (n.d.). Web site. Retrieved October 5, 2009, from http://www.imiaweb.org/default.asp

Luckman, J. (1999). *Transcultural communication in health care*. Clifton Park, NY: Delmar Cengage Learning.

MedlinePlus. (n.d.). Health information in multiple languages. Retrieved October 5, 2009, from http://www.nlm.nih.gov/medlineplus/languages/languages.html

National Council on Interpreting in Health Care. (n.d.). Web site. Retrieved October 5, 2009, from http://www.ncihc.org

The 24 Languages Project. (n.d.). Consumer health brochures in multiple languages. Retrieved October 5, 2009, from http://library.med.utah.edu/24languages

Index

Wait...There's More!

SLACK Incorporated's Health Care Books and Journals offers a wide selection of books in the field of Physical Therapy. We are dedicated to providing important works that educate, inform and improve the knowledge of our customers. Don't miss out on our other informative titles that will enhance your collection.

Gait Analysis:
Normal and Pathological Function, Second Edition
Jacquelin Perry, MD, ScD; Judith Burnfield, PhD, PT

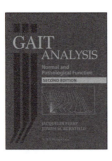

576 pp, Hard Cover, 2010, ISBN 13 978-1-55642-766-4, Order# 47662, **$92.95**

The *Second Edition* to *Gait Analysis* offers a re-organization of the chapters and presentation of material in a more user-friendly, yet comprehensive format. Essential information is provided describing gait functions, and clinical examples to identify and interpret gait deviations. Learning is further reinforced with images and photographs.

Patient Practitioner Interaction:
An Experiential Manual for Developing the Art of Health Care, Fourth Edition
Carol M. Davis DPT, EdD, MS, FAPTA

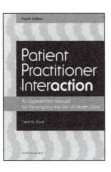

304 pp, Soft Cover, 2006, ISBN 13 978-1-55642-720-6, Order# 47204, **$47.95**

The updated fourth edition of *Patient Practitioner Interaction*, by Dr. Carol Davis, will guide health care professionals to promote the healing process in patients and their loved ones through sensitivity and improved communication. This renowned text is a proven essential and belongs on the bookshelf and in the minds of every physical therapy student and health care professional.

Cultural Competence: A Lifelong Journey to Cultural Proficiency
Ronnie Leavitt, PhD, MPH
288 pp, Soft Cover, 2010, ISBN 13 978-1-55642-876-0, Order# 48760, **$49.95**

Physical Therapy Documentation: From Examination to Outcome
Mia Erickson PT, EdD, CHT, ATC; Rebecca McKnight PT, MS; Ralph Utzman PT, MPH, PhD
224 pp, Soft Cover, 2008, ISBN 13 978-1-55642-782-4, Order# 47824, **$47.95**

Cardiovascular/Pulmonary Essentials: Applying th Preferred Physical Therapist Practice Patterns(SM)
Marilyn Moffat PT, DPT, PhD, FAPTA, CSCS; Donna Frownfelter DPT, MA, CCS, FCCP, RRT
328 pp, Soft Cover, 2007, ISBN 13 978-1-55642-668-1, Order# 46682, **$58.95**

Integumentary Essentials: Applying the Preferred Physical Therapist Practice Patterns(SM)
Marilyn Moffat PT, DPT, PhD, FAPTA, CSCS; Katherine Biggs Harris PT, MS
160 pp, Soft Cover, 2006, ISBN 13 978-1-55642-670-4, Order# 46704, **$50.95**

Musculoskeletal Essentials: Applying the Preferre Physical Therapist Practice Patterns(SM)
Marilyn Moffat PT, DPT, PhD, FAPTA, CSCS; Elaine Rosen PT DHSc, OCS, FAAOMPT; Sandra Rusnak-Smith PT, DHSc, OC!
448 pp, Soft Cover, 2006, ISBN 13 978-1-55642-667-4, Order# 46674, **$58.95**

Neuromuscular Essentials: Applying the Preferred Physical Therapist Practice Patterns(SM)
Marilyn Moffat PT, DPT, PhD, FAPTA, CSCS; Joanell Bohmert PT, MS; Janice Hulme MS, PT, DHSc
320 pp, Soft Cover, 2008, ISBN 13 978-1-55642-669-8, Order# 46690, **$58.95**

Culture in Clinical Care
Bette R. Bonder PhD, OTR/L, FAOTA; Laura Martin PhD; Andrew W. Miracle PhD
208 pp, Soft Cover, 2002, ISBN 13 978-1-55642-459-5, Order# 34590, **$49.95**

Please visit **www.slackbooks.com** to order any of the above titles!
24 Hours a Day...7 Days a Week!

Attention Industry Partners!

Whether you are interested in buying multiple copies of a book, chapter reprints, or looking for something new and different — we are able to accommodate your needs.

MULTIPLE COPIES

At attractive discounts starting for purchases as low as 25 copies for a single title, SLACK Incorporated will be able to meet all your of your needs.

CHAPTER REPRINTS

SLACK Incorporated is able to offer the chapters you want in a format that will lead to success. Bound with an attractive cover, use the chapters that are a fit specifically for your company Available for quantities of 100 or more.

CUSTOMIZE

SLACK Incorporated is able to create a specialized custom version of any of our products specifically for your company.

Please contact the Marketing Communications Director for further details on multiple copy purchases, chapter reprints or custom printing at 1-800-257-8290 or 1-856-848-1000.

*Please note all conditions are subject to change.

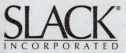

SLACK®
INCORPORATED
Health Care Books and Journals • 6900 Grove Road • Thorofare, NJ 08086

1-800-257-8290
Fax: 1-856-848-6091
E-mail: **orders@slackinc.com**   **www.slackbooks.com**